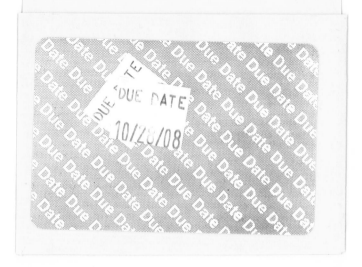

Topics in Environmental Physiology and Medicine

edited by Karl E. Schaefer

The Circadian System of Man
Results of Experiments
Under Temporal Isolation

Rütger A. Wever

With 181 illustrations

Springer-Verlag   New York   Heidelberg   Berlin

Rütger A. Wever
Max-Planck-Institut für Verhaltensphysiologie
8131 Andechs
West Germany

Library of Congress Cataloging in Publication Data

Wever, Rütger A
   The circadian system of man.

   (Topics in environmental physiology and medicine)
   Bibliography: p.
   Includes index.
   1. Circadian rhythms. 2. Human biology. I. Title.
QP84.6.W48   612   78-11543

Printed in the United States of America.

9 8 7 6 5 4 3 2 1

ISBN 0-387-90338-0   Springer-Verlag New York Heidelberg Berlin
ISBN 3-540-90338-0   Springer-Verlag Berlin Heidelberg New York

Preface

Biological rhythmicity has been a subject of scientific research for a relatively short time. In the special case of daily, or circadian rhythms, it is only during the past twenty years that rapidly increasing efforts have been undertaken in evaluating properties and mechanisms. As a consequence of these efforts, the study of biological and, in particular, circadian rhythmicity is no longer a somewhat dubious occupation but rather a serious branch of science which combines the interdisciplinary efforts of numerous researchers around the world. The general result of these efforts is that many features of circadian rhythms of many different species of living beings are well known today.

In addition to studies with lower organisms, the evaluation of human circadian rhythms was originally more or less a compulsory exercise done in order to extend the "catalogue of species"; of course, the work was of unusual importance due to the special position of man in biology. In the course of the very first experimental series, it became clear that humans possess an "internal clock" as had been established in various organisms, protists, plants, and animals, and that human circadian rhythms fit the general regularities of biological rhythms known at that time. However, it soon became apparent that circadian rhythmicity of man shows, additionally, particularities of great general interest, for practical and theoretical reasons. In other words, studies on humans do not only lead to practically applicable consequences but also have the capacity to contribute in a special way to our general knowledge about biological rhythmicities. It was, therefore, the inevitable consequence of the first preliminary human studies to continue this work with special emphasis.

Most of the results compiled in this book are from experiments that have been conducted for more than a dozen years at the Max-Planck-Institut für Verhaltensphysiologie in Andechs. The series includes many studies with different experimental designs which all contribute to the evaluation of general properties of the human circadian system. All these different types of experiments have in common the necessity for conditions of complete long-term isolation—conditions that might seem unreasonable to impose on humans. In fact, however, all volunteering subjects reported that they enjoyed participation in the experiments. There is some evidence (though hardly to be expressed in figures) that the subjective well-being of the volunteers is a prerequisite for the expression of 'good' rhythms. Special efforts, therefore, have been focused to create an atmosphere of comfort and ease. It may be that the local color of Andechs is conducive to this pleasant atmosphere; the nice village of Andechs, which is situated in a beautiful landscape, includes a famous monastery with a recommended brewery (a typical Bavarian combination). Moreover, in most experiments, the decision was made to give preference to the careful measurement of only a few, well-selected variables which did not trouble the subjects too much, instead of utilizing all technical possibilities; in some cases the measurement of certain variables was omitted in order to maintain the well-being of the subject. Of course, it was possible to operate in this way only in the evaluation of general rhythm properties which is now more or less completed; the treatment of special questions needed special methods.

The laboratory of Andechs has been one of the few laboratories studying circadian rhythms in man. Several of these used natural caves to isolate the subjects from environmental time cues. All experiments performed in caves have been very successful and have had important results. It is evident that the comparison between these results and those of the Andechs series is of particular interest because the experiments have been performed under very different circumstances. It is, however, quite natural that, due to the difficulty of the cave studies, they include only occasional controlled experiments and neither systematic repetitions under identical conditions nor systematic variations in the experimental conditions. Other laboratories have used artificial isolation units like those used in Andechs but have rarely performed controlled experiments. To my knowledge, results of series including more than 4 experiments are available only from two other places. However, these experiments were performed for other purposes, lasted only half as long as the Andechs experiments, and hence, were unable to address many of the questions which form the subject matter of this book. It may, therefore, be pardonable that the author deduces the general properties of the human circadian system mainly from his own studies, and that he refers to other studies only comparatively. At present, some excellent experimental series are in progress elsewhere which promise to extend the results given here; results of these studies, however, cannot yet be utilized.

In spite of the restriction to human rhythms, this book is intended for all those who are engaged in the study of circadian rhythmicity; not only physiologists and psychologists but also biologists, in general. The book does not require detailed knowledge of rhythm regularities; the glossary will help in understanding the special terminology of the field. Although major emphasis is placed on the theoretical deduction of system properties, practical aspects are not ignored. This book may, therefore, also be of interest to those engaged in applied aspects, such as medicine in general, or industrial medicine, aerospace medicine, or applied psychology in particular. Other aspects of practical importance are the possible occurrence of rhythm disorders which may be more common than is presently acknowledged. The knowledge of these disorders, as a prerequisite for restabilization, should be of interest for all fields of medicine, in particular psychiatry.

It is of primary importance to me to thank all subjects who volunteered for the experiments under such apparently strange conditions. Without their ready cooperation, the performance of the studies would have been impossible. My further thanks are due to my coworkers (in temporal order), P. Rieger, E. Poeppel, H. Giedke, R. Lund, C. Goertzen, and J. Zulley, who dealt with special details of the studies but also assisted generally in the performance of the experiments. Without their continuous help, the experiments would not have been feasible. It is worth noting that most of them applied to work at the institute after having volunteered as a subject; all others participated in an experiment during their stays. I also wish to thank all the technical assistants who simultaneously worked as the "good genii" of the experiments, taking care of the subjects and providing them with food and all other living necessities, and thus, guaranteeing the well-being of the subjects: (in temporal order) Sigrid Ludorf, Roswitha Hauenschild, Claudia Sievers, Traude Prenzel, Renate Helfrich, and Gertrud Wacker. For the preparation of all drawings, I thank my wife, Renate Wever.

My very special thanks apply to Ursula Gerecke; without her continuous supervision of all practical details and her careful analyses of all recorded data, the task could never have been completed. Last but not least, I wish to acknowledge gratefully the steady support of Prof. Dr. Dr.h.c. J. Aschoff. He had, many years ago, introduced me to the rhythm research, and he has attended all my work with invaluable advice based on his comprehensive knowledge in a field of science of which he was one of the initiators. Without numerous discussions with him, and also with the other colleagues of our institute, it would have been very hard to complete this work. Moreover, I thank him for his critical review of this manuscript.

Finally, it is a pleasure to acknowledge the support of the Deutsche Forschungsgemeinschaft.

Contents

1
Introduction

Rhythmicity is a ubiquitous biological phenomenon. Like homeostasis, it is one of the basic manifestations of living systems (Aschoff and Wever, 1962b). Within the broad spectrum of biological rhythms, circadian rhythmicity, for several reasons, assumes a special position. Its periodicity is quite unusual in that it corresponds to an external rhythmicity, and thus it seems to possess both internal and external components. Knowledge of the basic properties of the circadian system is of special interest for practical and theoretical reasons.

1.1. The Circadian System

Circadian rhythms have been studied in species as diverse as unicellular organisms and man. The rhythms of various organisms seem to have similar properties. However, the choice of an experimental species for the evaluation of these properties may be influenced by pragmatic factors. In this regard the study of human circadian rhythms offers advantages. Studies on human subjects allow simultaneous measurement of a variety of rhythmic variables, and the results obtained can be of increasingly practical significance, as, for example, in medicine. There are, however, disadvantages to experiments with human subjects: for example, the limitations in the type and duration of reasonable experiments, and the possible influence of motivation which may distort the results obtained. Nevertheless, human experiments are necessary and must be employed in addition to animal experiments.

The objective of this book is to evaluate properties of the human circadian system. It does not deal descriptively with the great variety of rhythmic phenomena known. There are many excellent recent papers reviewing 24-hour variations of nearly all measurable variables, physiological (Aschoff, 1970, 1971, 1973; Aschoff et al., 1974b; Conroy and Mills, 1970; Halberg, 1969; Scheving et al., 1974) and psychological (Colquhoun, 1971, 1972; Hildebrandt, 1976) and responses of the organism to external stimuli (Moore Ede, 1973; Reinberg, 1967, 1974, 1976). In this book the author deals with underlying mechanisms as deduced from studies in which the circadian system was

1

experimentally manipulated. The objective is to elucidate the basic mechanism of circadian rhythmicity. It should be understood that in such studies experimental measurements may be restricted to only a few variables from the great variety mentioned; but these variables should possess functional differences as great as possible.

The difficulty in evaluating properties of the circadian system is that this system cannot be observed directly. Only overt rhythms of more or less arbitrarily defined variables are accessible to direct measurements. It is the established hypothesis that the overt rhythms are controlled by an oscillatory system. This hypothesis assumes a coupling between the oscillatory system and the overt rhythm, and this coupling influences the overt rhythms as well as the underlying oscillatory system. The possibility cannot be excluded that stimuli applied experimentally in order to influence the oscillatory system likewise may affect the interlinked coupling forces. It could be misleading, therefore, to transfer conclusions drawn from properties of measured overt rhythms to properties of the hypothetical oscillatory system, or to apply conclusions from experimentally elicited alterations of overt rhythms to corresponding alterations of the basic oscillators, without having additional information concerning the coupling.

It is characteristic that a coupling between an oscillatory process and an overt rhythm can change each parameter except the frequency or the rhythm period. This means that the overt rhythm period is the only parameter clearly reflecting the corresponding parameter of the underlying controlling oscillator. (There is a hypothesis under consideration which assumes that coupling capacity may transform the frequency of an underlying oscillation into another frequency of an overt rhythm (Brown, 1972); however, since there are good reasons to argue that this hypothesis neglects basic features of the circadian system (Wever, 1974a), the hypothesis may well be dismissed.) In order to evaluate properties of the oscillatory system underlying circadian rhythmicity, experiments must involve the period in some way. Only measurements of alterations in the overt rhythm period permit clear conclusions concerning equal alterations in the period of the underlying oscillator. Measured alterations in all other overt rhythm parameters may or may not reflect equal alterations in corresponding underlying oscillator parameters because of the additional effects of interlinked couplings.

For the investigation of circadian rhythms, it is desirable, however, to have more information than only that concerning the period. Information concerning additional oscillatory parameters (e.g., mean value, amplitude, and wave form) is necessary to obtain as much complete data as possible. Data on these associated parameters are required despite the difficulty of obtaining them. The best method of attaining this information is to observe the various parameters in many different mutually independent variables. According to the hypothesis, the basic oscillator remains the same in different overt rhythms, as long as the periods coincide, with only the couplings being different. Comparative measurement of these different rhythms is the preferred method of drawing conclusions about the influence of coupling. If different couplings could be coordinated with the different rhythms, there would be a difference in their influences, and no consistent regularities would be detected in a comparison of the different rhythms with regard to the parameters beside period. If the influence of the couplings, however, was negligible, consistent regularities could be detected with the different rhythms, based only on the properties of the oscillatory system. In this case, it should be possible to relate these regularities by application of oscillation theory. Finally, if the influences of different couplings on overt rhythms are great and identical in different rhythms, consistent regularities can be detected; the general system properties, in such cases, would be combined with properties of the coupling and those of the oscillator and would not be in agreement with postulates of oscillation theory. In order to distinguish the effects of the oscillatory system and those of the interposed couplings, the parameters of different overt rhythms must be compared with each other and with postulates of the oscillation theory. Comparative measurements of different rhythms can be performed with humans more effectively than with other organisms.

In summary, this book deals with properties of the human circadian system. The way to evaluate these properties is by comparative measurement of several different overt rhythms under experimental conditions essentially affecting the period of the circadian rhythms. From results obtained in different experiments, conclusions are drawn concerning mechanisms of the underlying oscillatory system separated from properties of couplings between this system and overt rhythms. This work does not deal expressly with the practical significance of the theoretical conclusions, although the applications, even in humans, are of increasing importance. Such applications presuppose theoretical mastery of all problems involved. Therefore, this thorough study is intended to prepare a basis for practical uses.

1.2. Human Circadian Rhythms

Diurnal rhythms in physiological variables were first described for pulse rate (Autenrieth, 1801), gas exchange during respiration (Prout, 1813), and evaporation (Reil, 1822). Later, measurements of deep body temperature were added. Figure 1 shows measurements prepared by Gierse (1842) using himself as the subject. From other measurements, it has been known for more than a century that the rhythmicity of physiological variables is not only due to ordinary changes between activity and rest. For example, with constant bed rest, the time course of deep body temperature continues to be rhythmic. Even while fasting, the same is true, as shown in figure 2, taken from Juergensen (1873). This indicates that rhythmicity of physiological variables is un-

likely to be simply a reaction to activity rhythm or rhythmic food intake.

More than 100 variables have been shown to change their values rhythmically with a 24-hour period. All these variables, physiological and psychological, readiness for single events (e.g., birth, death), and responses to external stimuli follow daily rhythmic courses. They show correspondingly a maximum and minimum value within a 24-hour day, but they are different in amplitudes and temporal positions of their extreme values. Description of the rhythmic character of the different time patterns can be summarized in "phase maps" demonstrating the temporal sequence in the rise and decline in different variables as a function of objective time (Aschoff, 1963a, 1966, 1967b; Halberg, 1965; Halberg and Reinberg, 1967). Figure 3 is an example of a "phase map" including rhythms of different variables which are chosen arbitrarily.

A "phase map" has meaning only if the rhythmicities are of sufficient reliability. In fact, it has been shown that the rhythms of physiological variables are satisfactorily reproducible when the measurements are repeated with the same subjects over a period of time (Krieger and Krieger, 1966; Krieger et al., 1971; Reinberg et al., 1967) or when comparing measurements obtained in differ-

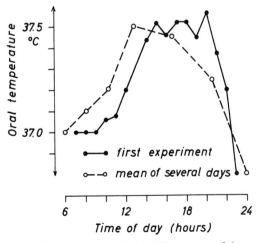

Figure 1. First record of a daily course of deep body temperature (i.e., oral temperature). After Aschoff (1955), with data from Gierse (1842).

4   Introduction

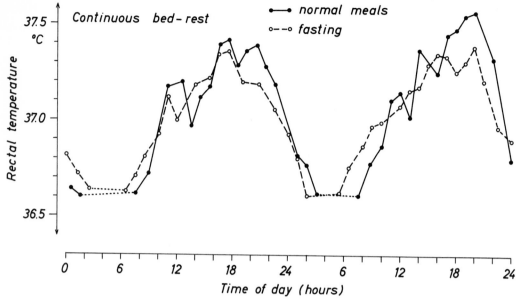

Figure 2. First record of a daily course of deep body temperature (i.e., rectal temperature) during continuous bed rest, with normal meals and while fasting. After Aschoff (1967a), with data from Juergensen (1873).

ent laboratories using different subjects. Figure 4 summarizes data on cortisol measurements, plasma concentrations (above) and excretion in urine (below) obtained by six different groups of authors. Generally, there is agreement among the time courses including the main episodes in plasma cortisol. The time courses of the urine curves are delayed in comparison to the plasma curves by about 3 hours (Aschoff, 1973). The evidence for sufficient reliability also extends to psychomotor variables. Figure 5 shows measurements of computation speed in children; these data were obtained by different authors, and separated in time by a fifty-year period.

Thus one must conclude that the different rhythms exhibit highly reliable temporal patterns. A high degree of temporal order in the functioning of organisms complements the spatial order manifested in structure. The maintenance of this temporal order in organisms, concomitant with many different biological processes conditioning each other, is one of the significant aspects of diurnal rhythmicity. The other significance is the temporal integration of steadily changing bi-

ological processes in an environment steadily oscillating between day and night.

Ordinary "phase maps" obtained from healthy subjects living in an undisturbed natural environment are, of course, valid under such conditions. However, obtained under such conditions, their validity becomes doubtful after being disturbed either internally (within organisms) or externally (in the environment). It is to be expected, after these disorders, that phase maps becomes altered in either temporary or permanent ways. To understand the influences of disorders on the temporal organization of biological processes, the setting up of a purely descriptive "phase map" is not sufficient. Investigations of the underlying circadian system are needed to understand such influences. These investigations, however, cannot be performed by measuring parameters of undisturbed systems but only by measuring disorders established experimentally.

The investigation of the human circadian system began with the first experimental series performed under constant environmental conditions, excluding all natural time cues (Aschoff and Wever, 1962a). The first

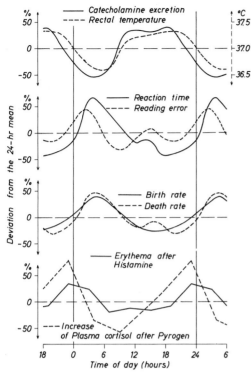

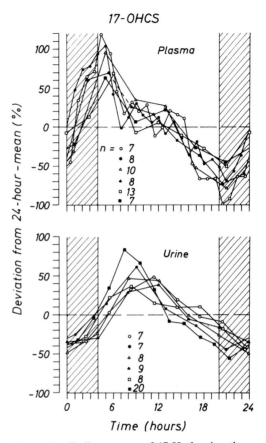

Figure 3.   Example of a "phase map" with aver-aged courses of eight arbitrarily choosen varia-bles. Physiological variables: catecholamine ex-cretion (Wisser et al., 1973) and rectal temperature (Aschoff et al., 1972). Psychological variables: reaction time (delay time in teleprint responses; Browne, 1961) and reading error (Bjerner and Swensson, 1953). Single events: birth rate (Gauquelin, 1971), and death rate (Wi-gand, 1934). Responsiveness: against histamine (Reinberg, 1965) and pyrogene (Takebe et al., 1966). The courses of some of the variables de-pend on the special sample arbitrarily chosen; it may be subject to variations in detail but not in general.

Figure 4.   Daily courses of 17-Hydroxicorticos-teroids in plasma (above) and urine (below), each from six different groups of investigators with averages from several subjects each (n: number of subjects in the respective investigation). From Aschoff (1973).

experiment of this series, performed in an artificial isolation unit, indicated a period deviating from 24 hours that was consistent in all variables measured (Fig. 6). The mea-sured period was 25.1 hours and resulted in a total phase shift against local time of 9 hours. The experiment was too short to de-cide whether a steady state period was at-tained indicating autonomy of the system, or whether the rhythm was still in the transient process of reentrainment to an overlooked zeitgeber, resulting in a temporarily changed period.

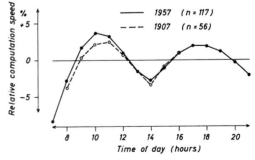

Figure 5.   Computation speed of school chil-dren, measured twice, with an interval of 50 years. From Baade (1907) and Rutenfranz and Hellbruegge (1957).

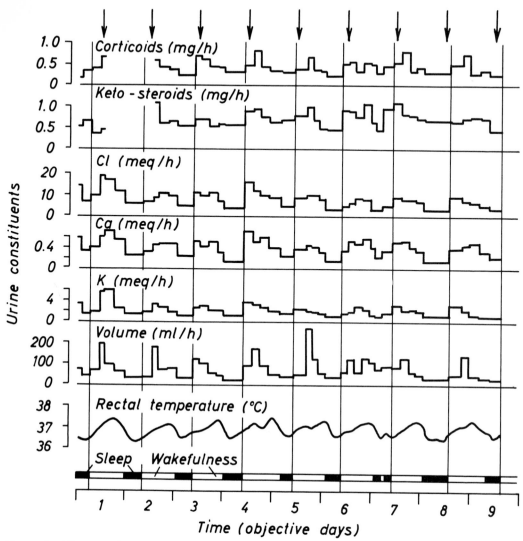

Figure 6. First experiment showing a free running human circadian rhythm, measured under constant conditions without environmental time cues. Longitudinally presented, from bottom to top, are the courses of the activity and rest cycle, rectal temperature (measured continuously), and six urine constituents (i.e, mictions taken at self-selected intervals). The arrows at the top indicate noon in local time. From Aschoff and Wever (1962a).

In subsequent experiments, it became clear that subjects felt a state of well-being during the isolation period and, therefore, the length of the experiments could be extended. Results of these experiments were fundamentally the same as those of the first one. The period was always close to 25 hours instead of 24 hours. In one experiment of sufficiently long duration, the total phase shift between the biological rhythm and local time exceeded 24 hours, proving the autonomy of the human circadian rhythm (i.e., its generation by endogenous processes). The course of this experiment is shown in figure 7. On the third day of the experiment, the subject's watch was taken away, and all environmental time cues were omitted. The subject then showed a rhythmic period of 25.9 hours continuing for 17.5 cycles (19 objective days), again being consistent in all

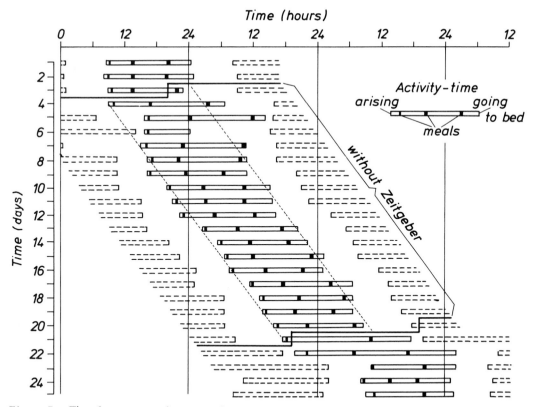

Figure 7. First human experiment, under constant conditions, proving the endogenous origin of circadian rhythms. Presented are successive activity periods, one beneath the other, as a function of local time (abscissa). From Aschoff and Wever (1962a).

measured variables. After reestablishing contact with the environment, the subject's rhythm was nearly reversed in comparison to the normal phase relationship to local time. This rhythm resynchronized, in about 4 days, by lengthening the rhythmic period again so that he deviated from real time after finishing the total experiment by 2 days. This shows the ability of the human circadian system to be rhythmically independent of environmental changes of day and night.

With these experiments, the endogenous origin of human circadian rhythms had been demonstrated just as had been done earlier with non-human species. These experiments also demonstrated that examination of human rhythms can open new insights into the circadian system because of the possibility of making comparative measurements of a great variety of physiological and psychological variables simultaneously. The most im-

portant rhythms have been measured either continuously (e.g., rectal temperature) or integratively (e.g., urine constituents such as electrolytes and hormones). The resulting continuous time series allow the study of interactions between the rhythms of different variables. Suggestions of mutual temporal dissociation of the circadian system had been included in the results of the first experimental series mentioned. The discovery of internal dissociation was the first step to the multioscillatory concept having an important position in the understanding of the human circadian system. The first series of human experiments under constant environmental conditions eventually resulted in their confident reliability for human subjects. All nine subjects stated that they generally felt quite well except for some initial discomfort at the beginning of the experiment. Most of the subjects agreed, without

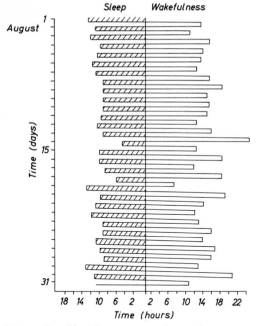

Figure 8.   First human experiment in a cave without environmental time cues. Presented, one beneath the other, are the durations of sleep (left) and wakefulness (right) of the subject, as determined outside the cave from his telephone calls (section). From Siffre (1963).

hesitation, to participate in another experiment, of even longer duration.

The first long-term studies concerning autonomous circadian rhythms in man were conducted 1 year later. One experiment was conducted in a natural cave for 2 months (Siffre, 1963). Another was conducted in an artificial isolation unit for 5 months (Findley et al., 1963). The results of these experiments were essentially the same as those of the shorter experiments. The subjects exhibited comparatively regular rhythms with periods clearly longer than 24 hours. Because of their long durations, both experiments resulted in phase shifts against local time of several days, once again confirming the endogenous origin of human circadian rhythms. These experiments also showed that there was no general temporal trend in the autonomous period or in any other parameter measured. Both experiments confirmed that the isolation, both spatial and temporal, did not result in serious adverse effects, even when isolation lasted several months.

In the cave experiment, change between wakefulness and sleep was the only variable measured during the total experiment. It resulted in a true oscillatory period of 24.6

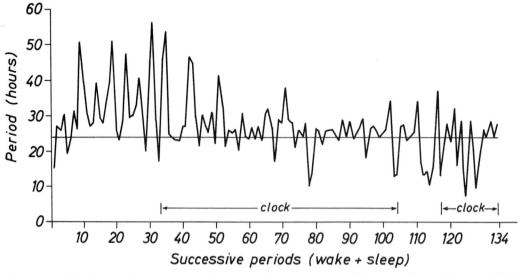

Figure 9.   First human long-term experiment, under constant conditions, performed in an artificial isolation unit. The subject temporarily had a watch, but no other environmental time cues. Presented are the durations of full cycles, including wakefulness and following sleep. From Findley et al. (1963).

hours. Figure 8 shows original activity data available from this experiment; unfortunately, this is only a portion of the total experiment. In this experiment, occasionally pulse rate had been measured and an estimate of the 120-second period was made by the subject while arising and retiring (during the 57 periods, 99 pulse rate measurements and 168 time estimations were performed). Only after a complicated mathematical procedure was established could a period estimation be possible. The result was consistent with the period of 24.6 hours (Halberg et al., 1965).

The 5-month experiment in the isolation unit was performed originally disregarding rhythm problems; its purpose was to evaluate endurance of complete isolation. This experiment resulted in an average activity period of 27.2 hours. Figure 9 shows original data from this experiment. As can be seen from figure 9, the day-to-day variations in activity data are much larger than in all ex-

periments mentioned previously (Figs. 6–8). Formally computed standard deviation of successive activity cycles exceeds ±8.6 hours. Only in this experiment, and in contrast to all other experiments discussed to this point, is any serial correlation of successive activity data missing. It cannot be ascribed to an oscillatory process but rather to a stochastic process. The subject (Fig. 9) had a watch temporarily available, and there are indications that he tended to be synchronized to local time during this portion of the experiment. Therefore, because of a lack of consistent data, definite unambiguous conclusions concerning the tendency to external or internal synchronization cannot be drawn.

After these pilot studies, investigations on human circadian rhythms, under experimentally controlled conditions without natural time cues, were systematically performed in caves and artificial isolation units. In the following survey (Tables 1/I and 1/II)

Table 1/I. Isolation Experiments in Natural Caves

No. of experiment	Year	Subject	Stay underground in isolation (days)	Authors
1	1962	M.S. ♂	62	Halberg et al., 1965b; Mills, 1967b; Siffre, 1963; Siffre et al., 1966
2	1963	G.W. ♂	105	Mills, 1964a, 1964b, 1967b
3	1964/1965	T.S. ♂	125	Ghata et al., 1969; Mills, 1967b; Siffre et al., 1966
4	1964/1965	J.L. ♀	88	Ghata et al., 1969; Mills, 1967b; Reinberg et al., 1966; Siffre et al., 1966
5	1965	Seven ♀♀	15	Apfelbaum and Nillus, 1967; Apfelbaum et al., 1969; Nillus, 1967
6	1966	D.L. ♂	127	Mills, 1966, 1967b; Mills et al., 1974
7	1966	J.M. ♂	182	Colin et al., 1968; Fraisse et al., 1968; Jouvet, 1968; Mills, 1967b
8	1968/1969	P.E. ♂	136	Chouvet et al., 1974
9		J.C. ♂		Jouvet et al., 1974; Siffre, 1972
10	1972	M.S. ♂	205	Siffre, 1975

Table 1/II. *Isolation Experiments in Artificial Units**

No. of experiment	Place	Number of experiments (subjects)	Average (longest) stay in isolation (days)	Kind of experiments	Authors
1	München	9 (9)	14 (19)	Free running	Aschoff and Wever, 1962a
2	College Park	1 (1)	152	Free running (temporarily with watch)	Findley et al., 1963
3	Erling-Andechs	205 (232)	29 (89)	Free running and zeitgeber	Aschoff, since 1965 Wever, since 1965
4	New London	1 (2)	9	Free running	Clegg and Schaefer, 1966
5	Marburg	4 (4)	12 (18)	Free running	Hildebrandt, 1966 Schaefer et al., 1967 Hildebrandt et al., 1968 Holleck, 1972 Kess, 1972 Lucas, 1973
6	Minneapolis	1 (1)	18	Free running	Kriebel, 1970
7	Manchester	9 (15)	9 (13)	Free running	Elliott et al., 1971a Mills et al., 1973, 1974
		8 (23)	9 (14)	Zeitgeber (phase)	Elliott et al., 1971b, 1972 Mills, 1973
		? (25)	?	Zeitgeber (period)	Mills et al., 1976
8	Gainesville	14 (14)	12 (14)	Free running	Webb and Agnew, 1974a
		8 (8)	20 (20)	Zeitgeber (phase)	Webb and Agnew, 1974b
		14 (14)	11 (14)	Zeitgeber (period)	Webb and Agnew, 1975
9	Moffett Field	2 (6)	21	Zeitgeber, temporarily free running	Winget, 1975

*For supplementation, see note on p. 24.

the two types of experiments are studied separately for clarity. Cave experiments mostly lasted longer than experiments in artificial isolation units. One long-term isolation experiment mentioned (Fig. 9) was an exception and was not really successful regarding evaluation of the basic oscillatory process. Physical conditions were very different in the two types of experiments. The artificial units were appropriately furnished for the most part to guarantee a comfortable stay of the subjects. The caves were inhospitable (the ambient temperature was about 7°C), and the subjects lived in small tents. It is likely, for these reasons, that the subjects participating in cave and isolation unit experiments differ regarding personality data. Finally, the facilities for recording many different biological variables, continuously if possible, were much easier to install in artificial units specifically constructed for isolation experiments than in natural caves where technical problems are difficult to overcome (e.g., the usually long distance between the location of any subject and the measuring equipment).

1.3. Operations and Methods

1.3.1. Facilities and Subjects

Because homogeneity of data is the prerequisite for consistent deductions of regularities of human circadian rhythms, emphasis was placed on one experimental series consisting of more than 200 isolation experiments under varying conditions. The experiments were performed in two units of an underground building especially constructed for the purpose of isolation experiments. To exclude environmental noise which varies greatly with time of day and, therefore, constitutes time information, each unit was double walled with separate floors, walls, and ceiling, so that each unit floated individually in glass wool within the outer building. Noise from the outside, or from the other unit, could not be heard unless it was sufficiently loud to surpass pain threshold (130 dB). In addition, one of the units was shielded against electric and magnetic fields but was equipped to introduce these fields artificially. The other unit was unshielded, allowing both fields to enter naturally (orientation by magnetic compass as well as radio reception is impossible in the "shielded" unit and can be nearly unattenuated in the "non-shielded" unit). Details of the construction and measurements of the shielding coefficients were given in Wever (1967c, 1969b, 1974d). Figure 10 shows the outline of the total building. Each of the units consisted of a living room with a bed, small kitchen, and toilet with shower. The entrance from the control room into the experimental unit was only through a lock, the two doors of which were magnetically latched. The rooms were furnished like comfortable apartments so that the subjects had no feeling of living in a laboratory. Figure 11 shows an interior view of one unit.

The series includes 205 experiments up to the end of 1976, performed under varying conditions but all isolated from natural time cues. 184 of these experiments were performed with singly isolated subjects, 18 experiments with two subjects together, and 3 experiments with four subjects together. The average length of the experiments ($\pm$ standard deviation) was 29 ± 5 days, with a range of 10 to 89 days. The greater majority of subjects felt they remained in good health during the experimental period. It is important to emphasize that all subjects knew they were not confined and could leave the isolation units without contacting the experimenter. The majority of subjects spontaneously asked to participate in another experiment after completing their initial isolation. 21 subjects participated in two subsequent experiments; two subjects participated in three subsequent experiments. Seven of the 232 subjects left the experiment before the agreed time. Only three left because they could not endure the isolation; the remaining four left for unanticipated personal reasons.

All subjects who participated in the isolation experiments were volunteers, and, therefore, were probably not a representative sample of the total population. It must be assumed that subjects volunteering for such an unusual experiment deviated from the average population in many respects, including some possible deviation of the circadian system itself. It was apparent that the results obtained in the experiments could not be accepted as totally representative, therefore emphasis was placed on qualitative factors. On the other hand, the subjects were psychologically examined before and after each experiment, and, as the general result, they did not deviate significantly from the average student population. The experimental data obtained during the different experiments showed remarkably small interindividual variations, in spite of the great variability in basic personality data of the volunteers. Therefore, results obtained from volunteers, to a certain degree, can be expected to reflect results representative of the greater population.

1.3.2. The Measurements

In the selection of variables to be recorded, preference was given to those that could be

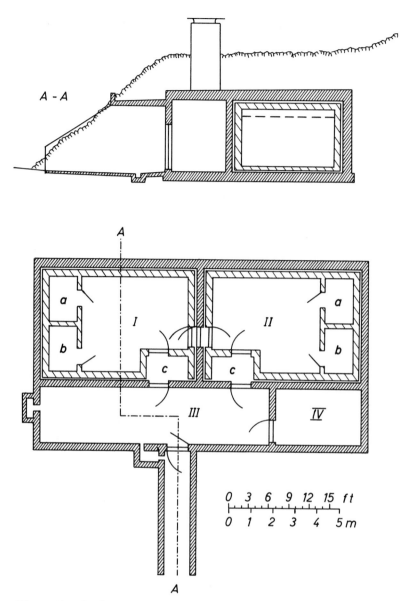

Figure 10. Outline of the isolation station: floor plan (below) and cross section (above). Narrowly shaded areas: reinforced concrete. Widely shaded areas: brick walls. *I* and *II:* experimental units (a = kitchen; b = toilet with shower; c = lock). *III:* control room. *IV:* special experimental chamber. From Wever (1969b).

measured continuously. Primarily, this was deep body temperature which was measured by means of a rectal probe (resistance thermometer). A sufficiently long wire connected the probe with the recording system outside the experimental unit. Like all other relevant measurements, rectal temperature data were acquired simultaneously (1) by a continuously running recorder for direct visual inspection, and (2) by a computer system for subsequent objective analyses (10 measurements per second; averaged data stored in minute intervals). It is worthwhile to note that the subjects were in no case aware of

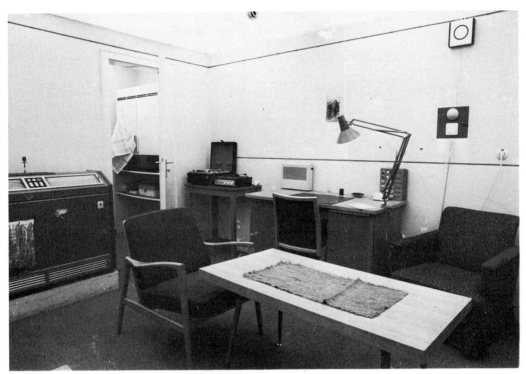

Figure 11.   View into one of the experimental units. From Wever (1969b).

the actual values of the measured variables thereby avoiding irregular influences of biofeedback on the rhythms.

The next most important variable was the activity of the subjects, recorded in different ways which complemented each other. The subjects indicated subjectively whether it was "day" or "night" and, from their responses, activity time and rest time were separated. In a few cases where, normally inadmissible, naps were unavoidable, the beginning and end of the naps were indicated. The locomotor activity of the subjects was recorded continuously by contact plates on the floor invisible under carpets. Bed movements were recorded by contacts which indicated sleeping behavior of the subjects. In some experiments, sleep was recorded by continuous polygraphic sleep recordings, using common techniques (i.e., EEG, EOG, EMG). In these experiments, the alternation between wakefulness and sleep was determined clearly as well as various sleep stages. In figure 12, the four types

of activity recordings, one subjectively scored and three objectively measured, are presented comparatively together with the rectal temperature, resulting from an experiment performed under constant conditions. This figure introduces the two preferred methods of presenting original data.

The longitudinal presentation (Fig. 12/I) shows the rhythmic course of the variables. Because of the compressed time scale, only smoothed time courses of the different variables are presented for clarity, but not the actual measured minute values. As can be seen in figure 12/I, activity time coincides with time of locomotor activity, and rest time with time of bed movements and objectively recorded sleep respectively, with small overlaps. There is only one short interval with bed movements during activity time (5th day), but it does not indicate a nap because locomotor activity is high (the subject possibly stored some heavy items on his bed at that time). In this special experiment, the course of rectal temperature does not

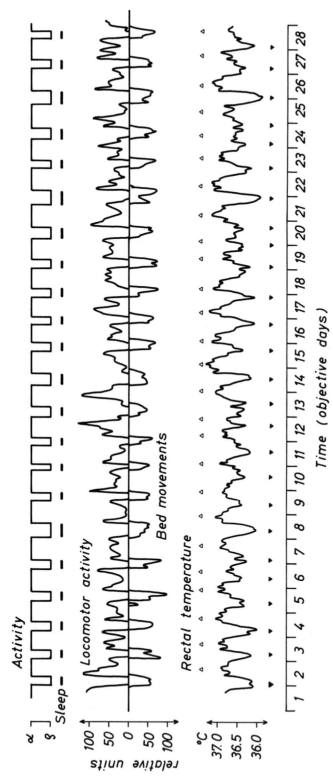

Figure 12. Comparison of four different types of recording activity of a subject (A.F., ♂ 24 y) living under constant conditions without time cues. (1) Subjective scoring of activity and rest (i.e., "day" and "night"). (2) Locomotor activity recorded from contact plates under the floor of the experimental room. (3) Sleep movements recorded from a contact in the bed. (4) Sleep, as determined from a polygraphic EEG record. **I:** Longitudinal presentation. The four types of activity recordings are presented longitudinally, one beneath the other, as a function of local time. From top to bottom: Subjectively scored activity, polygraphically recorded sleep, locomotor activity, and bed movements with reversed ordinate scale. For comparison, in the lowest row, the course of rectal temperature is presented. The temporal positions of maximum, and minimum values of rectal temperature, scored from the smoothed course, are given as triangles.

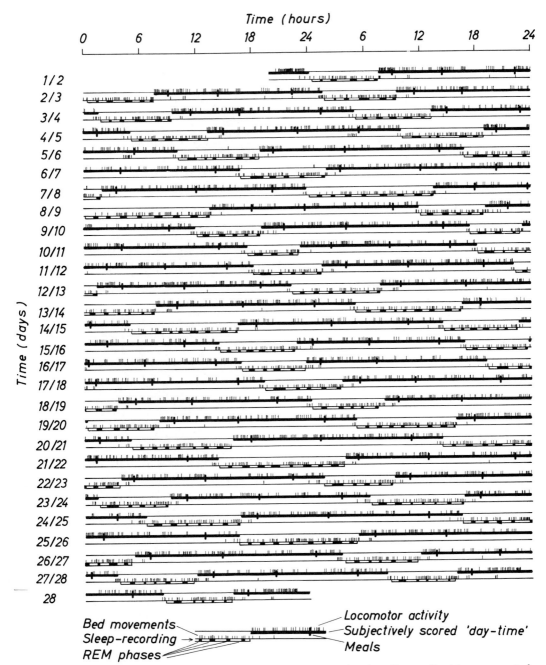

Time (hours)

Figure 12/II. Successive presentation. The records from successive days (i.e., ordinate) are presented, one beneath the other, as a function of local time (i.e., abscissa). For clarity, two successive days are presented after each other, so every day appears twice in the presentation. From each day, the upper row includes the subjective activity scoring, with an indication of the meals, and the computer plot of locomotor activity. The lower row includes the polygraphically recorded sleep, with an indication of the REM phases, and the computer plot of bed movements.

coincide with the activity course (internal desynchronization; cf. 2.2.1). This is especially clear from the inspection of triangles indicating the instances of maximum and minimum values (the triangles are taken simply from the inspection of the longitudinal temperature course).

In the vertical presentation (Fig. 12/II), successive days are drawn one below the other. The temporal resolving power is much greater than in the longitudinal presentation because of the extended time scale. The actual minute values can be separated. The number of variables presented is limited for the sake of clarity. Figure 12/II shows, at the upper line of each day (the total plot is doubled so 2 successive days are presented in each line), the subjectively scored activity time with the times of meals marked (there was no requirement to have three meals per day or cycle, respectively, but in this case, the subject did so) and the objectively recorded locomotor activity. At the lower line of each day, figure 12/II shows the sleep of the subject, as determined from polygraphic recordings (with the REM phases marked), together with the bed movements (the computer plots of locomotor and bed activity indicate for every minute whether there was activity or not). As can be seen in figure 12/II, the subject went to sleep several minutes after he scored termination of activity time (the average ± standard deviation was 10 ± 6 minutes), and he scored activity onset several minutes after awakening (mostly from a REM phase). Only on the 19th day, this delay exceeded half an hour (the average was 13 ± 9 minutes). While the locomotor activity is restricted to the activity time, bed movements are recorded not only during rest time but also for some time before and after rest time. This mainly may be caused by preparation of the bed for sleep and making the bed after awakening. Bed movements clearly increased when the subject was lying in bed but not asleep and during the REM phases.

It can be determined from figure 12 that the different kinds of recording activity coincide. Even the simplest type of recording,

the subjective scoring, gives a sufficient statement about the activity of the subject. This remains true although, for this example, an experiment was selected showing internal desynchronization during the total experiment (Fig. 13). The determination of activity is more irregular in these cases than with internally synchronized rhythms, meaning that discrepancies between the different kinds of activity recordings must be expected during internal desynchronization rather than during internal synchronization. Nevertheless, this coincidence is present even in this experiment. In most of the following presentations, therefore, activity is represented by subjective scorings, especially for the period determination, which, in all these cases, results in equal values based on all four activity recordings mentioned. It only must be considered that rest time (in this example: 9.08 ± 2.21 hours) is consistently longer than true sleep time (8.69 ± 2.25 hours) and activity time (21.2 ± 1.37 hours) is consistently shorter than true wake time (21.5 ± 1.40 hours) respectively. As a consequence, the true ratio betwen wakefulness and sleep is, in principle, larger than the activity rest ratio (2.48 against 2.33). The different activity recordings are not considered separately except in the very rare experiments where discrepancies between the different kinds of activity recordings lead to different periods (Fig. 82).

In addition to rectal temperature and activity, the measurement of urine constituents (e.g., volume, electrolytes, catecholamines, steroids) is meaningful. It supplies integrative values (the actual time course of the kidney excretion cannot be determined, but at least the average excretion value can be) reflecting a continuous course, although smoothed. In contrast to this, values that can only be measured occasionally, and where the real time course (and even the average value) between two measurements is unknown, are less useful because the conclusions from these values for a continuous time course require an interpolation. The only type of interpolation free of arbitrariness is the linear one but this type is, of necessity, connected with a flattening of the rhythm, if present. All other types of interpolation (including a sinusoidal shape) assume hypotheses about the rhythm shape to be expected which need special foundation. This normally will not be possible because the shapes of the rhythms vary from subject to subject, variable to variable, condition to condition, and, partly, from day to day (Wever, 1973d).

The applied type of interpolation becomes increasingly important if the measuring intervals are nonequidistant. The practicability of determining a rhythm depends less on the number of measuring points than on the width of the largest interval between successive measurements. It is a common belief that a rhythm needs at least 8 equidistant measuring points for its establishment; only in special cases 6 points are sufficient. With nonequidistant intervals, the largest regular interval between 2 successive measurements determines the practicability of the computation. The rhythm determination based on nonequidistant measuring intervals is equivalent to a number of equidistant intervals resulting from the complementation of the largest regular interval by equal intervals to the full cycle. For example, if there is, in the 24-hour day, a regular night gap between successive measuring points of 8 hours, the rhythm determination, based on the day values, corresponds in its reliability to a rhythm determination, based on only 3 equidistant measuring points, independent of the actual number of measuring points during the daytime. This means that the rhythms determination of those variables, of which the measurement is possible only at discrete instants (e.g., psychological variables, performance data, hormone concentrations in blood), is possible only when at least one or two values are measured during the sleep time of the subjects. Normally this means that subjects have to be awakened for the measurements. Without the sleep interruptions, meaningful statements about rhythm parameters (e.g., amplitude, mean value, phase) cannot be given even in a rhythm with a predetermined period. If the

shape of the rhythm underlies temporal fluctuations, not even the rhythm period can be derived with certainty. This means that, if sleep interruptions are not practicable for any reason (e.g., during constant conditions), only continuously gained data (e.g., rectal temperature) or integratively gained data (e.g., urine constituents) enable a sufficient computation of any rhythm endpoint.

1.3.3. The Analyses

In the presentation of the measurement results, preference must be given to the presentation of the original data because each mathematical pretreatment uses a more or less arbitrarily chosen model. Only the presentation of the original data guarantees an unprejudiced picture of what has really been measured. The two preferred methods of presenting original data have been illustrated (Fig. 12). The second (vertical) presentation especially demonstrates the period (or phase) of the rhythm. Its limitation to only a few variables mainly is not a serious handicap because frequently the great variety of measured variables can be represented sufficiently by only two (e.g., activity and rectal temperature). However, the presentation of the raw data cannot substitute for extensively computed analyses of the data. First, the simple inspection of complex data does not allow for strong conclusions. For example, if a time series simultaneously includes more than one periodicity (in addition to the unavoidable "biological noise"), the inspection of the raw data may result in misleading interpretations. Only the presence of a single periodicity in a time series, combined with small perturbations by superimposed noise, allow clear, direct statements. Second, quantitative statements about rhythm parameters can be raised only on the basis of objectively computed analyses. The knowledge of those quantitative statements is required if the dependency of the rhythm on experimental conditions may be evaluated. It, however, has to be considered that some of these rhythm endpoints are meaningful

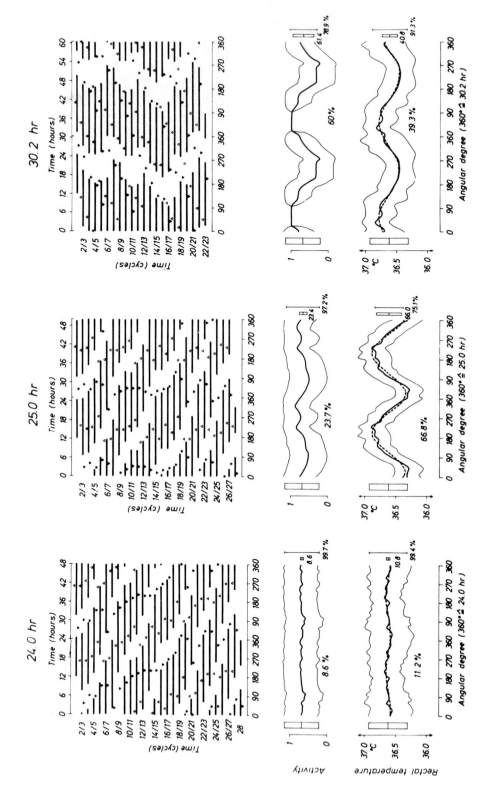

Figure 13/I

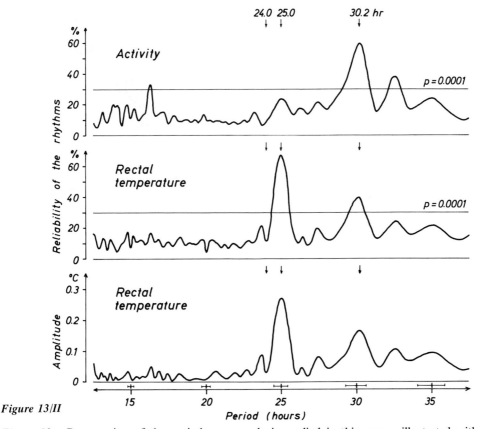

Figure 13/II

Figure 13. Presentation of the periodogram analysis applied in this paper, illustrated with data of subjectively scored activity and rectal temperature, from the experiment shown in figure 12. *I.* Special presentation for three separate periods. In the upper diagrams, successive periods are drawn, one beneath the other, and, for clarity, two periods, one after another. The presentation, with $\tau = 24.0$ hours, is identical to that in figure 12/II. The bars indicate subjectively scored activity, the triangles indicate temporal positions of maximum (Δ) and minimum values ($\blacktriangledown$) of rectal temperature (Fig. 12/I). In the lower diagrams, the average cycles are presented, as pooled from the upper diagrams, with the three averaging periods mentioned. The thick lines give the averages, corresponding to the upper diagrams, from activity (1 = activity; 0 = rest) and rectal temperature; not only from the extremum values, but also from the complete courses. The thin lines give the formally computed standard deviations around the averages. Especially from the activity computations, it is clear these "standard deviations" are meaningless when taken separately, since their ranges can exceed the range between 0 and 1, outside of which activity is not defined. The dotted lines in the rectal temperature poolings give the fundamental periods. At the left side of each pooling diagram, mean and formally computed standard deviation of the total time series is presented (broad bars; identical with all averaging periods). At the right side, means and formally computed standard deviations of the average cycles (narrow bars) and the averaged range of the formally computed standard deviations around the average cycles (limited lines) are presented. The small numbers indicate the percentages of the standard deviations (right) in relation to the overall standard deviation (left). The large numbers indicate the "standardized" reliabilities (i.e., standard deviation of the average cycle in relation to the overall standard deviation, standardized with regard to a "normal circadian time series," including 25 successive cycles with measuring intervals of 1 hour).

Figure 13/II. Complete periodograms of activity and rectal temperature, based on reliability analyses, as illustrated in figure 13/I, computed with a variety of periods (abscissa = period; ordinate = standardized reliability). The three characteristic periods, exemplified in figure 13/I, are indicated by arrows. The thin line at 30% indicates the "borderline reliability," above which true rhythmicity, in contrast to random fluctuations, can be assumed with high probability. In the lowest diagram, Fourier analysis of rectal temperature is given, presenting the amplitudes (i.e., ordinate) of the fundamental periods (dotted lines in Fig. 13/I) coordinated to the different period values (i.e., abscissa). At the abscissa scale, the period inaccuracies are indicated as inherent in every mathematic period analysis.

19

only with a definite hypothesis. For example, "amplitude" or "acrophase" are meaningful values only if the sinusoidal course of the rhythm can be established. If rhythms of different shapes have to be compared, statements concerning differences in endpoints like "amplitude" or "acrophase" can be misleading (Wever, 1973d). Third, statistical statements are desirable for quantitative analyses in order to test the significance of the results evaluated. One of the most important statistical problems which can be solved only by quantitative analyses is determining whether a seemingly regular variation, included in a time series, is caused by a true underlying periodicity or only by random fluctuations.

Frequently, longitudinal statistics have been applied to obtain statistical statements. This method is useful if successive events within the time series can be shown to be serially independent of each other. The mutual independence of the units used, or the fulfillment of the ergodic theorem, is a necessary prerequisite in the applicability of these statistics. In human circadian rhythms, this prerequisite can be shown, in corresponding analyses which will be mentioned in detail later, to be unfulfilled; therefore, longitudinal statistics are meaningless from the strict convention. They do not enable a statement of statistical probabilities to be made. The reliability of a rhythm determination, computed longitudinally from a single time series, however, depends on the length of the time series, in a similar manner, as the significance of a statistical statement depends on the number of events summarized in the statement. This reliability must not be confounded with statistical significance in the strict sense, although it may lead to statements of probability at another level. Statistical terms (e.g., standard deviation) can be of great descriptive value when computed formally from only longitudinal statistics. To keep the fundamental difference in mind, the term "statistical significance" will be restricted to results of transverse statistics which can be applied without reservations. If longitudinal statistics are applied formally, the results will be mentioned in terms of "reliability."

Rhythm statistics frequently are based on least square methods, comparing raw data with mathematical functions (normally sine or cosine waves). This method is useful if the special presupposed shape (e.g., the sinusoidal shape) can be established by a meaningful hypothesis. In human circadian rhythms, however, the shape of the rhythms varies from subject to subject, variable to variable, and condition to condition (Wever, 1973d). The necessary prerequisite in the applicability of this method is largely violated. As a consequence, confidence intervals, computed by applying the least square methods indicated, do not depend only on superimposed noise but also on the deviation of the real shape from the presupposed shape. Most critically, the deviations last mentioned, in principle, are not distributed randomly but systematically. Randomly distributed deviations are, however, a further necessary prerequisite in the applicability of the statistics. It follows that confidence intervals computed by applying these methods which, of course, are correct in themselves cannot have real statistical relevance. Even their descriptive relevance is small because of the ambiguity mentioned; therefore, other statistical methods must have preference which do not precondition any definite rhythm shape or any other definite rhythm parameter. Only in special cases that need foundations, least square methods, presupposing definite (e.g., sinusoidal) rhythm shapes, may be applied.

In this study, analytical methods will be applied which are free of the restrictions mentioned. These are transversable statistics that compare interindividual differences between rhythm parameters obtained under different experimental conditions. Preference is given primarily to nonparametric (rank order) statistics that must not presuppose any distinct distribution of the values concerned. In other words, if statistical conclusions are drawn in any way, only values originating from different subjects, computed as endpoints of separate time series analyses, will be taken for statistical units. In estimating parameters of a rhythm included in a single time series, a modified periodogram analysis will be applied which must not presuppose any distinct shape of the rhythm or any other restricting precondition. The periodogram analysis itself is well known (Schuster, 1898; Whittaker and Robinson, 1924; Kendall, 1946; Enright, 1965; Lamprecht and Weber, 1970). Its modification enables, among other things, statements of 'reliability' allowing conclusions for probabilities by simulating the assumed rhythmicity by random fluctuations and will be described briefly here.

The periodogram analysis is based on the superimposition of successive, but arbitrarily defined, periods of equal duration or "longitudinal pooling" with a constant averaging period. For example, figure 13 shows results of this procedure with data of subjectively scored activity and rectal temperatures from the experiment shown in figure 12. Figure 13/I illustrates the procedure in detail, with three different averaging periods. The left-hand diagram repeats the presentation of figure 12/II with additional indications of the temporal positions of maximum and minimum values of rectal temperature taken from the smoothed longitudinal presentation of the rectal temperature course (Fig. 12/I). The activity rhythm and the rectal temperature rhythm shift continuously in relation to the 24-hour time scale. In the "pooling procedure," the instantaneous values of all 28 successive days are averaged. With rectal temperature, the total time series is considered in the averaging procedure and not only the extreme values which are included in the above diagram. With neither activity nor rectal temperature is any average period recognizable but only random fluctuations. This indicates that a rhythmicity with the 24.0-hour period is not included in one of the time series presented. The middle diagram of figure 13/I shows the same procedure but with an averaging period of 25.0 hours. As can be seen with this period, the extreme values of the rectal temperature rhythm are positioned

vertically one beneath the other, but not the activity periods. The pooling procedure with the 25.0-hour period results in an average rectal temperature period of considerable oscillation range. The pooling of the activity data does not result, with this period, in a clear periodicity. The right-hand diagram of figure 13/I shows the same procedure once more but with the 30.2-hour period. This period best fits the activity rhythm, as is evident in the vertical coincidence of successive activity periods, though superimposed by more or less regular fluctuations over a period of many days. The extreme values of rectal temperature shift continuously in relation to the abscissa scale, similar to the 24.0-hour period, but with a slight accumulation of the maximum values in the range between 0° and 90° and of the minimum values between 180° and 270°. The pooling procedure resulted in an average activity period that is more strongly marked than with other period values, and in an average rectal temperature period with a range of oscillation larger than that with a 24.0-hour, but smaller than with a 25.0-hour period.

Next to the average periods (lower diagrams of Fig. 13/I), some different deviation measurements are indicated. At the left side of each diagram, mean and standard deviation of all measurements included in the total time series are presented; at the right side, mean and standard deviations of all values included in the average period, and the average of all standard deviations around the average period (average width of the band accompanying the average period) are presented. The two variability measurements last mentioned are expressed as percentages of the variability of the total time series. The two resulting proportions can be taken for the fraction of true rhythmicity included in the time series and the fraction of random noise or systematic but nonperiodic trend. The squares of both these proportions complement each other regarding the unit. The formally computed standard deviations themselves cannot be taken for statistical measures because they are not based on mutually independent measurements. Instead of computing standard deviations, any other measure of variability can be taken (e.g., parametric or nonparametric). It is necessary only to apply the same measurement of variability to the single mean as to the overall mean. It is appropriate, in practice, for uniform computations to divide the period selected, independent of its length, into a fixed number of equidistant classes (e.g., 24 classes according to "circadian hours") and to distribute the measured values into these classes according to their temporal order; then, for each of the classes, mean and standard deviation have to be computed from all values within the respective class. For special cases, the averaging period and, therefore, the classes need not have constant values but systematically varying values. With such a procedure, even analyses of rhythms with systematically varying periods are possible (Fig. 94/II).

By comparing the rhythmic fraction or the "reliability" of the rhythm with correspondingly computed fractions in series of random numbers, the probability can be stated indicating the accidental generation of the rhythm with the selected period by random fluctuations. These empirical evaluations have been confirmed recently by exact analytic computations (Dörrscheidt and Beck, 1975). To be precise, the probability for accidental generation of a rhythmicity depends not only on the computed "reliability," but also on the number of periods within the time series, the number of classes per period, and the number of measured points per class. In order to facilitate the comparison, the rhythm reliabilities can be normalized to parameters which are characteristic in circadian investigations. In all the following computations, 25 successive periods per time series, measuring intervals of 1 hour, and 24 classes per period are taken arbitrarily for the "standard circadian time series." With these values, a "normalized reliability" of 20% means that it is equally probable that the time series is based on a true rhythmicity with the selected period, or on random fluctuations or other non-periodic variations (e.g., systematic trend). A

"normalized reliability" of 24% means a probability of $p = 0.05$ that the rhythmicity is simulated, by chance, by random fluctuations, and a "normalized reliability" of 30% means a random probability for rhythmicity of only $p = 0.0001$. The latter value normally is taken for the "borderline reliability," to discriminate between true rhythmicities and random fluctuations.

The procedure exemplified in figure 13/I with three characteristic averaging periods must be repeated with a variety of periods. A complete period analysis then results by plotting the normalized reliabilities as a function of the period, as shown in figure 13/II. This procedure can be applied with steadily varying values (e.g., body temperature) as well as variables that can accept only discrete values (e.g., the subjectively scored activity (activity = 1; rest = 0)). Beside the normalized reliabilities of the rhythms, figure 13/II includes, for comparison, the result of a conventional period analysis from rectal temperature (Fourier analysis) (i.e., the amplitude of rectal temperature rhythm plotted as a function of the period). As seen with rectal temperature, both kinds of analyses coincide with positions of peak periods; however, only the computation of reliabilities allows a decision on whether or not a peak period corresponds to a true rhythmicity. Furthermore, only the computation of reliabilities allows comparison of rhythms of different variables regarding their qualities. In this special example, the rectal temperature includes a highly reliable rhythmic component with a 25.0-hour period and, additionally, a secondary rhythmic component with a 30.2-hour period; activity includes a primary rhythmic component with a 30.2-hour period and a secondary component at 32.5 hours (another peak at 16.25 hours represents the 2nd harmonic of 32.5 hours). As the general result, rectal temperature and activity show primary peaks at different periods (indicating "internal desynchronization"; cf. 2.2.1) but they show peaks, if at all, at equal periods. The primary period of activity (30.2 hours) coincides with the secondary period of rectal temperature. At the primary period of rectal temperature (25.0 hours), activity shows a small peak with a reliability of 24%, indicating a probability for accidental simulation of this period by random fluctuations of $p = 0.05$. At the secondary period of activity (32.5 hours), rectal temperature shows a small peak with another reliability of 24%, indicating another probability for random generation of $p = 0.05$.

In other examples, simple Fourier analyses are given. In those presentations, only period values are plotted which are defined as submultiples of the total time series. Simultaneously, this kind of presentation clearly shows the accuracy in periods which cannot be improved by any period analysis. The reason is that each period estimation (τ) includes, independent of the special mathematical method applied, an inaccuracy ($\Delta\tau$) which is given by $\Delta\tau \geqslant \tau^2/T = \tau/n$, where T is the length of the total time series and n is the number of successive periods (τ) within this time series. In figure 13/II, these inaccuracies are indicated based on the 660-hour time series. They correspond to the broadnesses of the peaks at the respective periods. This inevitable inaccuracy in the period estimation, which is based on the length of the time series, is often confused with the variability in phases, which can be much smaller, and does not depend on the length of the time series. This variability in phases, which is meaningful only with regard to a specified period, can be calculated either from the intervals between successive corresponding phases (e.g., activity onset, maximum of rectal temperature), or from the deviations of those phases from a computed regression. The variability in phases can be a useful quality in describing properties of a rhythm. It is, however, crucial that this variability does not enable specific statistical statements be made about the period (e.g., about the deviation of an estimated period from a fixed value (e.g., 24 hours)).

Applying Fourier analysis, the period values computed are defined as harmonics of the total time series; therefore, in these cases a two-step method is used. First, with a great variety of periods, the period that has the largest amplitude is determined. Second, the time series is limited to a multiple of that period. As a consequence of this concept, the centers of gravity of the different periods included in the spectrum are in integral relationship. If more than one relevant period is included in one time series (Fig. 13), this concept may give rise to the suggestion that those periods are, in principle, in an integral relationship. This interpretation, however, is a product of the procedure applied and the actual relationship between the periods needs additional investigation (in figure 13 the different relevant periods are not in an integral relationship). Finally, with this procedure the period with the largest amplitude is taken as 100% for clarity and better comparability.

The analyses mentioned allow the possibility of describing the time series measured quantitatively. They even allow statistical statements about whether or not a rhythm, with a predetermined period, is included in the time series. The analyses do not allow statements concerning the mechanism of a proven rhythmicity which can be based on either an oscillatory process (with superimposed background noise), or a stochastic process (of limited band width). There are many similarities between these two processes although they are based on very different mechanisms. For example, the distribution of successive periods (better: equivalent intervals) included in the time series, as indicated in a period histogram (better: interval histogram), may be the same, or all kinds of period analyses may lead to similar results in both processes. A discrimination between both processes is possible, however, by inspecting the serial correlation between successive events within the time series. These successive events may be successive periods which are defined by any arbitrarily selected phase. In a stochastic process, successive periods are mutually independent of each other and the serial correlation between one period and the following one, one period and the next but one, or to any distinct later period is zero. In an oscillatory process, the serial correlation between successive periods usually is negative. If this correlation happens to be zero or positive, the serial correlation between one period and the next but one, or to a later period is negative. Generally, in an oscillatory process, the serial correlations between one period and a later period alternate with increasing distances between the compared periods, between negative and positive values. In an activity rhythm, additionally, the correlation between complementary activity and rest times can be considered. In a stochastic process there can be a serial correlation between activity time and following rest time or between activity time and preceding rest time, but there cannot be serial correlations between activity time and both the following and preceding rest time. If such an 'overlapping' serial correlation is present, the underlying mechanism must be oscillatory.

The discrimination mentioned between oscillatory and stochastic processes, based on the serial correlation, is not conclusive in the strictest sense. A negative serial correlation only states that the overt rhythm considered is controlled by an underlying rhythm of a variability that is smaller than that of the overt rhythm. This underlying rhythmicity may be an external zeitgeber which normally has a great precision; therefore, each overt rhythm under the influence of a zeitgeber shows negative serial correlations independent of its endogenous origin. If an overt rhythm, which can be shown to run autonomously, shows negative serial correlations, an underlying rhythmicity of a smaller variability must be present. Normally, such an underlying rhythmicity is meaningful when termed an oscillatory process. However, it cannot be fundamentally disproved that this underlying control rhythm is based on a stochastic process with a band width smaller than that of the overt rhythm considered. The terms melt into one another, and the discrimination becomes more a question of definition than of principle. In the following, basic rhythms of very small variabilities, controlling overt rhythms of larger variabilities, will be called "oscillators" according to conventional nomenclature.

Note added in proof:

Only after completion of this book (September 1977), an excellent study in human circadian rhythms appeared (C. A. Czeisler: Human circadian physiology: internal organization of temperature, sleep-wake and neuroendocrine rhythms monitored in an environment free of time cues. Dissertation, Stanford Univ. 1978). This study, performed in an artificial isolation unit in Bronx N. J., includes 11 isolation experiments with singly isolated subjects, lasting for 16 to 103 days (average: 34 days). The results of these experiments harmonize in many respects with the results discussed in this book, including the temporary occurrence of real internal desynchronization in 4 subjects. The agreement concerns the rhythms of activity and rectal temperature; in addition, however, the study mentioned includes, in most of the subjects, evaluations of Plasma Cortisol and Somatotropin (Human Growth Hormone). The agreement, moreover, concerns the structure of sleep which has not been described in detail in this book but elsewhere (J. Zulley: Der Einfluss von Zeitgebern auf den Schlaf des Menschen. Dissertation, Univ. Tübingen 1978. R. Wever: Schlaf und circadiane Rhythmik. In: Schlaf und Pharmakon (Herausg.: G. Harrer und V. Leutner); Schattauer-Verlag, Stuttgart—New York 1979).

2
Autonomous Rhythms

2.1. External Synchronization and Desynchronization

In order to recognize the specialties of autonomous rhythms, a long-term study of externally synchronized rhythms is considered for comparison. Figure 14 shows the courses of some variables measured for 1 week in a young man living on a strict 24-hour routine. Besides the change between wakefulness and sleep (activity rhythm), two physiological and two psychological rhythms are presented. The time courses have been measured either continuously (e.g., rectal temperature), in an integrating fashion over regular intervals (e.g., potassium excretion in urine) or by spot checking at regular intervals (e.g., psychological variables). During nighttime, the subject was awakened for urine mictions and tests. Figure 14/I shows the remarkable regularity in the rhythmic courses of all variables. The longitudinal pooling of the data (Fig. 14/II) shows the high reliability of all rhythms. A more detailed inspection of Figure 14 indicates that in the physiological rhythms all data contribute to the rhythmicity in nearly equal

amounts. In the psychological rhythms, however, the relevance of the rhythmicities mainly is based on the sharply decreased night values; the plateaus during daytime would hardly constitute reliable rhythms.

2.1.1. Free Running Rhythms

When a subject does not live under a 24-hour routine but is isolated from all environmental time cues, the rhythms persist autonomously. Figure 15 shows long-term courses of some physiological variables measured in a young man living under isolation. To continue the constancy of the conditions, dates for tests could not be given externally at regular intervals but had to be selected by the subject himself; inevitably at irregular intervals. Tests and urine mictions could not be done during the sleep time of the subject; therefore, under constant conditions, only variables that are measurable either continuously (e.g., rectal temperature) or integratively (e.g., urine constituents) can be used efficiently. This means that psychological

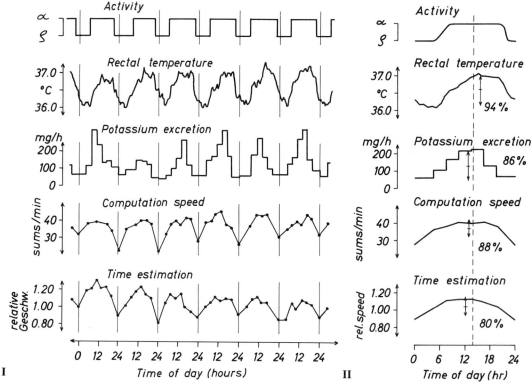

Figure 14. Rhythm of a subject (J.P., ♂ 31 y) living under standardized conditions under the influence of a strict 24-hour routine. Presented, from top to bottom, are the courses of the activity and rest cycle (α = wakefulness; ρ = sleep), rectal temperature (measured continuously), potassium excretion with the urine (from mictions at regular intervals), maximal computation speed (measured, after the urine mictions, with an automatic Pauli-test maschine), and time estimation (production of a 10-second interval measured, after the mictions, with an electric stopwatch). *I.* Longitudinally presented courses of the variables during 1 week. *II.* Longitudinally pooled courses of the rhythms, shown in I, presenting average cycles. The dotted line is midpoint of activity time. Mean value and amplitude of the fundamental periods of each rhythm are presented at the position of the respective acrophase. I from Wever (1973c).

rhythms cannot be obtained efficiently under constant conditions.

Figure 15/I shows that all variables oscillate diurnally and synchronously to each other. A closer inspection shows that the phases of the biological rhythms shift gradually relative to local time. At the beginning of the experiment, the phase relationships were normal (e.g., onset of activity at about 8.00 AM; end of activity at about midnight; maximum of rectal temperature during the late afternoon). These phases are reversed, regarding local time, in the middle of the experiment and have nearly normal values again at the end of the experiment. As a result of the continuous phase shift, the sub-

ject subjectively had experienced only 25 days during the 26 objective days of the experiment. This means the periods of all rhythms have values of 25 hours instead of 24 hours. This observation is confirmed by the result of computed period analyses (Fig. 15/II). All spectra clearly show single peaks at the same period of 25.0 hours. In the next step, the different rhythms are pooled longitudinally based on this computed period. Figure 15/III shows that the reliability of all rhythms is sufficient although they are autonomous, or free running, and not forced, or even stabilized, to a fixed period as in figure 14.

The deviation of the free running period

from 24 hours can be seen more clearly using another method of presenting the data. Figure 16 shows results from another experiment of the same type. For clarity, only rhythms of activity and rectal temperature are presented. In figure 16/I, the deviation of the oblique dotted line, computed as the regression combining the midpoints of successive activity times, from the vertical line demonstrates the deviation of the period from 24 hours. As seen in figure 16/I, this subject had a very regular activity rhythm with a period of 25.3 hours, resulting in a total phase shift against local time of nearly 2 days. The subject also had not perceived the deviation of his subjective time from the objective time. After the experiment, he was confused completely when his carefully kept calendar was incorrect by 2 days. The rhythm of rectal temperature (represented by the triangles) had the same period (i.e., it ran synchronously to the activity rhythm during the total experiment). The period analyses given in Figure 16/II confirm this result. In the rhythm of activity, as well as rectal temperature, only one sharp "spectral line" is present, with the center of gravity at 25.3 hours. Because of the length of the respective time series, the peaks are remarkably small. The analyses of the rhythms of all other variables measured result in similar spectra with only one sharp peak each at 25.3 hours. The longitudinal pooling of the rhythms (Fig. 16/III) indicates the high reliability of the free running rhythms. The reliability of the rectal temperature rhythm can be taken from the percent value and, more obviously, from the width of the standard deviations around the average period.

2.1.2. Criteria for Autonomy

In the experiments demonstrated in figures 15 and 16, there is no doubt that the rhythms were not synchronized by a 24-hour zeitgeber. This is indicated by the total phase shifts against local time of more than 360°, or 24 hours, respectively. In the computed period analyses, this is indicated by the fact

that the 24.0-hour period is clearly outside the "spectral lines." In the second example (Fig. 16), even the 24.8-hour period (apparent revolution of the moon) is outside the spectral line. In this case, it can be excluded that the rhythm is synchronized by the apparent revolution of the moon. In our environment, external rhythmicities in the 'circadian' range can be present only with periods of 24.0 hours and 24.8 hours (the latter period being very weak, at best). If a rhythm shows a period sufficiently deviating from these values, it cannot be induced by an external rhythmicity and, therefore, runs free autonomously (i.e., it is of endogenous origin).

The proof that a rhythm is autonomous and not induced by 24-hour zeitgeber can be furnished only if the period deviates sufficiently from 24 hours. If a period is very close to 24 hours, a total phase shift of more than 24 hours from local time would need an experiment of impracticable duration; therefore, to prove the autonomy of the rhythm, based on the total phase shift, is impossible. It cannot be excluded that the free running rhythm of a subject is very close to 24 hours. In such cases, it would be especially interesting to decide objectively whether a rhythm is really free running or induced by a zeitgeber. It would be desirable to have criteria for the autonomy of a rhythm that is independent of the total phase shift against possible zeitgebers. Such an independent test can be derived from the determination of internal phase angle differences between different rhythms.

The internal phase angle difference between the rhythms of activity and rectal temperature, derived from the pooled periods, differs considerably, when obtained under constant conditions (Figs. 15/III and 16/III), from those obtained in a 24-hour day (Fig. 14/II). For example, the maximum rectal temperature occurs in the late afternoon or early evening, when measured in a natural 24-hour day, and occurs in the first half of the activity time, (i.e., in the subjective morning), when measured under constant conditions (Aschoff et al. 1967a). This state-

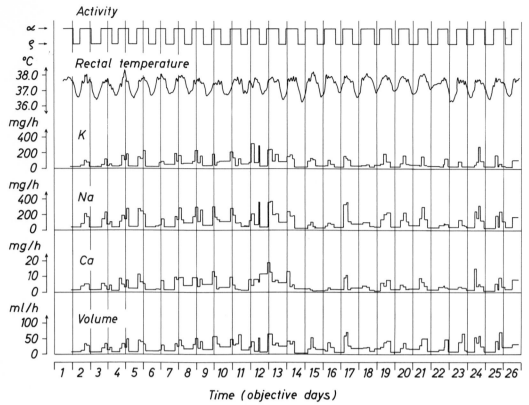

Figure 15. Autonomous rhythm of a subject (J.E., ♂ 25 y) living under constant conditions without environmental time cues. Presented from top to bottom, are the rhythms of activity (i.e., alternation between wakefulness α and rest ρ), rectal temperature (measured continuously), and four urine constituents (i.e., mictions taken at self-selected intervals). *I.* Longitudinally presented courses of the six variables during the total experiment.

ment, derived from the few examples demonstrated, can be generalized. It has been shown that the phase relationships of the rectal temperature extreme values, relative to the activity period when measured under constant conditions, differ from those measured under entrainment to the natural 24-hour day, to a high statistical level, when averaged from many subjects. It also has been shown that the phase positions of the maximum rectal temperature, when compared in the two conditions mentioned, differ from each other more than those of the minimum. Consequently, the shapes of the rectal temperature rhythm, or its temporal courses, are different from each other in the two conditions to a high statistical level. These differences can be seen in figure 17

which summarizes results originating from many subjects. When circadian rhythms are entrained to a 24-hour day, the rectal temperature rhythm lags behind the activity rhythm by a statistical significance of $p < 0.001$. This remains true for the relationships between temperature maximum and midpoint of activity, temperature minimum and midpoint of rest time, and the acrophases of the two rhythms. On the contrary, in autonomous rhythms measured under constant conditions, the rectal temperature rhythm leads the activity rhythm, with a statistical significance of $p < 0.001$, with all three phase relationships mentioned. This result suggests the possibility that the internal phase angle difference between the rhythms of activity and rectal temperature can serve

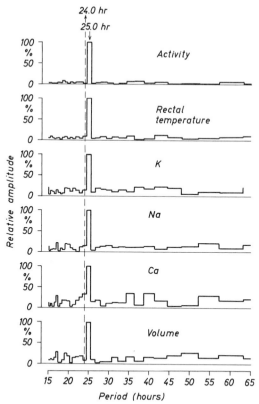

Figure 15/II. Period analyses of the six time series presented in I.

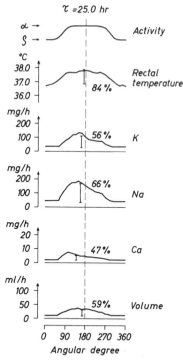

Figure 15/III. Longitudinally pooled courses of the six rhythms, with an averaging period as derived from II. Mean value and amplitude of the fundamental periods of each rhythm are presented at the position of the respective acrophase. From Wever (1975a).

as a criterion for the state of rhythm (whether synchronized or free running).

Not only the temporal relationship, between the activity rhythms and rectal temperature, alters with the transition from the entrained state to the free running state but also the internal phase relationships between other rhythms. Figure 18 shows results from an experiment in which a young man was partly restricted to a 24-hour routine but, for another part of the same experiment, lived under constant conditions. During both parts, he lived in the same standardized spatial environment and was measured for numerous different variables. In figure 18, the temporal positions of the maximum and minimum of 12 of these rhythms, presented relative to the activity rhythm, are compared from the two parts. Nearly all extreme values shift to earlier phases of the activity

rhythm with the transition from the entrained to the autonomous state. Moreover, the extreme values of different rhythms shift for different quantities, indicating internal phase shifts between the different rhythms. Finally, the maximum and minimum of most rhythms shift for different quantities, indicating alterations in the shapes of the rhythms. The total organization of the circadian system, therefore, is different in the two rhythm states.

The sign of the internal phase angle difference between the rhythms of activity and rectal temperature has been discussed as possible criterion for the autonomy of circadian rhythms; however, it has not yet been shown that this criterion is independent of the period, which is the basis for the primary criterion (phase shift against local time). To demonstrate this, it must be proven that the

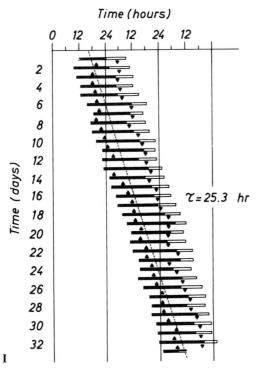

Time (hours)

Figure 16. Autonomous rhythm of a subject (A.G., ♂ 26 y) living under constant conditions without environmental time cues. *I*. Temporal course of the rhythm. Presented are the successive periods, one beneath the other, as a function of local time (i.e., abscissa). The activity rhythm is represented by bars (black = activity; white = rest). The rectal temperature rhythm is represented by triangles, indicating the temporal positions of maximum (▲) and minimum values (▼). The ordinate is the sequence of the subjective days.

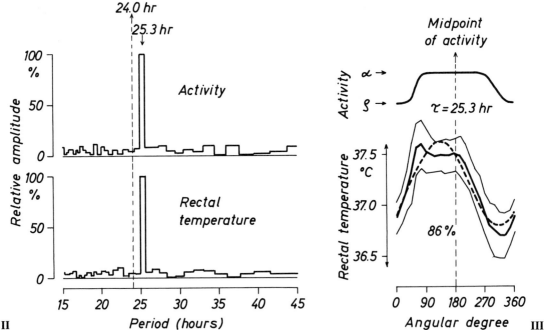

Figure 16/II. Period analyses of the two time series presented in I. *III*. Longitudinally pooled courses of the two rhythms, with an averaging period, derived from II. With the activity rhythm, the steepnesses of the transitions between activity (α) and rest (ρ) indicate the intraindividual variability around the mean onset and end of activity. With the rectal temperature rhythm, the thick line gives the average cycle and the thin lines give the range of the formally computed standard deviations around the average cycle. The dotted line gives the course of the fundamental period. From Wever (1973a).

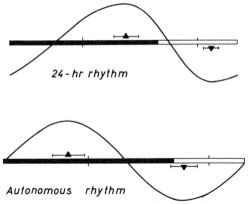

Figure 17. Average course of the rectal temperature rhythm, relative to the average activity rhythm (black = activity; white = rest), in rhythms entrained to the natural 24-hour day (above) and autonomously running rhythms (below), each averaged from many subjects. From the rectal temperature rhythm, mean temporal position of the extremum values and standard deviations are indicated. From Wever (1968b).

internal phase angle difference mentioned is not correlated to the rhythm period. In figure 19, the internal phase relationship between the two rhythms is drawn as a function of the period, computed from 31 experiments in which the autonomy of the rhythm has been proven by a total phase shift against local time of more than 180°, and no significant correlation was found. The computed correlation coefficient cannot be differentiated from zero statistically. The computed regression, though not deviating significantly from zero in the statistical analysis, is negative; therefore, the linear extrapolation of the internal phase angle difference to a period of 24 hours would result in a value deviating even more from the value measured in the entrained system than the average of the values measured in the free running system. This means that the criterion for autonomy of circadian rhythms, based

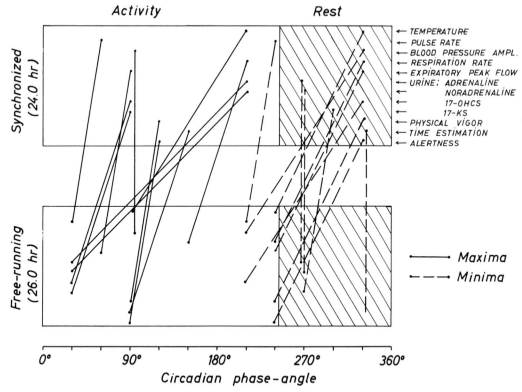

Figure 18. Temporal positions of the extremum values in the rhythms of twelve different variables, physiological and psychological, relative to the activity cycle, in the rhythm entrained to the 24-hr day (above) and the autonomously running rhythm of a subject (below) (J.K., ♂ 29 y). Data from Kriebel (1971).

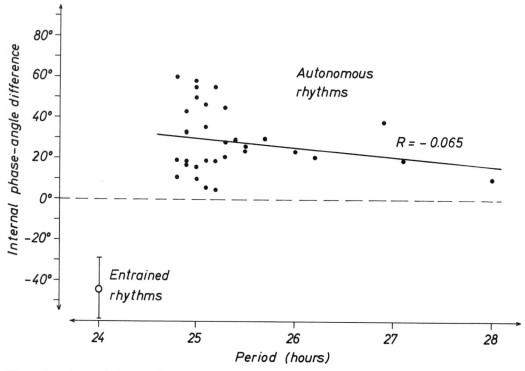

Figure 19. Internal phase angle difference between the rhythms of rectal temperature and activity (i.e., acrophases) in autonomously running rhythms (i.e., ordinate), plotted as a function of the period (i.e., abscissa). The coefficient of rank correlation (Spearman) is indicated. For comparison, the internal phase angle difference, in rhythms entrained to the 24-hour day (Fig. 17), is indicated.

on the internal phase angle difference between the activity rhythms and rectal temperature, has been proven to be independent of the period and independent of the other criterion based on the total phase shift against local time. This second criterion is derived only emperically and needs a foundation (and possibly a restriction) which will be given later (cf. 4.2.1).

2.1.3. Criteria for Oscillatory Origin

With criteria discussed already, it can be tested whether or not a rhythm is entrained to an external zeitgeber. The application of these criteria proves, in the examples shown, that this is not the case. It establishes the autonomous origin of the rhythms considered. The question arises whether the underlying mechanism is an oscillatory or a

stochastic process. To distinguish these two processes in autonomous rhythms, serial correlations must be computed. These computations will be given extensively with the examples of autonomous rhythms shown in figures 15 and 16.

In the experiment shown as the first example of an autonomous rhythm (Fig. 15), there is a clear dependency between successive periods. In the rhythm of rectal temperature, successive periods, when measured from one maximum to the next, are correlated with $r = -0.486$ and, from one minimum to the next, with $r = -0.479$. From conventional statistics, these correlations deviate significantly from zero ($p < 0.05$). The correlations between one period and the next but one (or to the one before but one) are also negative, but smaller, in amount ($r = -0.147$ with the maximum, for reference, and $r = -0.153$ with the minimum). From conventional standards, the deviations of these values from zero are not significant. Almost the same results are true with the activity rhythm. The correlation between successive periods, when measured from the beginning of activity to the next action, is significantly negative ($r = -0.395$; $p < 0.05$), whereas the correlation between one period and the next but one is nearly zero ($r = -0.039$). The correlation between successive activity periods, when measured from one termination of activity to the next, is again significantly negative ($r = -0.539$; $p < 0.01$) and the correlation between one period and the next but one is again close to zero ($r = +0.021$). The negative correlation between successive periods means that a period that is, by chance, longer than the average of all periods during this experiment, is preferably followed and preceded by a period that is shorter than the average. Consequently, deviations of a period induced by superimposed noise are corrected, on the average, by the next period. This statement is true for the two overt rhythms and for all reference phases considered. With this result, the oscillatory origin of the rectal temperature rhythm and the activity rhythm have been shown.

In the activity rhythm of this experiment, the overlapping correlations between the durations of successive activity times and rest times also indicate the oscillatory origin of the rhythm. The correlation coefficient, computed from the durations of activity time and each following rest time, is $r = -0.516$ (significant with $p < 0.01$). This means that an activity time longer than the average of all other activity times normally is followed by a rest time that is shorter than the average of all other rest times, and an activity time shorter than the average normally is followed by a rest time longer than the average. This correlation alone does not indicate the oscillatory origin; therefore, the correlation between activity time and preceding rest time also is considered. In this case, it is again negative ($r = -0.240$), although not significant from conventional standards. These correlations together confirm the oscillatory origin and disprove the stochastic

origin of the rhythm. These correlations also relate to the distribution width of the periods. The formally computed standard deviations of the activity periods, taken from the beginning of activity to the next action ($s_\tau = \pm 1.53$ hours), is smaller than the deviation computed from the combined deviations of activity time and rest time, with the predetermination of a random combination [$(s_\alpha^2 + s_\rho^2)^{1/2} = \pm 2.16$ hours]. This confirms that the control of the total period has preference over the control of activity time or rest time.

In the other example of an autonomous rhythm (Fig. 16), the result is generally the same but deviates in detail. In the rhythm of rectal temperature, the correlation between successive periods is $r = -0.418$, when measured from one maximum to the next, $r = -0.473$, when measured from one minimum to the next. Both correlations deviate significantly from zero ($p < 0.01$). The correlations between one period and the next but one are nearly zero ($r = -0.019$ and $r = -0.078$). In the activity rhythm, the correlation between successive periods, when measured from one onset of activity to the next, is $r = -0.196$, and between one period and the next but one is much stronger, being $r = -0.508$. Only the latter value can be guaranteed statistically to deviate from zero ($p < 0.01$). This means that deviations of a period from the average of all periods, induced by superimposed noise, are corrected, in the overt rhythm of rectal temperature, preferably by the following period. In the overt activity rhythm, however, these occasional deviations are corrected preferably by the following but one period. This is true only if the activity period is measured from one activity beginning to the next; and the result differs if the terminations of activity are considered for determining the activity period. In this case, the correlation between one period and the next is much stronger than between one period and the next but one ($r = -0.488$ versus $r = -0.057$). The oscillatory origin also has been shown in this experiment, with the two overt rhythms considered, but the results also indicate differences in the oscillatory processes underlying the two overt rhythms.

In the second example of an autonomous rhythm, the oscillatory origin of the activity rhythm is confirmed additionally by the overlapping correlations between the durations of successive activity times and rest times. The correlation between activity time and the following rest time is negative ($r = -0.691$) at a high level of significance ($p < 0.001$). The correlation between activity time and preceding rest time, however, is positive ($r = +0.397$) and also statistically significant ($p < 0.01$). These results indicate a process that is oscillatory. The positive correlation to the preceding rest time indicates that this process deviates from the other example of an autonomous activity rhythm (Fig. 15). This difference in the processes controlling the activity rhythm was previously indicated by the correlations of successive periods, as mentioned above. It, however, cannot be differentiated from the results obtained from the computed correlations, whether the properties of the underlying oscillators themselves or the couplings between the underlying oscillators and the overt rhythms are different. The overlapping correlations diminish again the formally computed standard deviations of the periods, in comparison to the combined deviations of activity time and rest time [$s_\tau = \pm 1.19$ hours; $(s_\alpha^2 + s_\rho^2)^{1/2} = \pm 2.03$ hours].

The oscillatory origin of the rhythms has been proven, with the computations given above, by the serial dependencies within the rhythms. The statements are based on correlations that deviate, by applying conventional statistics, significantly from zero. This means that the other hypothesis, which supposes mutual independency of successive events within the time series, has been disproven significantly. The proven serial dependency rules out the application of longitudinal statistics within the time series because the basic presupposition of each statistic, the mutual independency of the units used, has been disproven by the significant statement concerning the serial dependency. Statistical statements, therefore, taken from successive events within a time

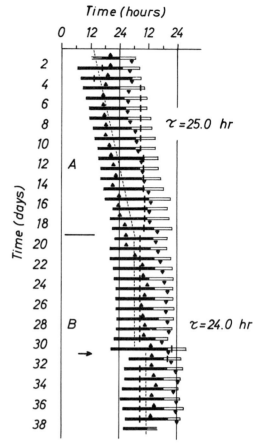

Figure 20.   Rhythm of a subject (A.S., ♂ 26 y) who was intended to live continuously under constant conditions without time cues. The experiment is divided arbitrarily into two sections (A and B) for further analyses. *I.* Temporal courses of the rhythms of activity and rectal temperature, presented successively with one period beneath the other. Indications are the same as in figure 16/ I. Marks at the bars indicate instances of servicing the lock. The arrow indicates an obvious phase shift of 5 hours, as considered in subsequent analyses. From Wever (1969b).

series, are useful if the time series is based on a stochastic process but useless if the time series is based on an oscillatory process.

2.1.4. Application of the Criteria to Critical Experiments

With the different criteria mentioned above, it is possible to decide whether a rhythm runs autonomous or is entrained by a 24-

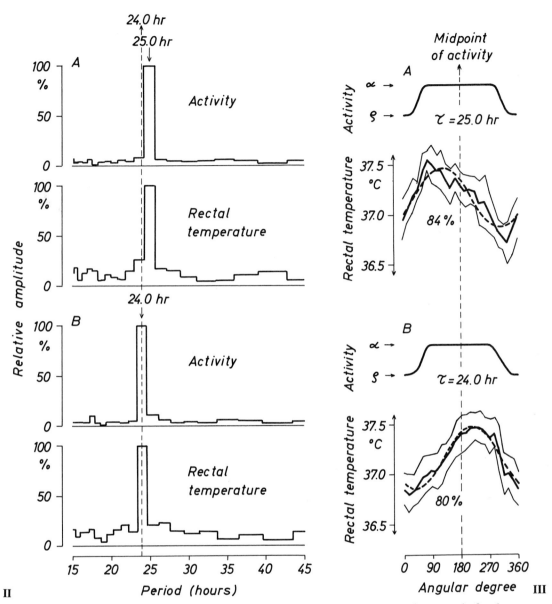

Figure 20/II. Period analyses of the two time series presented in I, computed separately for the two sections (A and B). *III.* Longitudinally pooled courses of the rhythms, computed separately for the two sections (A and B), with averaging periods derived from II. Indications are the same as in figure 16/III.

hour zeitgeber, and whether a rhythm is based on a stochastic or an oscillatory process. The first decision is possible even in experiments in which the period deviates so little from 24 hours that the resulting total phase shift against local time is less than 12 hours. The second decision is possible even in experiments in which the rhythm has been proven to run autonomously. With these criteria, some examples will be considered in

the following which seem to be unclear at first glance but the usefulness and the limits of the criteria can be tested.

Figure 20 shows results originating from an experiment where the subject was to remain under unchanged conditions during the total experiment. The course of the rhythm, however, shows a clear change in the period after about 18 days (Fig. 20/I); the subject showed a period of 25.0 hours to that time but his period was very close to 24 hours thereafter. This result could be interpreted as a consequence of an unknown change in what were considered constant conditions. On the other hand, the about 24-hour period in the second part could be due to entrainment to an unknown zeitgeber; however, no zeitgeber had been introduced deliberately. Before speculating about the nature of the zeitgeber, it has to be tested whether the rhythm was, during the second part, autonomous or entrained. In the following computations, the arbitrarily sectioned parts A and B have been treated separately. To get a more consistent result, 5 hours have been eliminated at day 30 because, on that day, a phase shift occurred with the activity rhythm and rectal temperature rhythm. Figure 20/II shows the results of the period analyses which confirm the conclusion from the raw data. The longitudinal pooling (Fig. 20/III) indicates, by the sign of the internal phase relationship between the two rhythms, the rhythm was autonomous, or free running, during part A but entrained to a 24-hour zeitgeber during part B. During both parts, the rhythms are reliable enough to guarantee the correctness of this statement. The result of testing the serial correlations, moreover, proved that the rhythms, during both parts, were based on oscillatory processes.

After entrainment of the rhythm, during part B, has been shown, the question arises concerning the nature of the effective zeitgeber. In this special case, the zeitgeber could be found subsequently. The assistant, who was responsible for checking the subject, went into the connecting lock every morning at the same time (Fig. 20/I), contrary to the instruction to go into the lock only during the sleep time of the subject. Additionally, she left letters with the subject on these occasions. During part A, the time coincided with the sleep time but not during part B. The subject confessed that, during his afternoon tea, he often went into the lock to see whether the assistant had left a letter there and finished his tea only after he had found the letter. After he had missed these indirect contacts for 2 days (during the weekend another assistant had checked the subject ac-

cording to instructions), he found the contacts had shifted to his dessert after lunch. He had not perceived, during the 2 day interval, the contact times had not shifted but his own rhythm had. This experiment was not successful, regarding the original purpose, but did show the effectiveness of social contacts as zeitgebers.

Figure 21 shows results from another experiment with a period deviating from 24 hours during the first section but with a period of 24.0 hours during the second section. In this experiment, the conditions were changed after 10 days in a manner (withdrawal of Lithium) where a shortening of the autonomous period had to be expected (Engelmann, 1972, 1973). The period, in fact, was shorter during the second section than during the first (Fig. 21/II) but the internal phase relationship between the rhythms of activity and rectal temperature (Fig. 21/III) indicated autonomy during the first section and synchronization to 24 hours during the second. It can be concluded from these results that withdrawal of Lithium shortened the period. This shortening did not result directly in an autonomous period of 24 hours but in a period so close to this value that the rhythm became synchronized to exactly 24 hours. There must have been an unknown zeitgeber that was too weak to synchronize the rhythm, as long as its period was 24.7 hours, but was strong enough to synchronize the rhythm after its period was shortened. The only other possibility is that the withdrawal of Lithium did not affect directly the autonomous period but increased the sensitiveness of the rhythm against a continuously present 24-hour zeitgeber so that it became effective. Independent of the hypothesis to be preferred, the result of this experiment leads to the conclusion that a 24-hour zeitgeber had been present; the modality of which could not be evaluated. The experiment was not fully successful regarding its original purpose because its result did not show the effect of Lithium on the autonomous period. The result of this experiment, however, is of interest because it proves the presence of a weak unidentified 24-hour zeitgeber in spite of strict isolation (this experiment had been performed in the nonshielded

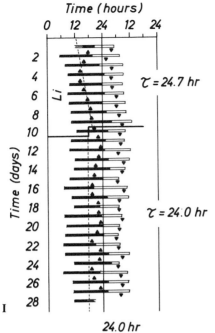

Time (hours)

$\tau = 24.7\ hr$

$\tau = 24.0\ hr$

Time (days)

I

Figure 21. Rhythm of a subject (W.E., ♂ 41 y) who was intended to live continuously under constant conditions without environmental time cues, with regular administration of Lithium-carbonate during the first section and without Li-administration during the second section. *I.* Temporal courses of the rhythms of activity and rectal temperature, presented successively, one period beneath the other. Indications are the same as in figure 16/I.

Figure 21/II. Period analyses of the two time series presented in I, computed separately for the two sections with and without Li-administration. *III.* Longitudinally pooled courses of the two rhythms, computed separately for the two sections with and without Li-administration, with averaging periods derived from II. Indications are the same as in figure 16/III.

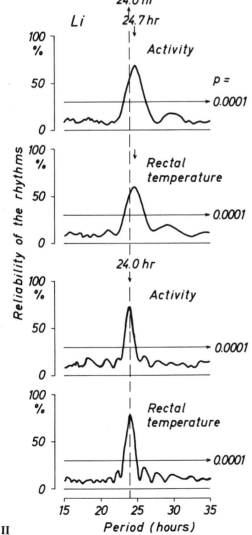

Reliability of the rhythms

II   Period (hours)

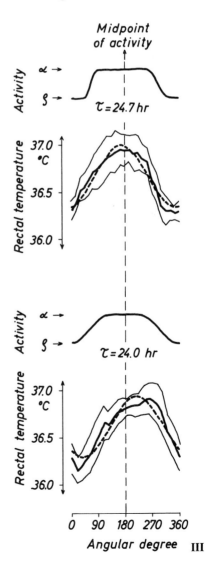

III   Angular degree

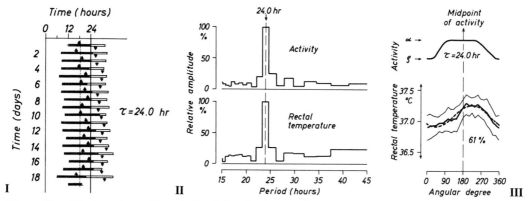

Figure 22.   Rhythm of a subject (P.R., ♂ 25 y) who was intended to live under constant conditions without environmental time cues. *I.* Temporal courses of the rhythms of activity and rectal temperature, presented successively one period beneath the other. Indications are the same as in figure 16/I. From Wever (1969b). *II.* Period analyses of the two time series presented in I. *III.* Longitudinally pooled courses of the two rhythms, with an averaging period derived from II. Indications are the same as in figure 16/III.

unit; cf. 2.4.4 and 3.2.3). The presence of this zeitgeber also has to be considered in all other experiments. Other subjects, however, were in the same experimental unit and under equivalent conditions (e.g., without Lithium administration) not synchronized to a 24-hour period, even with autonomous periods deviating from 24 hours by only 0.2 hours. It must be assumed, therefore, that this subject was especially sensitive to the unidentified zeitgeber.

Figure 22 shows results from the only experiment in which the subject showed a period of 24 hours during the total experiment although all environmental time cues were intended to be excluded. The determination of the internal phase angle difference from the longitudinal poolings (Fig. 22/III) proved that the rhythm was entrained to a 24-hour zeitgeber. The search for the nature of this zeitgeber was especially difficult because the subject was a student of the institute engaged in the human isolation studies and was familiar with many details of the performance of the experiments. After exclusion of all other possible sources of error, there remained the fact that the equipment for stabilizing the line voltage feeding the illumination (Wever, 1967c, 1969b) was in operation during nearly all experiments but not during this experiment. It may be sug-

gested, therefore, that this subject was entrained to 24 hours by the diurnal variations of the illumination because of fluctuations in the line voltage, which also has been suggested in some animal experiments (Wever, 1967b).

Of more than 150 subjects with presumably autonomous periods, only two subjects showed periods that might be shorter than 24 hours. Figure 23 shows the course of the experiment with the shortest period. It lasted only for 10 days, with a period of 23.5 hours (Fig. 23/II). A total phase shift against local time of only 5 hours resulted. Unfortunately, the testing of the internal phase angle difference from the longitudinally pooled rhythms (Fig. 23/III) did not give an answer whether or not the rhythm ran autonomously. The two rhythms were exactly in phase; the rectal temperature rhythm neither leads the activity rhythm, as in autonomous rhythms, nor lags behind the activity rhythm, as in entrained rhythms. It cannot be determined from this experiment whether or not, in a healthy subject, an autonomous rhythm with a period shorter than 24 hours is possible. The only other subject with an autonomous period shorter than 24 hours (τ = 23.8 hours) showed, in a later experiment under equivalent conditions, a period longer than 24 hours (τ = 24.2 hours; Fig. 38).

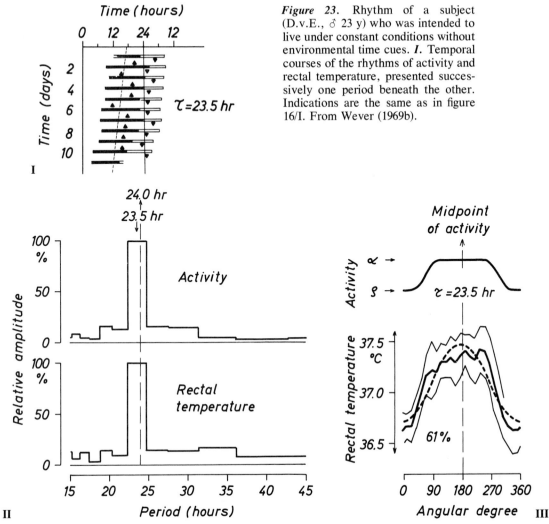

Figure 23. Rhythm of a subject (D.v.E., ♂ 23 y) who was intended to live under constant conditions without environmental time cues. *I.* Temporal courses of the rhythms of activity and rectal temperature, presented successively one period beneath the other. Indications are the same as in figure 16/I. From Wever (1969b).

Figure 23/II. Period analyses of the two time series presented in I. *III.* Longitudinally pooled courses of the two rhythms, with an averaging period derived from II. Indications are the same as in figure 16/III.

The period of the rhythm shown in figure 23 was close to, but shorter than, 24 hours. In figure 24, the course of a rhythm is shown in which the period is close to, but longer than, 24 hours. The resulting total phase shift against local time is too small to allow a decision whether this rhythm is autonomous or entrained. The computed period analysis (Fig. 24/II) confirms a period of 24.3 hours. The inspection of the temporal relationship between the rhythms of activity and rectal temperature from the longitudinally pooled rhythms (Fig. 24/III) clearly proves, in this

experiment in contrast to the preceding example (Fig. 23/III), that the rhythm runs autonomously. The rectal temperature rhythm clearly leads the activity rhythm.

2.1.5. *Summary of Free Running Rhythms*

To the present, 150 subjects have been isolated under constant conditions with the intention that their rhythms run externally desynchronized. The experiments averaged 29

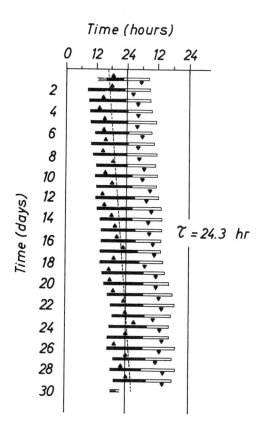

Time (hours)

τ = 24.3 hr

Figure 24. Autonomous rhythm of a subject (D.P., ♀ 25 y) living under constant conditions without time cues. *I.* Temporal courses of the rhythms of activity and rectal temperature, presented successively one period beneath the other. Indications are the same as in figure 16/I.

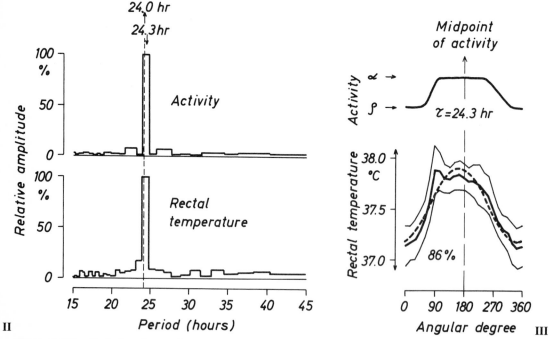

II

III

Figure 24/II. Period analyses of the two time series presented in I. *III.* Longitudinally pooled courses of the two rhythms, with an averaging period derived from II. Indications are the same as in figure 16/III.

days. With the criteria just discussed, it can be tested whether or not this intention always was realized (i.e., whether the rhythms ran autonomously) and whether the rhythms were based on oscillatory or stochastic processes. In the following, both of these tests will be applied.

Of the 150 subjects, only one subject clearly had been synchronized externally to a 24-hour zeitgeber, unintentionally, during the total experiment (Fig. 22). In one other subject, both criteria together did not allow a decision whether the rhythm ran autonomously or externally synchronized (Fig. 23). Data of these experiments have been eliminated from further consideration of autonomous rhythms. Four more subjects showed rhythms that were running autonomously during one part of the experiment but synchronized unintentionally to a 24-hour zeitgeber during another part (Figs. 20 and 21). The first parts of these experiments can be included in further considerations concerning autonomous rhythms. Circadian rhythms of 148 subjects, isolated under constant conditions, can be summarized to evaluate properties of autonomous circadian rhythms in man (five of the six experiments that were not fully successful regarding the original purpose of the experiments, originated from the 1st year of the experimental series). Additionally, there are rhythms of 15 more subjects that were exposed to a weak artificial zeitgeber but showed autonomous rhythms since the zeitgeber failed to be effective.

In the experiments discussed, the different overt rhythms ran synchronously (in other experiments, they did not; cf. 2.2). In these experiments, the basic mechanism can be tested to be either oscillatory or stochastic. In the following, the appropriate test, demonstrated earlier with two experiments, will be applied to a sample of 38 experiments.

Considering the overt rhythms of rectal temperature, the mean serial correlation for the 38 experiments (± standard deviation) between one period and the following one is, if computed with the maximum values for reference, $\bar{r} = -0.461 \pm 0.118$ (significantly

deviating from zero with $p \ll 0.001$). In a small part of the experiments, the serial correlation between one period and the next but one is larger than between one period and the next one; if the larger correlation of the two always is considered, an average serial correlation of $\bar{r} = -0.473 \pm 0.103$ follows (which deviates from zero with an even higher degree of significance). If, instead of the maximum values of the rectal temperature rhythm, the minimum values are taken for reference, nearly the same numbers of serial correlations result.

Considering the overt activity rhythms, the mean serial correlation for the 38 experiments between one period and the following one is (± standard deviation) $\bar{r} = -0.401 \pm 0.166$ (significantly deviating from zero with $p \ll 0.001$). In about 30% of the subjects, the serial correlation is better when computed between one period and the next but one than when computed between one period and the next. If the serial correlation that has the larger value of these two always is considered, an average correlation of $\bar{r} = -0.474 \pm 0.115$ follows (which differs from zero with an even higher degree of significance). These coefficients of serial correlation are valid if a period is defined from one beginning of activity to the following but nearly the same numbers result if the termination of activity (or the beginning of sleep) is taken for the limitation of an activity period.

In the activity rhythms, the serial correlation between activity time and rest time have been computed. When taken from each activity time and following rest time, it results in an average for the 38 experiments of $\bar{r} = -0.519 \pm 0.227$ and, when taken from each activity time and preceding rest time, $\bar{r} = -0.020 \pm 0.306$. The serial correlation first mentioned deviates significantly from zero ($p \ll 0.001$). The serial correlation last mentioned, on the contrary, cannot be differentiated from zero. This result, however, does not mean there is no serial correlation at all. Computation of the kurtosis shows that the distribution of single coefficients of serial correlation is bimodal with clear accu-

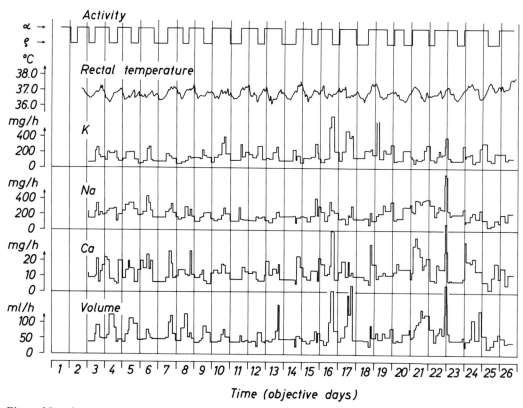

Figure 25. Autonomous rhythm of a subject (L.v.F., ♂ 24 y) living under constant conditions without time cues. Presented, from top to bottom, are the rhythms of activity (i.e., alternation between activity α and rest ρ), rectal temperature (measured continuously), and four urine constituents (i.e., mictions taken at self-selected intervals). *I.* Longitudinally presented courses of the six variables during the total experiment.

mulations of positive and negative values. The kurtosis, or the excess of a distribution (computed from the 4th moment), indicates the shape of this distribution. In particular, a negative kurtosis indicates a flattened distribution; a rectangular distribution shows a kurtosis of -1.22; and an even smaller kurtosis indicates bimodal shapes. Considering the serial correlations between activity time and preceding rest time, the computed kurtosis is -1.29, indicating the bimodal distribution mentioned (for comparison: the kurtosis of the distribution of the serial correlations between activity time and following rest time is -0.30). It is highly probable, therefore, that the serial correlations between activity time and preceding rest-time also deviate from zero but with an inconsistent sign, in contrast to the consis-

tently negative sign, of all other serial correlations mentioned. As a consequence of the serial correlations within the activity period, the combined standard deviations of activity time and rest time (average: $(s_\alpha^2 + s_\rho^2)^{1/2} = 2.00 \pm 0.45$ hour) are larger than the directly measured standard deviations of the periods (average: $\overline{s_\tau} = 1.32 \pm 0.32$ hour), on the average for 0.68 ± 0.32 hour (significantly deviating from zero with $p \ll 0.001$), or for a factor of 1.52. This indicates once more that the control of the total period has preference over the separate control of activity time and rest time.

In summary, with the great majority of subjects, the rhythms have been proven to run autonomously when all environmental time cues are excluded; the meaning is that human circadian rhythms evidently are of

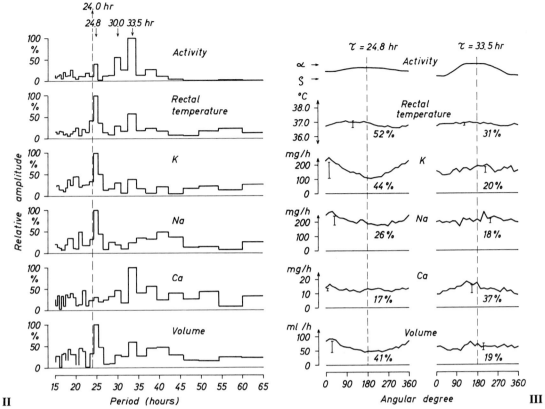

Figure 25/II. Period analyses of the six time series presented in I. *III.* Longitudinally pooled courses of the six rhythms, with two averaging periods derived as the two most prominent peaks from II. Mean value and amplitude of the fundamental periods are presented at the position of the respective acrophase. From Wever (1975a).

endogenous origin. Additionally, it has been shown the autonomously running rhythms are serially correlated, and are based on oscillatory, not stochastic, processes. This is true with the rhythms of activity as well as with rectal temperature. This means that human circadian rhythms are controlled by self-sustained oscillators.

2.2. Internal Synchronization and Desynchronization

In the previous chapter, only examples of free running rhythms were discussed where all measured variables oscillated synchronously to each other; meaning the rhythms of different variables within one subject were synchronized internally. This is the

case in most subjects, but not all. Some of the subjects showed internal desynchronization instead (a state where different variables oscillate with different periods in the steady state). Properties of the different manifestations of this state will be treated in the following.

2.2.1. Real Internal Desynchronization

As an example of internal desynchronization, figure 25 shows results from an experiment where a subject lived 26 days in strict isolation without any time cues, like the subject of the experiment shown in figure 15. The time series in figure 25, however, take courses which are very different from those in figure 15. The change between wakefulness and sleep or the activity rhythm shows only 19 periods, in contrast to the 25 activity periods in figure 15/I during the same span of objective time. The course of the activity rhythm is much more irregular in figure 25/I than in figure 15/I. The rectal temperature rhythm in figure 25/I includes 25 periods as in figure 15/I, but its amplitude is much more variable. The temperature amplitude seems to oscillate with a period of about 3 to 4 days. The difference in period numbers of different overt rhythms during the total experiment means that the periods of the different rhythms have different values. From figure 25/I, a period of the activity rhythm of 33.5 hours and of the rectal temperature rhythm of 24.8 hours can be derived. The other rhythms presented take nonuniform courses. The excretions of potassium and sodium oscillate more or less synchronously to the rectal temperature rhythm (i.e., likewise with a period of 24.8 hours). The rhythm of calcium excretion seems to run synchronously to the activity rhythm. The rhythm course of urine volume is not clear.

From the different rhythms, the subject had perceived only wakefulness and sleep. The subject was very confused when the experiment was finished on his 19th day whereas 26 days were planned. It was difficult to convince the subject, by showing him all records accumulated during the experiment, his calculation of time was incorrect. He did not realize that his subjective days were much longer than the objective days; in this case by 40% instead of 4% as, in the average, in case of internal synchronization (Fig. 15). He also did not realize that most of his physiological rhythms ran slower than the objective change between day and night but much faster than his psychologically scored time. In experiments with internal desynchronization, it must not be only differentiated between the courses of objective and subjective time but also between physiological and psychological time.

Clear answers to the question for the dominant periods of the different rhythms come from a period analysis (Fig. 25/II).

Although computed in the same manner as the period analyses shown in figure 15/II, the obvious picture is very different. In cases of internal desynchronization, not only one sharp peak is present, as in cases of internal synchronization, but several peaks with the dominant peak not being the same in different rhythms. In the activity rhythm, there is a dominant peak with the center of gravity at 33.5 hours, corresponding to the obviously observed activity period (Fig. 25/I). There are, however, additional smaller peaks at periods of 30.0 and 24.8 hours. The latter peak coincides with the period of the rectal temperature rhythm, as derived from the raw data (Fig. 25/I). The rectal temperature rhythm contains a dominant peak with the center of gravity at 24.8 hours, confirming the period determination given earlier. This rhythm also contains another peak at 33.5 hours (with the dominant period of the activity rhythm). The period with the third greatest amplitude is at 30.0 hours and is again present in the activity rhythm. In the four other rhythms presented, only the three peaks mentioned appear in the period analyses but with changing proportions and preferences.

The phenomenon of internal desynchronization constrains to the conclusion that the assumption of only one single oscillator controlling the variety of overt rhythms is insufficient. It has to be concluded, rather, that there are several different control oscillators. The inspection of the raw data may suggest the assumption that the different overt rhythms are controlled separately by underlying oscillators. For example, it is suggested from figure 25/I that the activity rhythm is controlled by an activity oscillator and the overt rectal temperature rhythm by a temperature oscillator running consistently with a shorter period. A closer examination of results of the computer analyses shows that this simple picture has to be modified. There are, in fact, different basic oscillators which are characterized by the different peak periods. These oscillators, however, do not correspond simply to the overt rhythms of different variables. The inspection of figure 25/II suggests, rather, that each of the different oscillators contributes to the control of the rhythms of many, or even all, of the different variables; or the overt rhythm of each variable is controlled simultaneously by many, or even all, of the existing oscillators. The simple 1:1 coordination between oscillators and overt rhythms of distinct variables is furthermore suspicious because the definition of a variable is more or less arbitrary and dependent on the measuring equipment. For example, body temperature can be taken for an autonomous variable which may be separately controlled by a feedback system, or considered as nothing more than the net effect of heat production and loss which are separately controlled by feedback systems. From this point of view, the rhythm of body temperature is caused by the interference between the rhythms of heat production and loss. Even these rhythms can be understood as induced by interactions between rhythms of underlying, more basic, variables. Following this concept, it has to be accepted that there exist coordinations between basic oscillators and chains of functions, which may manifest themselves by different measurable variables but are not described sufficiently by these variables.

Regarding the autonomy of the desynchronized oscillations, only the first criterion mentioned is applicable, based on the total phase shift against possible zeitgebers. The second criterion, which deals with the internal phase angle difference between different overt rhythms, can be applied only in internally synchronized rhythms where a constant phase relationship exists. According to the first criterion, not only the 33.5-hour period, but also the 24.8-hour period, deviates significantly from 24 hours, as can be seen from the comparison of the corresponding spectral lines with the dotted 24.0-hour line in the spectrum (Figure 25/II). This means that the oscillators assigned to all relevant periods mentioned run autonomously.

If data of a time series should be pooled longitudinally, the period used for averaging

is clear if the time series includes only one relevant period. In case of internal desynchronization, a time series, however, includes more than one relevant period (Fig. 25/II) and, therefore, the longitudinal pooling can be done with at least two different periods. In figure 25/III, the results of the longitudinal pooling of the rhythms, given in figure 25/I, are presented and were performed with the two dominant periods of 24.8 and 33.5 hours (Fig. 25/II). Corresponding to the multiplicity of periods included in each time series, the reliability of each period is much smaller than in cases of internal synchronization with only one period in each time series (Fig. 15/III). Only in the rhythms of activity and calcium excretion, the longer period is the more reliable. In all other rhythms, the shorter period is the more reliable. This discrimination, as shown in figure 25/III, corresponds to the conclusion drawn from the raw data (Fig. 25/I).

Of special interest is the determination of internal phase angle differences. From figure 25/III they can be determined with the two different periods presented. The internal phase angle difference, between the rhythms of activity and rectal temperature, is nearly the same with the two periods and also nearly the same as in free running rhythms when internally synchronized (Fig. 17). The internal phase angle difference between the four other rhythms to each other also is nearly identical with the two periods; but the phases of these four rhythms are nearly reversed with the two periods when compared with the rhythms of activity and rectal temperature.

The internal phase angle differences derived from figure 25/III are hypothetical values which are not observable directly from figure 25/I. The directly observable phase angle difference between the rhythms of activity and rectal temperature generally is not constant but continuously changing. This is a necessary consequence of the fact that these two rhythms show different periods. This means that on some days, the two rhythms show their normal temporal relationship with a temperature maximum dur-

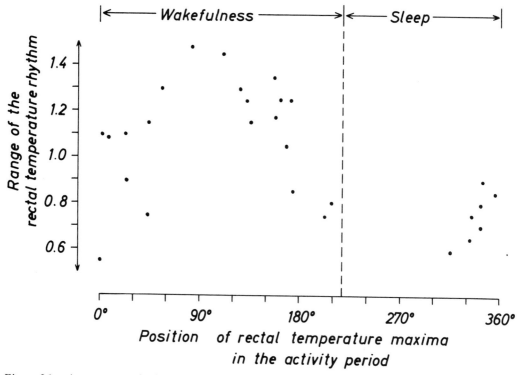

Figure 26. Autonomous rhythm of a subject (M.B., ♀ 22 y) living under constant conditions without time cues. The range of the rectal temperature cycles (measured from minimum to the following maximum) are plotted as a function of the temporal position of the temperature maximum within the activity cycle. The average activity cycle is taken for 360°. After Aschoff et al. (1967b).

ing activity time and a minimum during rest time. On other days, this temporal relationship is reversed; the temperature is maximum during rest time and the minimum during activity time. The amplitude of the rectal temperature rhythm alters, depending on the phase angle difference between the rhythms of activity and rectal temperature. On days with a normal mutual phase angle difference, the amplitude is large (e.g., at days 3/4, 7/8); however, the amplitude is small when the phase angle difference is reversed (e.g., at days 5/6, 9/10). Generally, there seems to be a discrepancy between the phase angle differences between the overt rhythms, which are continuously changing, and the fundamentally constant phase angle differences between the averaged periods. The disentanglement of this apparent discrepancy is based on the hypothesis that each overt rhythm can be described, in cases of internal

desynchronization, as a superposition of some oscillations with different periods, between which beat phenomena occur.

The correlation between the amplitude of the rectal temperature rhythm and the temporal position of this rhythm, relative to the activity rhythm, becomes more obvious with another type of presentation. The data in figure 26 originate from another experiment with internal desynchronization. During 31 objective days, the subject showed an activity rhythm with a mean period of 40.8 hours and a rectal temperature rhythm with a mean period of 24.7 hours. In figure 26, the oscillation ranges of single temperature cycles are plotted as a position function of the corresponding temperature maximum within the activity period. The temperature amplitude is large when the mutual phase relationship is normal (i.e., when the temperature maximum falls into the activity time) and the temperature amplitude is small when the phase relationship is reversed. As can be seen in figure 26, all phase angle differences between the two rhythms from 0° to 360° occur, but not with equal frequencies. Again, this behavior indicates mutual "relative coordination" (v. Holst, 1939a) or beat phenomena which will be discussed in detail later on (Fig. 112).

In the example of internal desynchronization (Fig. 25), internal desynchronization occurred from the beginning of the experiment. In other cases, internal desynchronization occurred spontaneously during the experiment after the rhythms were internally synchronized at the beginning. An example of such a case is presented in figure 27. During the first two weeks, all rhythms measured showed equal periods of 25.7 hours. On the 14th subjective (or 15th objective) day, the period of the activity rhythm lengthened to a mean of 33.4 hours without any environmental factor being changed. On the same day, the period of the rectal temperature rhythm shortened to 25.1 hours. The internal phase angle difference, between the two overt rhythms presented, is constant during the first section of the experiment but continuously changing during the second section; the courses of both rhythms, activity and rectal temperature, show scalloping patterns which again indicate the presence of mutual relative coordination or beats (Fig. 112). Also in this experiment, three different speeds during the time lapse must be considered. The experiment terminated after 33 objective days but the subject had realized only 27 days. During this time, rectal temperature had gone through 31 cycles.

For the subsequent computer analyses, the course of the experiment is divided into two sections, A and B, which will be treated separately. Figure 27/II shows the period analyses of the two sections. In section A, with internally synchronized rhythms, only one spectral line is present in each time series, with the center of gravity at 25.7 hours. The same picture also has been obtained from all other rhythms measured. This spectral line differs significantly from

24 hours, indicating autonomy of the rhythm. In section B, with internally desynchronized rhythms, the analysis results in a spectrum with two clearly separated peaks in each time series. In the activity rhythm, the peak at 33.4 hours is the dominant but there also is another reliable peak at 25.1 hours. In the rectal temperature rhythm, peaks at the same two periods are present, with dominance of the shorter over the longer period. The spectra of the other rhythms measured (but not presented) in this experiment, again show the same two peaks but, in contrast to the other example (Fig. 25/II), in most of the rhythms the longer period is the dominant. Generally, it is the result of the period analyses of section B that the spectrum includes the period of the respective overt rhythm as the highest peak, but the deviating periods of the other overt rhythms are also included, though with smaller amplitudes (or reliabilities). All peaks deviate clearly from 24.0 hours, indicating that the rhythms, which are assigned to the different periods, are autonomous.

Of special interest again is the determination of the internal phase angle difference between the two overt rhythms from the longitudinally pooled periods (Fig. 27/III). In section A, the pooling procedure is clear because there is only one possible scanning period. The rectal temperature rhythm leads the activity rhythm, as is characteristic for autonomous rhythms, in general. In section B, the rhythms can be pooled with two different averaging periods corresponding to the two peaks included in the period analyses (Fig. 27/II). The internal phase angle differences, obtained with the two periods, are equal, as seen in the other example (Fig. 25/III), and are also equal to the internal phase angle difference obtained in section A, where the overt rhythms ran synchronized internally. The combined results support the hypothesis that there are two different oscillators, which are characterized by the different periods in section B and which run synchronously to each other in section A. Each of the oscillators contributes to the control of many, or even all, overt rhythms, with an

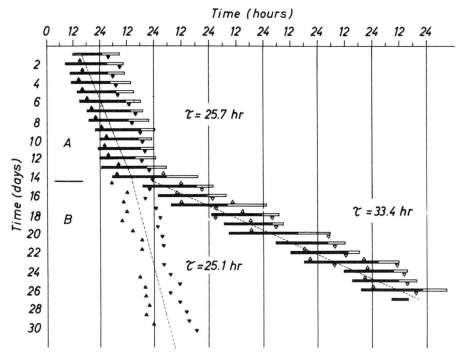

Figure 27. Autonomous rhythm of a subject (E.v.S., ♀ 24 y) living under constant conditions without time cues. The experiment is divided arbitrarily into two sections (A and B), for further analyses. *I.* Temporal courses of the rhythms of activity and rectal temperative, presented successively one period beneath the other. Indications are the same as in figure 16/I. White triangles are temporally correct redrawings of corresponding black triangles.

internal phase angle difference between the different rhythms, which is the same in all oscillators of one subject, independent of the period and whether the different overt rhythms are internally synchronized or desynchronized. Conversely, each of the many overt rhythms is controlled by some, or even all, existing, separated autonomous oscillators. Only the fractions, by which the different oscillators contribute to the control of the different overt rhythms, vary from variable to variable. The results derived from figure 27/III are in strict contradiction to the other hypothesis that each of the different oscillators controls the overt rhythm of one variable. The different oscillators must interact mutually, in this case, when separated by internal desynchronization in the sense of relative coordination. It would be a necessary consequence of this hypothesis that the mutual phase angle difference varies depending on the period; however, this is evi-

dently not the case. Figure 27/III shows the reliability of all rhythms concerned. As the numbers and drawn ranges of standard deviations around the average period show, this reliability is great in section A where only one period is present, and smaller, in section B where two periods are present. Each additional period included diminishes the reliability of the other periods.

There could be another possibility of interpreting the results concerning the occurrence of identical periods in the different rhythms (Fig. 27/II, B). It has been argued that this identity is due to only "masking effects" (cf. 4.3.2.). Masking is the result of a direct influence of one variable to another, or of a direct influence of an external stimulus to a variable, without reference to rhythmic processes. For example, each activity effects an increase in body temperature at any time and independent of rhythmicity. An activity rhythm, therefore, is

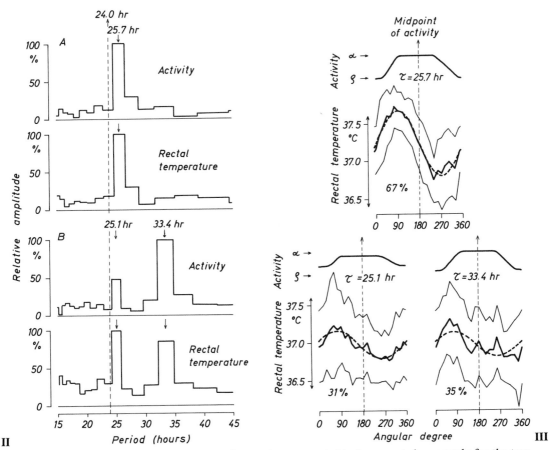

Figure 27/II. Period analyses of the two time series, presented in I, computed separately for the two sections (A and B). *III.* Longitudinally pooled courses of the two rhythms, computed separately for the two sections (A and B), with section A being an averaging period, derived from II, and B being two averaging periods, derived as the two most prominent peaks from II. Indications are the same as in figure 16/III. From Wever (1975a).

most likely reflected by a body temperature rhythm running parallel. If there is an activity rhythm with a period of 33.4 hours, a rhythm component of body temperature with equal period and phase can be expected due to masking; however, the inspection of the mutual phase relationship between the two rhythms measured shows that this picture is too simple. Figure 27/III B shows that the rhythms of activity and rectal temperature do not run parallel but with a leading phase of the temperature rhythm having a period of 33.4 hours, as with the other period (i.e., rectal temperature increases before the onset of activity, and hence, this increase in temperature cannot be the consequence of

masking because of an increase in activity). The internal phase of relationship measured between the different rhythms deviating from parallelism to the same amount with all different periods, during the state of internal desynchronization, rejects the assumption that mutual masking is involved essentially in the occurrence of multiplicity and identity of periods in the rhythms of each variable. The masking component which is present probably, is negligible rather in comparison to the oscillatory component.

In the experiments discussed as examples of internal desynchronization, the period of the separated rectal temperature rhythms always was close to 25 hours (i.e., close to the

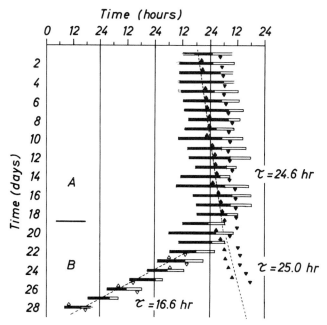

Figure 28. Autonomous rhythm of a subject (H.Z., ♂ 25 y) living under constant conditions without time cues. The experiment is divided arbitrarily into two sections (A and B), for further analyses. *1*. Temporal courses of the rhythms of activity and rectal temperature, presented successively one period beneath the other. Indications are the same as in figure 27/I.

value observed in internally synchronized rhythms), whereas the period of the separated activity rhythms always was considerably longer. This statement can be generalized regarding the rectal temperature rhythm but not the activity rhythm. In other experiments, internal desynchronization has been observed with an activity rhythm considerably faster than the temperature rhythm. Figure 28 shows the course of an experiment in which the different rhythms were synchronized internally in the first section (A) and internal desynchronization occurred spontaneously in the second section (B), but with an activity period being much shorter than the temperature period. It is the impression that after the sudden separation of the two rhythms presented at day 18, the activity rhythm becomes much faster and the temperature rhythm becomes slightly slower than before; the opposite of the other example (Fig. 27).

With this type of internal desynchronization, the subjective time does not pass slower, but faster, than the objective time.

The experiment was finished at the 26th objective day and the 28th subjective day. Physiologically, 25 rectal temperature periods had been passed during the experiment. This reversed difference, between the speeds of the objective and subjective time, had a great disadvantage. In the other experiments, the isolation was finished earlier than expected by the subjects but here the isolation lasted subjectively longer than objectively. In this special case, it originally was planned to perform the experiment for 28 objective days but the subject operated the alarm system for finishing the experiment 2 days earlier because he thought he was at the end of his 28th day and the experimenters had forgotten the agreed termination time.

The period analyses (Fig. 28/II) from section A resulted in one relevant peak with the center of gravity at 24.6 hours. The amplitudes of this period, when compared with the background level, are smaller than in the other spectra of internally synchronized rhythms shown. The period analyses from

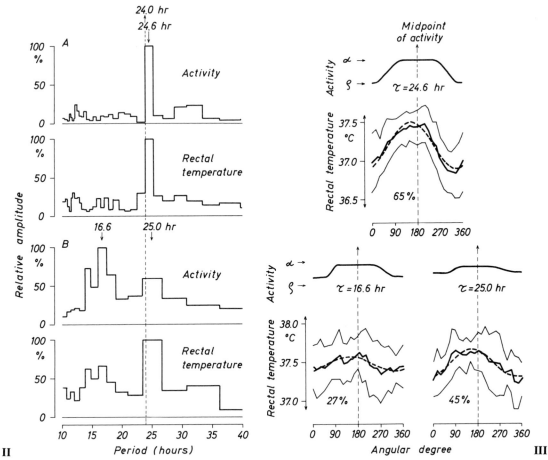

Figure 28/II. Period analyses of the two time series presented in I, computed separately for the two sections (A and B). *III.* Longitudinally pooled courses of the two rhythms, computed separately for the two sections (A and B), with section A being an averaging period, derived from II, and B being two averaging periods, derived as the two most prominent peaks from II. Indications are the same as in figure 16/III. From Wever (1975a).

the short section B resulted in spectra which were unclear but have at least two peaks each. The activity rhythm has a dominant peak at 16.6 hours, a secondary peak at 14.4 hours, and a third peak at 25.0 hours. The first period corresponds to the period of the overt activity rhythm and the last period corresponds to the period of the overt temperature rhythm. In the rectal temperature rhythm, there is one main peak at the period of the overt temperature rhythm (25.0 hours) but two small peaks are present at the same periods as in the activity rhythm. Also in these spectra, all peaks mentioned deviate from 24 hours and, therefore, all rhythms

occurring in this experiment are proven to be autonomous.

The determination of the internal phase angle difference between the two rhythms on the basis of pooling (Fig. 28/III) results in section A as a leading phase of the temperature rhythm, which is usual in autonomous rhythms. In section B, the pooling is computed with the two most important, and only reliable, averaging periods. The internal phase angle differences are nearly the same with the two periods, but a little greater than in the internally synchronized rhythms of section A. There is, however, a reason that the internal phase angle difference, with internal synchronization, deviates a little from that derived from section A. It is the impression, with an inspection of figure 28/I, that, before internal desynchronization started definitely at day 19, there were two beginnings of internal desynchronization at day 10 and day 14/15 which are not continued but cancelled. After exclusion of these cycles from the longitudinal pooling, the internal phase angle difference increases from 28° to 40°. This value is in full agreement with the other phase angle differences derived with the two periods of section B.

It could be argued that the differentiation between the two types of internal desynchronization mentioned, with activity periods much longer than temperature periods (Figs. 25 and 27) and with activity periods much shorter than temperature periods (Fig. 28), is only arbitrary, at least in experiments in which the subjects took naps. The distribution to one of the types would depend, following this argument, on the subjective scoring of sleep to be either a nap or a true night sleep. Normally, the subjects are asked to avoid naps, and, in the examples discussed so far, no naps were taken. In other experiments, however, subjects stated naps were unavoidable and, in these cases, it seemed to be more efficient to allow naps taken in bed instead of uncontrolled naps sitting in the chair. Also, in those cases, it is possible to discriminate objectively between internal desynchronization, with abnormally long and short activity periods, independent of the subjective scorings. This discrimination fundamentally is possible in all experiments including not only sections with internally desynchronized rhythms (section B in Figs. 27 and 28) but, additionally, sections with internally synchronized rhythms (section A in Figs. 27 and 28). In these experiments, with the occurrence of internal desynchronization, not only the activity rhythms alter their periods but also the rectal temperature rhythms. Such vegetative rhythms cannot be perceived consciously and do not depend, in any way, on subjective scorings.

In the experiment for figure 27, the drastic lengthening of the activity period is accompanied with a simultaneous slight shortening of the rectal temperature period. Conversely, in the experiment for figure 28, the drastic shortening of the activity period is accompanied with a simultaneous slight lengthening of the rectal temperature period. These period alterations, in opposite directions, are not accidental but systematic, as can be determined from the summarizing inspection of all corresponding experiments. In 26 experiments, internal desynchronization has been observed only in parts of the experiments but the rhythms were internally synchronized during other parts of the same experiments. Figure 29 summarizes results of all these experiments with regard to the periods. Because the periods of corresponding rhythms are distributed almost normally among the different subjects, only the respective normal distributions are presented for clarity.

The upper part of figure 29 includes results of 15 experiments in which the activity period drastically lengthened regarding the subjective scoring of an activity period. With the occurrence of internal desynchronization, the combined rhythms, with average periods of 25.55 ± 0.46 hours, split into separated rhythms with average activity periods of 34.04 ± 2.31 hours and average rectal temperature periods of 24.85 ± 0.30 hours. From the objective computations, the shortening of the rectal temperature period for 0.70 ± 0.38 hours statistically is significant with $p < 0.001$, as is the lengthening of the activity periods for 8.49 ± 2.13 hours. The lower part of figure 29 includes results of 11 experiments in which the activity period drastically shortened regarding the subjective scoring of an activity period. The combined rhythms here have an average period of 24.47 ± 0.15 hours which is significantly shorter (with $p < 0.001$) than the average period of the other experiments (upper part of Fig. 29). With the occurrence of internal desynchronization, they split again into separated rhythms with average activity periods of 17.91 ± 1.00 hours and average rectal temperature periods of 24.88 ± 0.13

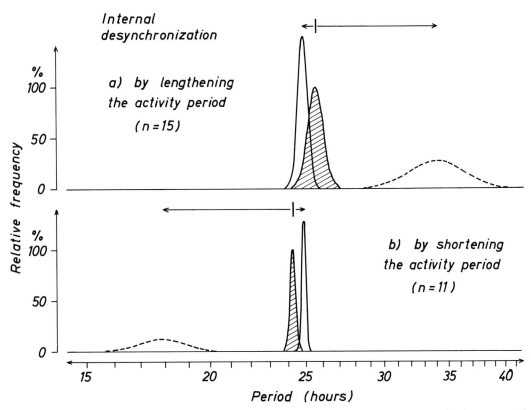

Figure 29. Summary of the results of all experiments where real internal desynchronization occurred during one section of the respective experiment (section B in Figs. 27 and 28), while the rhythms ran synchronized internally during another section of the same experiment (section A in Figs. 27 and 28). Above: results of 15 experiments where the activity periods, during the state of internal desynchronization, where longer than the rectal temperature periods (Fig. 27). Below: results of 11 experiments where the activity periods, during the state of internal desynchronization, were shorter than the rectal temperature periods (Fig. 28). All period distributions are given, for clarity, as the computed normal distributions. The actual distributions, in all cases, are very close to normal distributions. Hatched peaks: distributions of the combined periods of both rhythms, measured during the sections with internally synchronized rhythms. Empty peaks: distributions of the separated periods of the rectal temperature rhythms (solid lines) and activity rhythms (broken lines), measured during the sections with internally desynchronized rhythms. In each diagram, the ordinate is standardized in such a manner that the maximum of the (hatched areas) distribution of the combined periods is taken for 100%. From Wever (1975a).

hours. From the objective computations, the lengthening of the rectal temperature period for 0.41 ± 0.07 hour statistically is significant with $p < 0.001$ as is the shortening of the activity period for 6.56 ± 1.01 hours. Remarkably enough, the resulting periods of the separated rectal temperature rhythms equal each other in both cases. Implications of this conformity will be discussed later (cf. 3.4). Generally, the figures imparted an objective discrimination between the two types of internal desynchronization, with activity periods being either longer or shorter than the respective rectal temperature periods. This is possible even when the activity periods are disregarded. In some of the experiments included in figure 29, the direction of the alteration in the activity period may be unclear in the objective detection because of naps, which are scored only subjectively. The simultaneous alterations in the rectal temperature periods, which are independent of subjective scoring but are significant, qualify to unambiguous discriminations. Additionally, the rectal temperatures differ significantly in their periods as long as the rhythms run synchronized internally. The subjectivity of the scoring of sleep, to be either night sleep or nap, does not break the objectivity of the discrimination between the two types of internal desynchronization mentioned (i.e., with activity periods being either longer or shorter than the respective rectal temperature periods).

There are 12 experiments in which the rhythms remain desynchronized internally during the total experiment (Fig. 25). If the subject, in such an experiment, takes no naps, as is the case in the experiment for figure 25, an objective discrimination in the assignation to one of the two types of internal desynchronization again is possible. The objective activity recordings coincide with the subjective activity scorings. If, however, the subject takes naps, a discrimination between the two types of internal desynchronization mentioned can become impossible on the basis of only the objective measurements. This can be shown in figure 30. From his statements, the subject showed abnormally long activity periods during the total experiment, on the average of 33.4 hours. The result equals the activity periods of the other experiment (Fig. 25). With about half of the periods, however, the subject took naps which lasted, according to his subjective declaration, for about half an hour but were objectively nearly as long as the night sleeps. From the objective activity recording, which cannot differentiate between subjective declared naps and rest times, it must be stated that the subject altered between sections with abnormally long activity periods and those with abnormally short activity periods (i.e., between the two types of internal desynchronization). During both sections, the activity periods deviated drastically from the rectal temperature periods; therefore, the subjective scoring of the naps does not influence the classifying of the rhythm as being desynchronized internally. If one looks at the days the subject took naps, there is a general simple rule. On days when the temperature minimum falls into the nightsleep, the subject took no nap; however, on days when the temperature minimum falls into the subjectively scored activity time, the subject took a nap around the time of this minimum.

This relationship between rectal temperature and activity is more obvious in the longitudinal presentation of the original data given in Figure 30/II. It includes, in addition to the subjectively scored activity-rest cycle, data of locomotor activity obtained from the contact plates under the floor and data of sleep movements obtained from the contact in the bed. In general, every great change in locomotor activity is reflected by a parallel change in body temperature; the variations of both variables may indicate more or less regular, synchronously running ultradian rhythms (rhythms with frequencies higher than circadian). The amount of the sleep movements is, in comparison to locomotor activity, so small that body temperature cannot reflect these activities. In particular, there is a drop in body temperature every time the subject goes to sleep, and a rise in body temperature every time he stands up. These reactive changes in body temperature due to physical activities (masking effects; see Section 4.3.2) occur nearly independent of the phase of circadian variability, and in any case, they are small in amount in comparison to this variability. As can be seen in Figure 30/II, the subjectively scored "nights" coincide only rarely with rectal temperature minimum values; the positions of "night-sleeps" within the rectal temperature cycle vary from cycle to cycle. The subjectively scored "naps", however, coincide always clearly with a rectal temperature minimum, in remarkable contrast to the phase relationship between rectal temperature and night-sleep as just mentioned.

The period analysis of the subjective activity declarations (Fig. 30/III) shows a split period with the centers of gravity at 31.4 and 34.4 hours. Only the weighted mean of these two peaks results in the single overt activity period of 33.4 hours (Figs. 30/I and II). There is a small peak at the overt period of the rectal temperature rhythm (24.6 hours and further, a still smaller one (16.4 hours). The locomotor activity, recorded with the contacts under the floor, and the sleeping activity, recorded from the movements of the bed, show fundamentally the same spectra with the same peaks. The short period of 16.4 hours and the period of 24.6 hours, however, are much more pronounced and almost of the same amplitude as the long period. This can be understood from the described course of activity. The objective activity periods, with the recorded naps as rest time, alter between long periods, on the average of 33.4 hours, and periods of half this duration, whereas the naps are not relevant in the subjective activity declarations. It has been determined that the naps were closer to the temperature minimum than the real rest times. Finally, the period analysis of the rectal temperature rhythm shows one primary peak at 24.6 hours, and smaller secondary peaks at the other periods.

In this experiment, four prominent periods have been detected (Fig. 30/III). The longitudinal pooling can be done with four different averaging periods. In figure 30/IV, results of this procedure are shown not only for the subjectively declared activity but also for the locomotor activity and the sleeping movements. As can be seen, the objectively measured activities are less reliable but generally correlate to the subjectively stated activity. The locomotor activity is in phase with the subjective activity. With the period of 31.4 hours, the objective activity clearly lags behind the subjective one, for unknown reasons. In the locomotor activity, a bimodal course is recognizable (especially with $\tau = 24.6$ hours) because of the decreased performance around noon, which is found in many organisms. The sleeping activity passes, with all periods, reversed to the locomotor activity. The rectal temperature rhythm has the largest amplitude, at 24.6 hours, and, as usual in autonomous rhythms, it leads the activity rhythm with all periods. Only with the period 31.4 hours, the rectal temperature rhythm is in phase with the rhythm of subjective activity; however, when related to the objective locomotor ac-

tivity, it also shows a phase lead as with the other rhythm components.

Generally, from the objective activity recordings of this special experiment, no relevant difference can be stated in the amplitudes of activity periods, which are much longer than the rectal temperature periods, and those which are much shorter. In the subjective declarations, the longer activity periods have preference. It seems to be impossible, from only the objective measurements without regard to the subjective declarations, to decide to which type of internal desynchronization these results must be coordinated. The reverse seems to be true, in some experiments with internal desynchronization, in which the subjectively declared activity periods are very short (Fig. 28). The analysis of the objective activity recordings, in such cases, result in a spectrum which contains the short and long periods to almost equal amounts. The reason is that the subjective equally scored rest times alternate objectively in their quantitative pronounciation because of the alternating depth of sleep.

In summary, there are 38 cases in which the rhythms of the different variables measured in one subject show different periods in the steady state. In all cases, the overt rhythms of rectal temperature, and other rhythms, hold a period close to 25 hours. The activity rhythms, and other rhythms, alter their periods drastically (in the majority of cases to periods in the range between 30 and 40 hours, but in some cases to shorter periods in the range between 15 and 20 hours). Independent of the sign of the period alterations, these alterations may occur at the beginning of the experiment, or later on. All these different manifestations of internal desynchronization are characterized by continuously varying internal phase angle differences between the different overt rhythms. In the computed analyses, internally desynchronized rhythms are split into several rhythms with different period components which interfere with each other. The same periods are present in the rhythms of all different variables, with different propor-

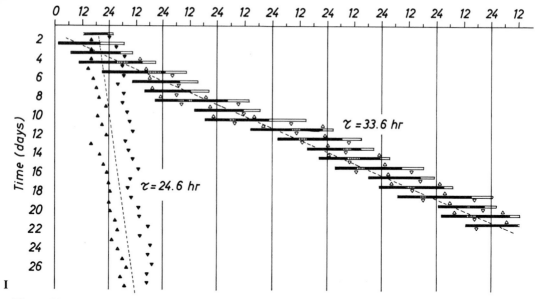

Figure 30. Autonomous rhythm of a subject (P.C., ♂ 23 y) living under constant conditions without time cues. *I.* Temporal courses of the rhythms of activity and rectal temperature, presented successively one period beneath the other. Indications are the same as in figure 27/I. Hatched areas within the black bars represent naps.

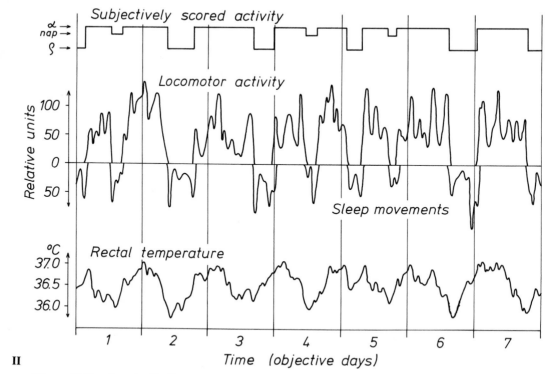

Figure 30/II. Longitudinally presented courses of subjectively scored activity, objectively recorded locomotor activity (from contact plates under the floor), sleep movements (from a contact in the bed; the scales of the two latter activity recordings are not comparable quantitatively), and rectal temperature. For clarity, the courses of the four time series are shown only from a section out of the total experiment (subjective days 15 to 19 from I) but with extended scales.

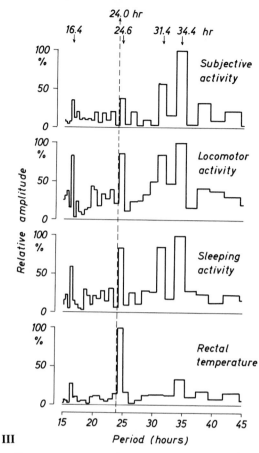

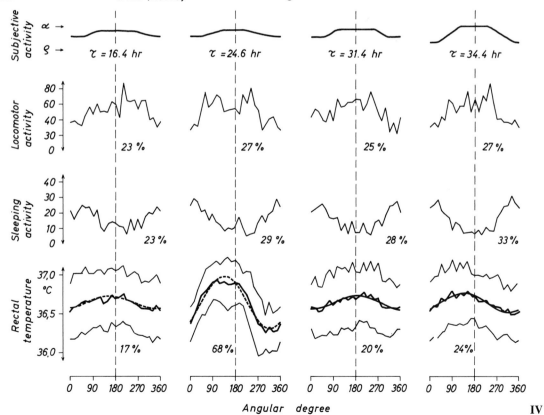

III

IV

Figure 30/III. Period analyses of the four time series presented in II, computed from the total experiment.

Figure 30/IV. Longitudinally pooled courses of the four rhythms in II, with four different averaging periods derived as the four most prominent peaks from III. Indications are the same as in figure 16/III.

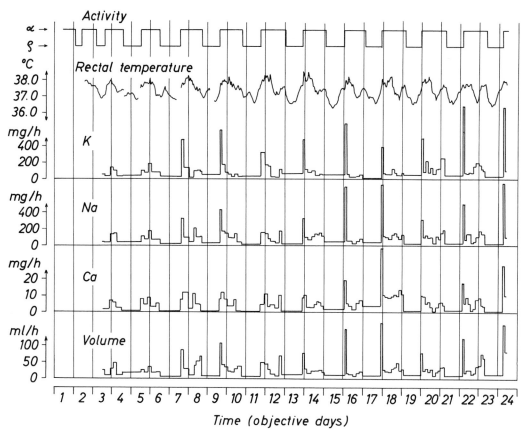

Figure 31.   Autonomous rhythm of a subject (N.Z., ♂ 24 y) living under constant conditions without time cues. Presented, from top to bottom, are the rhythms of activity (i.e., alternation between wakefulness α and rest ρ), rectal temperature (measured continuously), and four urine constituents (i.e., mictions taken at self-selected intervals. *I.* Longitudinally presented courses of the six variables during the total experiment.

tions and different preference periods in the different variables. In each of these period components, the internal phase angle differences, between the rhythms of different variables, are equal.

2.2.2. Apparent Internal Desynchronization

Internal synchronization is characterized by a temporally constant phase angle difference between different rhythms. This constancy does not include necessarily the different rhythms having equal periods. In some subjects, a rectal temperature rhythm with a period of about 25 hours is combined with an activity period of twice or half this value.

The phase angle differences between the two rhythms remain constant in such cases. The two rhythms are synchronized internally with each other. This mutual synchronization is, however, not the normal 1:1 mode, but a 2:1 mode or a 1:2 mode. Under rough inspection, this integral synchronization looks like internal desynchronization because of the obviously different periods of different rhythms; therefore, this state has been called "apparent internal desynchronization" in contrast to "real internal desynchronization," as discussed already (Wever, 1967c).

An example of this state is given in figure 31. This figure shows the temporal courses of six variables, measured with a young man living in strict isolation without time cues.

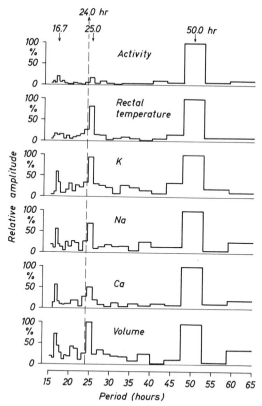

Figure 31/II. Period analyses of the six time series presented in I.

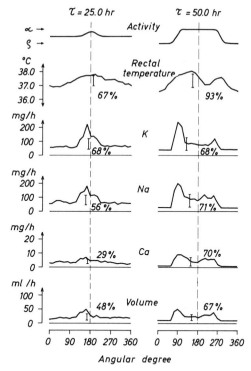

Figure 31/III. Longitudinally pooled courses of the six rhythms, with two averaging periods derived as the two most prominent peaks from II. Mean value and amplitude of the fundamental periods are presented at the position of the respective acrophase. From Wever (1975a).

His activity rhythm shows an unusually long period of, on the average, 50.0 hours; with an average activity time of 31.0 hours without a nap; and an average rest time of 19.0 hours without getting up. At the beginning, this behavior was very alarming to the experimenters because repeated sleep of such a long duration seemed to be very unusual in a healthy man. In comparison to the irregular course during real internal desynchronization (Fig. 25), the regular course of the activity rhythm is striking. Its regularity is similar to that during full internal synchronization (Fig. 15). The rhythm of rectal temperature is, during the first part, interrupted several times for technical reasons. During the second part, however, it shows a regular course with a period of 25.0 hours, which is half as long as the activity periods. In other words, one activity period comprises two

temperature periods. One maximum of rectal temperature occurs regularly at the beginning of each activity time and another at the end of each activity time. The internal phase angle difference between these two rhythms remains constant. In the rhythms of the substances excreted with the urine, the long lasting minimum values are conspicuous because of the long rest times without a break. During the activity times, the rhythms of all excretions show mostly bimodal courses, which is unusual during full internal synchronization.

The period analyses of the different time series (Fig. 31/II) show two relevant peaks; at 25.0 and 50.0 hours. A third peak at 16.7 hours is of no special meaning because it is caused by the special shapes of the rhythms (3rd harmonic of 50.0 hours). Only in the activity rhythm, the 50.0-hour period is included solely. This is true in the subjectively scored activity, as presented in figure 31/I as well as in the objectively recorded activity. In the longitudinally pooled rhythms (Fig. 31/III), the average period of 50.0 hours is of special interest because the reliability of the rhythms is much greater with this period than with 25.0 hours. With the period of 50.0 hours in all rhythms, except in the activity rhythm, bimodal courses of the averaged cycles, are recognizable with long lasting horizontal courses during rest time. The internal phase angle differences between the different rhythms correspond to values which are normal in autonomous rhythms. With the period of 25.0 hours, the phase angle differences against the activity rhythm deviate little from the normal to later phases but this cannot be of great meaning because the amplitude of the activity rhythm with this period is nearly zero. The mutual phase angle differences between the other rhythms are similar to those in autonomous rhythms (Fig. 15).

The state of apparent internal desynchronization, with lengthened activity periods, has been observed in 11 subjects; partly occurring from the beginning of the experiment shown in figure 31 and partly occurring spontaneously during the experiment. In all cases, the obvious period of the rectal temperature rhythm was close to 25 hours but the activity period was close to 50 hours; therefore, in contrast to the 'circadian' period near 25 hours, the period of the activity rhythm has been called 'circa-bi-dian' (Wever, 1967c). As in the state of real internal desynchronization, the subjects are aware only of the activity rhythm and are unable to realize deviations in the length of these periods from 24 hours. Although the subjective time passes with a speed of half the objective time, they do not notice this remarkable difference.

The observed cases of apparent internal desynchronization, or circa-bi-dian activity periods, can be separated into two different types. In the first type (four cases), activity time and rest time are uninterrupted and each is about twice as long as normal; the

activity time without naps and the rest time without breaks (Fig. 31). In one of these experiments, the unusual duration of sleep has been confirmed by polygraphic sleep recording. In the other type (seven cases), the rest time is about as long as normal and the activity time is interrupted by naps. These naps are short, in the opinion of the subjects, but objectively of about the same duration as the night sleeps. The first type shows circa-bi-dian activity periods even from computations using the objectively recorded activities. The second type seems to correspond to full internal synchronization when only the objective activity recordings are used. There are, however, essential differences as demonstrated in another example (Fig. 32).

In figure 32, results of an experiment are presented in which a subject lived under the same constant conditions as the other experiments without any external changes in the experimental conditions. From the beginning of the experiment, the subject stated naps were unavoidable. During the first 11 days, the objective duration of the naps corresponded to the subjectively scored duration of about 1 hour and the rhythms showed a normal internally synchronized course with a period of 25.0 hours. Beginning with day 12, the naps extended to an extraordinary duration but the subject did not score the duration as being any longer than the preceding days. As a consequence, the total activity period, as determined from the subjective statements of the subject, became twice as long as before. After three of those circa-bi-dian activity periods, the subject fell back to the normal rhythm. At subjective day 20, he again started the extraordinarily long naps and, with circa-bi-dian activity periods, remained in this state until the end of the experiment. It can be argued again that the very long naps correspond to objective rest times separating two periods. Following this argumentation, in figure 32 the activity rhythm is redrawn, in a shaded manner, with the long naps as additional rest times. With a rough examination, one could think of a normal circadian rhythm with full internal synchronization and constant internal phase re-

Time (hours)

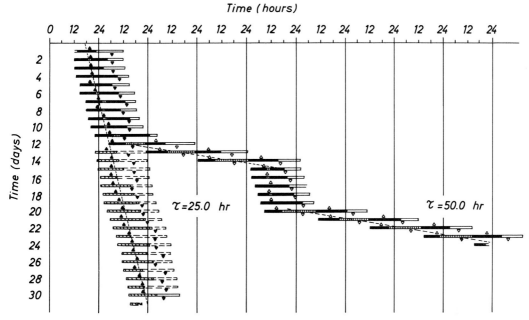

Figure 32. Autonomous rhythm of a subject (G.C., ♂ 23 y) living under constant conditions without time cues. Temporal courses of the rhythms of activity and rectal temperature, presented successively one period beneath the other. Indications are the same as in figure 30. Shaded bars: temporally correct redrawings of corresponding full bars, but with the long naps interpreted as rest times. From Wever (1975a).

lationships. This approach, however, can be rectified by a closer examination of the temporal organization of successive events within each activity period. On the days with the circa-bi-dian activity periods (12th to 14th and 20th to 24th subjective day), not only the naps were significantly longer than other days with circadian activity periods (15.51 ± 0.63 hours versus 1.30 ± 0.89 hours), but also some other intervals within each period. These differences concern the duration of the rest time (10,52 ± 1.32 hours versus 7.58 ± 1.86 hours). Additionally, on the days with the circa-bi-dian activity periods, the naps were even longer than the rest times (15.51 ± 0.63 hours versus 10.52 ± 1.32 hours). These differences concern, moreover, the temporal structure of the morning which passed objectively more slowly on the days with circa-bi-dian activity periods than on other days. This is indicated by the intervals between the beginning of activity and the beginning of the nap (8.75 ± 0.65 hours versus 7.08 ± 0.86 hours) and by

the intervals between breakfast and lunch (6.30 ± 0.83 hours versus 5.06 ± 0.94 hours). All differences stated, statistically are significant with $p < 0.01$ when the successive periods are taken as statistical units. This means that the drastic lengthening of the activity period on some days was not only due to the lengthened (and subjectively, possibly wrongly, interpreted) naps but already was predetermined objectively before the naps, indicating a change in the total internal organization. Corresponding results are true for all those experiments with apparent internal desynchronization in which the subjects took long naps. It is possible, generally, to differentiate objectively between circadian and circa-bi-dian activity periods, independent of whether or not the activity times are interrupted by naps (Figs. 31 and 32).

After considering the possibility of an internal 2:1 synchronization, the question arises concerning the inverted case (i.e., an internal 1:2 synchronization). In this case of apparent desynchronization, circadian rectal temperature periods, of about 25 hours, would be accompanied by circa-semi-dian activity periods of about 12.5 hours. This has been observed in only one subject. Figure 33 shows the course of the corresponding experiment. From the beginning, the subject showed activity periods averaging 12.3 hours. For clarity, the activity rhythm has been redrawn in figure 33, in a shaded manner, with circadian periods (i.e., with two circa-semi-dian periods successively). The subject did not perceive the abnormal shortness of her activity time, which averaged only 8.0 hours. During these short intervals, she took mostly three meals. From subjective day 10 to 12, and again from subjective day 16 to 24, she showed periods of normal length, without realizing the difference in the lengths of the activity cycles. The rectal temperature record, unfortunately, failed during the last part of the experiment. While the record was in operation it showed regular temperature periods of 24.5 hours. To compensate for the missing rectal temperature, the maxima of potassium excretions are included in figure 33. The rhythms of all other physiological variables showed regular periods of 24.5 hours. During the days with circadian activity periods, the phase angle differences, between the different rhythms, temporally were constant. Also, during the days with circa-semi-dian activity periods, the phase angle differences temporally were constant, although a maximum of rectal temperature or potassium excretion was present only in each second activity cycle. Because 26 days had been arranged for the duration of the experiment, it finished on the 26th subjective day but objectively, it lasted only 19 days. The result of this experiment confirmed that internal 1:2 synchronization is possible as well as internal 2:1 synchronization.

2.2.3. Internal Dissociation

As a result of all examples discussed, internal desynchronization can occur in the steady state (i.e., rhythms of different variables measured in one subject can show different periods as the experiment continues). The definition of internal desynchronization includes the steady state which only can be proven by a mutual phase shift between the different rhythms of more than 360°. In the period analyses, it is expressed by different peaks which are separated clearly from each other. In all examples of internal desynchronization discussed, this necessary presupposition was fulfilled. There are, however, other examples in which different rhythms accept different periods only temporarily. In the final state, they have equal periods again but with an internal phase relationship that differs from the original one. In the latter cases, the periods of the different rhythms differ from each other only during transients between different steady states. To differentiate this transient state from internal desynchronization, the term ''internal dissociation'' is used. It is defined by temporarily changing periods of different rhythms which characterize a transient behavior but not a steady state. The mutual phase shift between different rhythms is not more than 360°. It is obvious that internal desynchronization and internal dissociation can be differentiated only in experiments of sufficiently long duration.

In the previous chapter, it has been concluded that rhythms, which are synchronized to the natural 24-hour day, and autonomous rhythms, differ significantly in their internal phase angle differences (Figs. 17 and 18). This means that, at the beginning of each isolation experiment in which a subject lives under constant conditions, the transition from the synchronized state of the rhythm (before the experiment) to the autonomous state (during the experiment) is accompanied by a change in the internal phase angle differences (i.e., by internal dissociation). The necessary internal phase shift between the rhythms of activity and rectal temperature can be seen in all corresponding experiments. This again is demonstrated in figure 34. In the experiment shown at the left, the activity rhythm keeps, from the be-

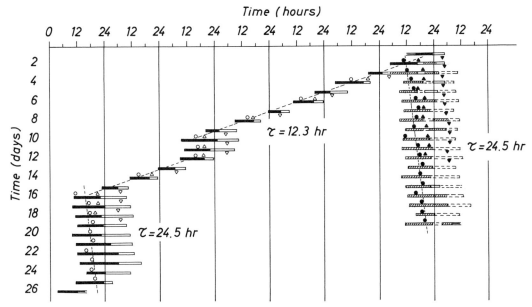

Figure 33. Autonomous rhythm of a subject (M.B., ♀ 20 y) living under constant conditions without time cues.Temporal courses of the rhythms of activity, rectal temperature, and potassium excretion (circles: indicating the temporal positions of the maximum values), presented successively one period beneath the other. Indications are the same as in figure 27/I. White circles: temporally correct redrawings of corresponding black circles. Shaded bars: temporally correct redrawings of corresponding full bars, but with some rest times interpreted as naps. From Wever (1975a).

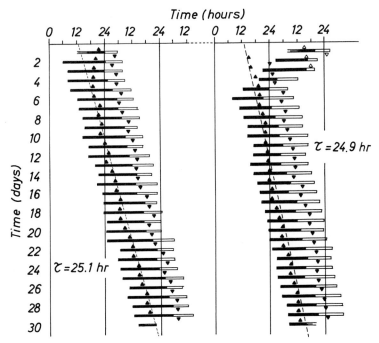

Figure 34. Autonomous rhythms of two subjects (M.S. ♂ 23 y. left; amd D.B., ♀ 21 y. right), in independent experiments, living under constant conditions without time cues. Temporal courses of the rhythms of activity and rectal temperature, presented successively one period beneath the other. Indications are the same as in figure 27/I.

ginning, a period of 25.1 hours but the rectal temperature rhythm reaches this steady state period only after about 6 days. During this time, the temperature period is shorter than the activity period. If the experiment had been finished after about 1 week, the conclusion would have been that the two rhythms have different periods and, further, that the activity period deviates from 24 hours while the rectal temperature period stays close to 24 hours. From the inspection of only the first week of the experiment, it is impossible to decide whether a steady state is reached. The inspection of the total experiment shows that the different periods, during the first week, are due to a transient behavior and that after that time, a steady state is reached with equal periods in the two rhythms. It has been concluded, from relatively short experiments, that human subjects frequently show internal desynchronization. It has been further concluded, from short term experiments, that the rectal temperature rhythm can hold a period of exactly 24 hours, even under constant conditions when the activity period deviates from 24 hours. These conclusions predetermine a steady state of the rhythms which could not be guaranteed in the respective experiments; therefore, it cannot be excluded that only transients have given misleading interpretations.

The alteration in the internal phase angle difference between the rhythms of activity and rectal temperature, which necessarily is connected with the beginning of each experiment containing autonomously running rhythms, must not occur by a mutual internal phase shift shown in the left part of figure 34. The same final steady state phase angle difference also can be reached by a phase shift in the opposite direction. This reversed, and necessarily greater, shift has been observed in a few experiments, with an example given in the right part of figure 34. In the greater portion of the experiments, the rectal temperature rhythm shifts, with the transition from entrained to free running rhythms, for about 90° to earlier phases of the activity rhythm, which holds its steady

state period from the beginning (Fig. 34, left). In a smaller portion of the experiments, the activity rhythm shifts, with this transition, for about 270°, to earlier phases of the rectal temperature rhythm, which holds its steady state period from the beginning (Fig. 34, right). It is evident that the last mentioned type of transition gives rise to misleading interpretations even more readily than the other type.

Internal dissociation occurs, as already discussed, at the beginning of each experiment in which human circadian rhythms run autonomously under constant conditions. It occurs further after various external alterations in the experimental conditions, which will be discussed later. It can occur spontaneously, however, during the experiment. The internal phase relationship between different rhythms may often be disturbed for any external or internal reason, known or unknown. These disturbances normally will be eliminated by returning to the original phase relationship due to phase shifts in the opposite direction to the releasing disturbance. The disturbance is difficult to detect because it is drowned by random noise. If, however, the phase shifting disturbance exceeds a certain amount, the system may prefer to return to the original phase relationship by continuing the disturbing phase shift and, therefore, completing a full cycle. The result is an internal phase shift between the two rhythms of 360°. In figure 35, two examples are shown which illustrate this special type of internal dissociation with disturbances in opposite directions. In both cases, the numbers of physiological and psychological days differ for 1 day but in opposite directions. By chance, in the case of 'forward jumping' of the activity rhythm (Fig. 35/I, right), the subjectively perceived time coincided with the objective time at the end of the experiment but deviated in the other case ('backward jumping') for 2 days from the objective time (Fig. 35/I, left). In all of these cases, external changes in the experimental conditions, or other known external disturbances, can be excluded as causes of the original deflection. In one of

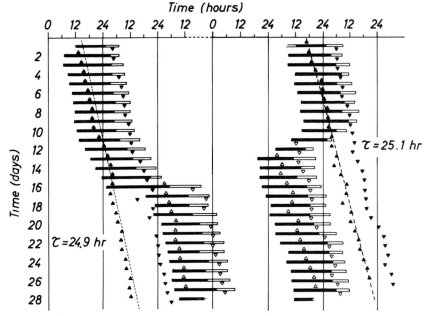

Figure 35. Autonomous rhythms of two subjects (H.D., ♀ 22 y, left; and H.B., ♂ 24 y, right) in independent experiments, living under constant conditions without time cues. *I.* Temporal courses of the rhythms of activity and rectal temperature, presented successively one period beneath the other. Indications are the same as in figure 27/I.

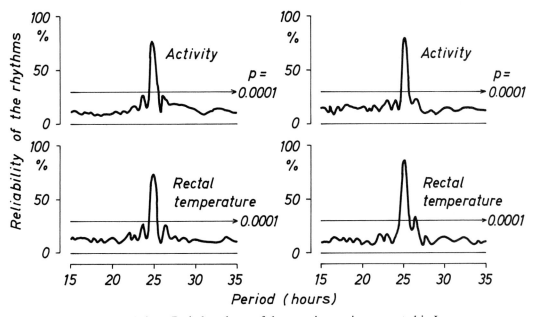

Figure 35/II.   Period analyses of the two time series presented in I.

the cases presented, however, an internal disturbance may be supposed. In the female subject, whose results are presented in the left part of figure 35, it was found later that the beginning of the internal dissociation (at subjective day 16) coincided with the first day of menstruation (there are other evidences that the duration of sleep may be disturbed during menstruation) (Hartman, 1967). In other similar cases, an internal factor releasing the disturbance could not be detected.

Internal dissociation, as examplified in figure 35, and internal desynchronization, as examplified in figures 25, 27, 28, and 30, must not be necessarily antagonisms. There can be continuous transitions between these states. In most cases of internal desynchronization, successive activity periods neither show equal values nor randomly varying values, but values which oscillate more or less around a mean in intervals of a few days (Fig. 27). From the multioscillator model as derived, these regular fluctuations in the activity period, and other periods are interpreted as beats between the two or more oscillators involved. In case of internal dissociation, there cannot be any meaningful reason not to describe the phase jumps of the activity rhythm as a beat phenomenon. For example, a formally computed regression of the activity rhythm in the experiments presented in figure 35 resulted in activity periods of 26.4 hours (left) or 23.9 hours (right) respectively. From these values, beat periods of 18.3 objective days (left; 24.9 hours versus 26.4 hours) or of 20.8 objective days (right; 25.1 hours versus 23.9 hours) would result. The experiments, however, did not last long enough to decide whether the phase jumps would have been repeated regularly enough to be compared to beats. Regarding the regularity it has to be considered with periods so close to each other, that the beat period changes drastically with small changes in the single original periods; therefore, it is more a question of definition than of principle if, in borderline cases of phase jumps at large intervals, it should be spoken of as internal dissociation

or desynchronization. This definition is supposed to be based on the result of computed period analyses. In a case of real internal desynchronization, period analyses result in at least two separate reliable periods (Figs. 25, 27, 28, and 30). In a case of internal dissociation, however, they result in only one reliable period. In the experiments underlying figure 35, the computed period analyses (Fig. 35/II) show only one reliable period is present in each experiment and they are the periods indicated in figure 35/I. The periods to be demanded, hypothetically, with the activity rhythms from the beat concept, at 26.4 hours (left) and 23.9 hours (right) respectively, are completely drowned out by random noise (i.e., they cannot be separated from values computed with any other period).

Between the clear cases mentioned, internal dissociation with one phase jump of the activity rhythm crossing other rhythms (Fig. 35) and internal desynchronization with regularly oscillating activity periods (Fig. 27), there are intermediate cases. These cases are characterized by phase jumps of the activity rhythm at more or less regularly large intervals. Besides some experiments with two jumps each, figure 36 shows an example with three jumps. This experiment is instructive especially because it shows a regular rhythm being fully internally synchronized during the first 4 weeks. The rhythm later becomes disturbed by some abnormally long activity periods numbered 27, 30, and 37. The first impression is that the activity rhythm runs, between the jumps, with the same period as before during the undisturbed section. This can be determined especially during the activity periods numbered 31 through 36 and 38 through 44. With a closer examination, however, this picture must be corrected. As seen from figure 36/I, the phase position of the rectal temperature rhythm gradually shifts, during these sections, to earlier phases of the activity rhythm, indicating different periods of the two overt rhythms during these sections. Correspondingly, the regressions, computed from successive activity periods during these sections, result in periods of 26.1 hours, which are clearly longer than the periods of the rectal temperature rhythm during the same sections (25.2 hours). In the examples presented in figure 35, the internal phase relationships are, before and after the phase jump, temporally constant and the computed periods of the two different overt rhythms coincide exactly. This observation favors, from the experiment concerning figure 36, the interpretation of internal desynchronization instead of internal dissociation.

This interpretation is supported by later computer analyses. The period analyses (Fig. 36/II) show, during the first section of 4 weeks, one reliable period in each time series at the coinciding value of 25.6 hours. During the second section, the analysis of the rectal temperature rhythm results in one reliable period, but in a period that clearly is shorter than that resulting during the first section. This change in period already justifies the interpretation as internal desynchronization (Fig. 29). The analysis of the activity rhythm results in a primary peak at the same period as the rectal temperature rhythm (25.2 hours). There is a secondary broad peak at a longer period of 29.0 hours that corresponds to the overt activity period indicated in figure 36/I. There is a third period at 33.5 hours which transgresses the threshold of reliability. This period originates from the first week after the occurrance of internal desynchronization (activity periods numbered 27 through 31) where the beat period obviously is shorter and the activity period longer. A sequential period analysis shows the separately successive occurrence of the periods at 33.5 hours and 29.0 hours. The period at 26.1 hours, as derived from the regressions of successive activity periods between the phase jumps, does not appear, in any way, in the analysis of the activity periods; justifying the beat concept again. In the analysis of the rectal temperature rhythms the periods included in the activity rhythm, as secondary peaks (29.0 hours and 33.5 hours), at least are suggested though not at a sufficient level of reliability. The longitudinal poolings of this

experiment (Fig. 36/III) do not show any specialty. During the first section, both rhythms presented show reliable average periods with a mutual internal phase relationship which is characteristic in autonomous rhythms. During the second section, the averaging process is meaningful only with the overt period of the rectal temperature rhythm (25.2 hours) since the other periods, which are relevant in the activity rhythm (29.0 hours and 33.5 hours), are not relevant in the rectal temperature rhythm. With the one period presented, the internal phase relationship equals that measured during the first section, but with another period.

In summary, there are transitions between internal dissociation and desynchronization which are characterized by phase jumps of the activity rhythm crossing the other rhythms in either direction. If a rhythm in an experiment of sufficient duration includes only one phase jump and if the computed period analysis includes only one relevant period (i.e., the overt period disregarding the phase jump), it should be termed internal dissociation. If, however, the course of the rhythm includes more than one phase jump and if the period analysis includes more than one reliable and clearly separable period, it should be termed internal desynchronization. In the latter case the activity period measured by regression in the intervals between successive phase jumps does not coincide with any period value resulting from the period analysis of the total time series. Therefore the interpretation of the phase jumps as beat phenomena is favored. The following conclusion can be drawn from the summarizing inspection of many experiments showing spontaneously occuring internal desynchronization. The longer the beat period (i.e., the smaller the difference between the two periods involved), the smaller the amplitude or the less the reliability of the rhythm component that differs more from 25 hours. In the activity rhythm this second rhythm component is significant only if the difference between the two periods exceeds 4 hours. In the rectal temperature rhythm the rhythm component

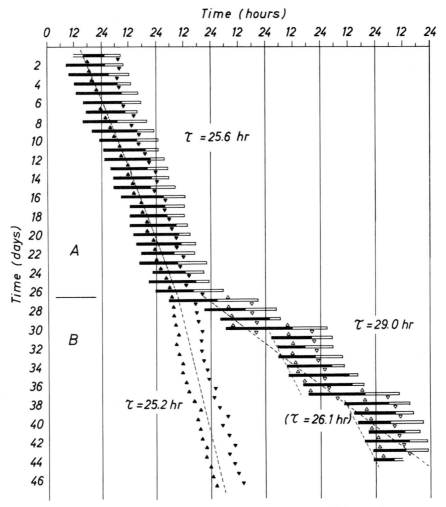

Figure 36. Autonomous rhythm of a subject (K.D., ♂ 26 y) living under constant conditions without time cues. The experiment is divided arbitrarily into two sections (A and B), for further analyses. *I.* Temporal courses of the rhythms of activity and rectal temperature, presented successively one period beneath the other. Indications are the same as in figure 27/I. Number in paranthesis: period of the activity rhythm during the short sections between two "phase jumps", computed by regression.

that differs in its period more than the other from 25 hours is always small in comparison to the 25-hour component.

2.2.4. Internal Desynchronization: Other Indications

Internal desynchronization, as previously described, seems to be unique in human experiments. In animal experiments, it sometimes has been observed that different rhythm components adopt different periods. In nearly all cases, however, this state is present only temporarily, until a phase shift between the two components of about 180° is reached. Thereafter, both rhythm components show coinciding periods (Pittendrigh, 1960, 1967; Hoffmann, 1970, 1971). In all these cases, the computed period analyses would result in only one reliable period. This "splitting phenomenon" corresponds to internal dissociation rather than to internal desynchronization. Beyond this state, there are only very recent indications that in monkeys real internal desynchronization may occur (Moore-Ede et al., 1976).

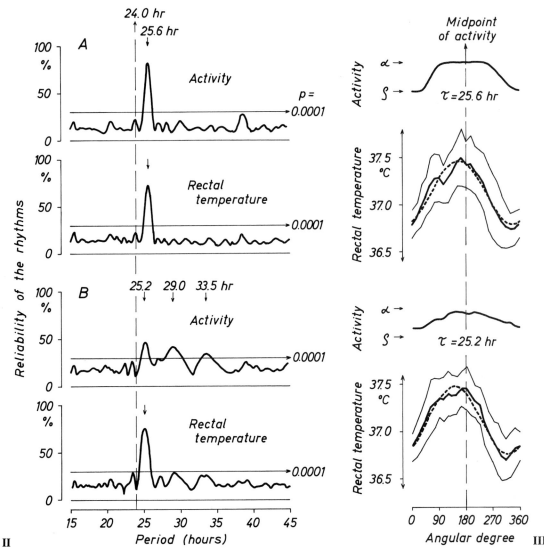

Figure 36/II. Period analyses of the two time series presented in I, computed separately for the two sections (A and B). **III.** Longitudinally pooled courses of the two rhythms, computed separately for the two sections (A and B), with section A being an averaging period, derived from II, and B being the averaging period, which corresponds to the most prominent peak in II. Indications are the same as in figure 16/III.

In human experiments performed by other investigators, internal desynchronization, with steadily varying internal phase relationships between different rhythms, seems to be a rare exception. From the long-term cave experiments, one case of real internal desynchronization has been stated (Mills et al., 1974). The subject (D.L.) showed, during 127 days in isolation, an average activity period of 25.1 hours and the authors stated a period, in some urine con-

stituents (sodium and chloride excretion), of 24.6 hours. Regarding the sodium rhythm, the authors state, "the steady drift in relation both to clock time and to the activity habits is clear," but there is a difficulty that casts doubt on this apparently clear result. This difficulty is based on the fact that true rhythms of the urine constituents had not been measured because urine was collected only intermittently; for nine spans each covering 22 to 48 hours and seven to twelve samples. For each of these "windows," the acrophase had been computed separately (with a period arbitrarily assumed to be 24 hours). The coordination of the nine urine acrophases to the activity periods, however, is arbitrary because the number of urine cycles between the separated windows is unknown. With the coordination chosen by the authors, a period of 24.6 hours follows. This coordination is based on the assumption that 20 cycles of 24.1 hours duration each are interposed between urine acrophases number 3 and 4. If, instead of this, the assumption is made that 19 cycles of 25.4 hours duration each are interposed, from the same data a mean period of 25.1 hours is computed, which coincides with the activity period. This second coordination is justified, even more than that chosen by the authors, because the average deviation of all measured acrophases around the computed regression is smaller with the period 25.1 hours than with the period 24.6 hours. There is no reason for a conclusion of internal desynchronization in this special experiment. It would be better to conclude that the rhythms ran synchronized internally, in contrast to the assumption of Mills et al. (1974).

There is another cave experiment (subject J.M.) which has sometimes been mentioned in this context (Colin et al., 1968; Fraisse et al., 1968; Jouvet, 1968). In a more recent paper (Jouvet et al., 1974), this experiment has been referred to as the first case of "total desynchronization"; however, in this experiment, only apparent desynchronization occurred. The subject adopted, during the first week of his stay of 153 days, a 'circadian' activity rhythm with a period of 24.8 hours. Later he spontaneously developed a circabi-dian activity rhythm for several months. At the beginning of this state there was one long-term activity time (about 34 hours) and one long term sleep time (about 15 hours) per period (Fig. 31). Later there were sleep times of normal durations but the activity time was interposed by naps which objectively lasted about as long as the real sleep times (Fig. 32). During the last section of the experiment, even circa-tri-dian and circa-te-tra-dian activity periods seemed to occur.

The rhythm of rectal temperature, which had been measured during limited sections of the experiment showed a period of 24.8 hours when extrapolated to the total experiment (Colin et al., 1968). The result of this experiment, therefore, corresponds exactly to the common picture of apparent internal desynchronization, as described earlier (Aschoff, 1965a; Aschoff et al., 1967b; Wever, 1967a, 1967c). There is no reason to conclude real internal desynchronization with independently running oscillators. In previous cave experiments, similar phenomena seem to have occurred. Siffre et al. (1966) reported the difficulty in deciding whether or not a subjectively declared nap, which lasted objectively 6 hours, should be graded as a real rest time. Closer reference to this phenomenon, however, is not given. Two more subjects (J.C. and P.E.) performing cave experiments, more recently, showed temporary circa-bi-dian activity periods, indicating the presence of apparent desynchronization (Jouvet et al., 1974; Chouvet et al., 1974).

From the experiments performed in artificial isolation units, one series has been stated to show commonly different periods in the rhythms of different variables (Mills et al.; 1973, 1974). In this series, 15 subjects spent 5 to 13 days in isolation from environmental time cues. Seven were alone and eight in groups of four. Applying the criteria used here, most of these experiments did not last long enough to allow a decision as to whether or not a steady state had been reached. A clear steady state, however, is necessary for the classification as internal desynchronization. In all experiments of this series, initial internal dissociation occurred as commonly in isolation experiments (Fig. 34): the completion of the transition from the entrained steady state to the free running steady state, either with internally synchronized or desynchronized rhythms, could not be observed. A decision whether or not internal desynchronization occurred, beyond the common initial dissociation, is not possible in most of the experiments. Only in two of the solitary subjects were there abnormally long activity periods (37 hours and 30 hours) and the analyses of the body temperature rhythms seem to result in two periods each, one normal 'circadian' period and another period coinciding with the respective activity period. The results obtained from these two subjects seem to correspond to results commonly obtained in cases of real internal desynchronization (cf. 2.2.1). Unfortunately, in these subjects, body temperature had been measured only intermittently during the wake time of the subjects, using the temperature of the urine, and original data were not presented, but only averaged endpoints. The reliability of the periods cited, therefore, cannot be estimated.

In the same experimental series (Mills et al., 1974), one of the two groups showed activity patterns with alternately long (14 to 16 hours) and short (3 to 7 hours) sleep times, with the short sleep times subjectively declared to be after lunch naps. The activity times between all sleep times were of normal lengths, averaging 14 hours. Considering the subjective declarations, the results seem to refer to apparent desynchronization with circa-bi-dian activity-periods (Fig. 32). Other cases of internal desynchronization of any type do not seem to be observed.

2.2.5 Conclusions

It is the conclusion of the summarizing inspection of all experiments discussed in this chapter that the assumption of only one single, endogenously driven oscillator controlling the circadian system is insufficient. There are several rhythmicities which have the capacity to oscillate independently. With this knowledge, it now must be concluded that in internally synchronized rhythms, different rhythmicities are present having the virtual capacity to oscillate independently. Because of their mutual synchronization, these different rhythmicities are not observable separately. Although it has been spoken of as oscillations, it is still an open question whether or not the different rhythmicities are controlled separately by oscillatory processes. It, indeed, has been shown that internally synchronized rhythms can be understood as being controlled by one endogenous oscillator (cf 2.1). This, however, does not mean necessarily that internally desynchronized rhythms are controlled by several endogenous oscillators. It cannot be excluded yet that some of the separated rhythms are based on rather stochastic processes. Therefore, the concept of the oscillatory origin of circadian rhythms must again be discussed, even regarding internally synchronized rhythms.

In the strict sense, a negative serial correlation proves an oscillatory origin of a rhythm only if this rhythm is not controlled by another rhythmicity with a smaller variability. This may be an external zeitgeber or another internal rhythm. If internally synchronized rhythms represent a system consisting of overt rhythms which synchronize each other mutually, the negative serial correlation of both of these rhythms proves, in the strict sense, the oscillatory origin only of that rhythm which has the smaller variability. In nearly all cases, this is the rhythm of the body temperature. The activity rhythm, which normally shows a larger variability, could be understood as controlled by the body temperature rhythm. Following this concept, it must show a negative serial correlation even if originally based on a stochastic process. Fortunately, the data available enables us to answer the question of the origin of the activity rhythm also, independent of the serial correlation between successive activity periods. This answer is given by the consideration of the 'overlapping serial correlation' between activity time and rest time. This latter serial correlation cannot be forced by the body temperature rhythm as it can be with the other serial correlation between successive periods. This latter serial correlation, therefore, only can be due to an oscillatory origin of the activity rhythm, independent of the body temperature rhythm.

In internally desynchronized rhythms, the problem is more intricate. It has been discussed, to this point in cases of internal desynchronization, different oscillators controlling the circadian system collectively exist. The intricacy is that the competent test (i.e., the serial correlation analysis) cannot be applied directly to the courses of the underlying periodical processes but only to the courses of the measured overt rhythms. These rhythms, however, are combined from the outputs of different periodic processes superposing each other, as had been concluded from the analyses of the different cases of internal desynchronization. This superposition results in beat phenomena which, unfortunately, make the application of the serial correlation analysis meaningless. Even if the different periodicities collectively underlying one overt rhythm would be based on separate stochastic processes, serial correlation would be simulated by the beat phenomena. This consideration concerns the serial correlation between successive periods, as well as the overlapping serial correlation between activity time and rest time.

As the result, a direct test for the oscillatory origin of the underlying periodicities cannot be applied when the circadian rhythms run desynchronized internally. This origin, rather, can be suggested only by analogy. In the majority of subjects, the circadian rhythms remain synchronized internally during the total experiment. In all the subjects, the oscillatory origin of the processes underlying the overt rhythms can be proven directly, as has been shown earlier. In the majority of those subjects who show internal desynchronization, moreover, this state is present only during parts of the experiments and, in those subjects, the oscillatory origin of the basic processes can be proven for those parts of the experiments where the rhythms run synchronized internally. It would be unlikely that in those subjects the basic processes alter, with the occurrence of internal desynchronization, from an oscillatory to a stochastic origin. The more simple hypothesis, therefore, is suggested that the measurable overt rhythms, in general are based on endogenous oscillators, whether or not internally synchronized or desynchronized. If we accept this hypothesis, the circadian system of man is controlled by different basic oscillators which are selfsustained separately, jus-

tifying the term "multioscillator system," The different oscillators mostly run mutually synchronized. The circadian system, then, can be understood as controlled by only one single oscillator. In some cases, however, the oscillators separate from each other so, in the steady state, they run with different periods. Such a system, by no means, can be understood as controlled by only one oscillator.

With the knowledge of the multioscillatory origin of human circadian rhythms, the ground is prepared to review the autonomous rhythms of all subjects, examined so far, together; independent of whether or not the rhythms run internally synchronized or desynchronized. In this summarizing inspection, however, it must be differentiated between overt rhythms, which can be measured directly, and oscillators, on which the overt rhythms are based hypothetically but which cannot be observed directly. Each of the underlying oscillators is not responsible simply for the control of one overt rhythm but, rather, for the control of all overt rhythms (though with different fractions). To simplify matters here, the period of the activity rhythm or the rectal temperature rhythm will be discussed in the following. It, however, must be kept in mind that this means, more precisely, the period of the oscillator which is dominant in the control of the overt activity rhythm, or the period of the other oscillator which is dominant in the control of the overt rectal temperature rhythm. The overt rhythms often include more than one relevant period (i.e., secondary periods other than the one primary or dominant period). The consideration of the two overt rhythms mentioned above is sufficient to represent the different oscillators and, therefore, the complete multioscillator system. The following presentations frequently are restricted to only these two rhythms for clarity.

2.3. Review of Autonomous Rhythms

After the consistency of rhythms, running under constant experimental conditions, has been proven, regarding their autonomic and oscillatory origin, these rhythms can be considered as summarizing. Because of the occurrence of internal desynchronization in a portion of the experiments, it would not be meaningful to summarize, in such a review, the periods of different overt rhythms collectively. It is more appropriate, as representatives of the great variety of overt rhythms, to summarize the rhythms of rectal temperature and activity separately. In the following review, from each experiment only one pe-

riod value for each will be considered, even if more than one subject participated. The reason for this method is the mutual synchronization within groups, which abolishes the statistical independence of period values of different subjects within the group (cf. 2.4.8.). Conversely, if personality data are considered, values of all subjects will be summarized, independent of testing in single or group experiments.

The upper part of figure 37 presents the histogram of periods of rectal temperature

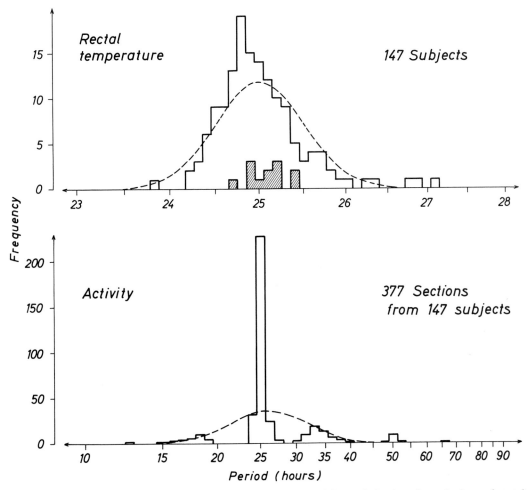

Figure 37. Summary of autonomous rhythms. Distributions of the period values from rhythms of rectal temperature (above) and activity (below), with logarithmic period scales (i.e., abscissa). In the histogram of rectal temperature periods, results from group experiments are indicated separately (hatched areas). This histogram includes one period value per subject, or per group in the group experiments, each averaged over the total experiment, independent of the experimental conditions. The histogram of the activity periods includes period values from two to three sections per subject, or per group in the group experiments, each section lasting 8 to 12 days, not including drastic changes in the period. Each period value is averaged over one section, independent of the experimental conditions. Dotted lines: formally computed normal distributions.

rhythms obtained in all experiments where rhythms ran autonomously. The 147 period values stem from 135 singly isolated subjects and 12 groups of two subjects each. From each experiment, the period is averaged from the total time series, independent of the experimental conditions. Apart from a few deviating values, the distribution of periods shown is remarkably small, in spite of the fact that the diagram includes data obtained under very different experimental conditions which could have influenced the period (cf. 2.4.). It also includes data of rectal temperature rhythms influenced by interactions with other rhythms and those which run independent of other rhythms (Fig. 29). The averaging of results for all experiments which are included in the diagram leads to a mean period ($\pm$ standard deviation) of 25.00 $\pm$ 0.50 hours. The normal distribution computed from these data (dotted line), however, really does not fit the experimental distribution, which is rather asymmetric. It is more meaningful, therefore, to compute the median of the periods instead of the mean. This method results in 24.93 hours, with a 95% confidence interval between 24.85 and 25.01 hours or a 99% confidence interval between 24.82 and 25.04 hours. The mean of the autonomous periods differs significantly from the period of the earth's rotation (24.00 hours; $p \ll 0.001$) as well as from the period of the apparent revolution of the moon (24.83 hr; $p < 0.001$). Applying nonparametric analyses, the median of the period likewise differs from the two environmental periods mentioned which are not covered by the confidence intervals.

If, instead of the mean rectal temperature periods from all experiments, only those periods that stem from experiments with internal desynchronization are averaged, the picture is somewhat different. It was shown in figure 29 that both types of real internal desynchronization, with activity periods being either much longer or much shorter than the rectal temperature periods, result in identical values of the desynchronized rectal temperature periods. This is true in spite of the significant difference in the rectal tem-

perature periods in internally synchronized rhythms. If all 38 experiments with internal desynchronization are considered (26 experiments with temporarily desynchronized rhythms according to figure 29 and 12 experiments with internal desynchronization during the total experiment) the mean period ($\pm$ standard deviation) is 24.88 $\pm$ 0.19 hours. The equality between the mean and the median of this distribution of 38 periods (24.87 hours) indicates a symmetric distribution. This distribution of only desynchronized rectal temperature periods is, in fact, much smaller than for all rectal temperature periods. The mean of this distribution likewise deviates significantly from the period of the earth's rotation ($p \ll 0.001$) but not from the period of the apparent revolution of the moon. Only after discussing the mode of synchronization by external zeitgebers (cf. 3.5.), can it be decided if this coincidence in the periods is due to a general external synchronization of internally desynchronized rectal temperature rhythms to the lunar rhythm or if it is only accidental.

The lower part of figure 37 presents the histogram of the activity rhythms of all subjects who were tested under constant conditions. It would be meaningless here to give periods averaged over a total experiment because of the drastic change in the period that could occur during an experiment due to internal desynchronization (Figs. 27, 28, 32, 33, and 36). It is appropriate, therefore, to compute periods of the activity rhythms for sections of each experiment in a manner where a section (lasting for about 8 to 12 days) never includes a drastic change in the activity period. The histogram includes periods of 377 sections originating from all 147 experiments. Each of the periods is averaged over one section, independent of the experimental conditions. Because the covered range of periods is much larger than with the rectal temperature periods, the classes of periods are broader than in the histogram of the rectal temperature periods. The abscissa scale is compressed for clarity.

As can be seen immediately, the distribution of the activity periods deviates greatly from the rectal temperature periods. It shows a multimodal distribution with clearly separated peaks. It only is meaningful here to compute, for statistical purposes, the median instead of the mean of the periods. Using this method, we obtain a result of 25.19 hours, with a 95% confidence interval between 25.11 and 25.26 hours (or a 99% confidence interval between 25.08 and 25.29 hours). For descriptive comparison only, the formally computed normal distribution is plotted in the histogram based on a mean of 26.04 hours and a range of standard deviations between 21.37 and 31.74 hours (the parameters are computed from the logarithms of the period values). The periods of the autonomously running activity rhythms are, on the average, significantly longer than those of the rectal temperature rhythms and they likewise differ significantly from the two environmental periods mentioned. From the different peaks in the distribution of the activity periods, the main peak represents internally synchronized rhythms, while other peaks originate from internally desynchronized rhythms. The two broad peaks adjoining the main peak (15 to 20 hours and 30 to 40 hours) correspond to rhythms with real internal desynchronization. The next small peaks (around 12.5 and 50 hours) correspond to rhythms with apparent internal desynchronization with internal 2:1 and 1:2 synchronization while one pe-

riod, with 65 hours, again corresponds to real internal desynchronization. All these different states of the rhythms are separated from each other with regard to their periods and there are no continuous transitions between these states.

After summarizing the periods, the next step will be the discrimination of the periods with regard to personality data. This discrimination, however, is meaningful only after it has been guaranteed that the differences in the periods, included in the histograms, primarily are due to interindividual and not to intraindividual variations. The difference between inter- and intraindividual variability can be tested in subjects who repeated isolation experiments under equivalent conditions. Of the 21 subjects who participated in more than one experiment, nine have performed two single experiments under constant conditions successively under identical experimental conditions (at least during relevant parts of the experiments). The other subjects participated at one time in single experiments, at another time in group experiments (Fig. 50), and in experiments with heteronomous rhythms (for an example, the results presented in figures 79 and 86 originate from the same subject). The results of the experiments referred to here are summarized in table 2.

Table 2 indicates that experimental condi-

Table 2. *Experiments with Autonomous Rhythms as Repeated under Equivalent Conditions*

Subject	Experimental condition		Interval between the experiments (months)	Autonomous period		
	Illumination	Shielding		1st experiment	2nd experiment	Difference
H.R., ♂ 67/69 y	constant	yes	15	25.3 hr	25.0 hr	−0.3 hr
B.D., ♀ 22/24 y	constant	yes	33	25.0	25.2	+0.2
H.Z., ♂ 24/25 y	constant	yes	5	24.9	24.6	−0.3
K.D., ♂ 25/26 y	constant	yes	13	25.7	25.6	−0.1
W.N., ♂ 29/30 y	constant	yes	12	24.9	24.8	−0.1
J.S., ♂ 29/31 y	constant	yes	23	24.5	24.7	+0.2
H.H., ♂ 27/31 y	constant	yes	50	24.9	25.1	+0.2
D.M., ♀ 28/28 y	self-control	no	2	24.9	25.2	+0.3
H.S., ♀ 61/62 y	self-control	yes	13	23.8	24.2	+0.4
			Mean	24.88 hr	24.93 hr	+0.05 hr
			Standard deviation	±0.52 hr	±0.41 hr	±0.26 hr

Statistical analysis concerning the difference in the standard deviations (F-test): 1st experiment versus difference in periods, $F = 4.00$; $p < 0.05$.

tions were not identical in all experiments. It shows that most of the subjects were exposed (coinciding in each experiment) to constant illumination instead of selfcontrolled illumination (cf. 2.4.2) and also most of the subjects were tested (again coinciding in each experiment) in the 'shielded' instead of the "nonshielded" experimental unit (cf. 2.4.4). Both of these experimental conditions have shown an influence on the autonomous period, and, therefore, may have an influence on the intraindividual variability. All referred experiments, furthermore, were performed with selfcontrolled ambient temperature, instead of a constant temperature (cf. 2.4.3), and without an artificial electromagnetic field (cf. 2.4.5.). Both of these conditions likewise have been shown to influence the autonomous periods. Table 2 also indicates the autonomous periods (of internally synchronized rhythms only) resulting from the experiments. It shows that the individual periods coincide in the mean and also the standard deviation (which represents the interindividual variability) with results of the much greater sample of all experiments with autonomously running rhythms (Fig. 37; upper part). Both samples, therefore, can be assumed to originate from the same basic sample (the results of table 2, which also are included in figure 37, constitute only a negligible part of the total sample). Additionally, table 2 shows the differences in periods between successive experiments. The mean indicates that there is no systematic trend. The standard deviation, which represents the intraindividual variability, is only half as large as the interindividual standard deviation of the autonomous periods of the first experiment. In the statistical analysis, the standard deviations of the individual experiments, and those of the differences between successive experiments with the same subject differ significantly. This indicates that inter- and intraindividual variability do not originate from the same basic sample.

In detail, it can be concluded, from table 2, that subjects showing periods deviating especially far from the mean, in subsequent experiments show periods closer to the mean. Even in those subjects, the differences in period are not greater than in subjects with periods very close to the mean in the first experiment. As an example, figure 38 presents results originating from two successive experiments of the subject, whose periods deviate farthest from the mean. The two experiments have been performed at an interval of 1 year under identical experimental conditions; expressly to examine if the remarkably short period of the first experiment was accidental or due to an individual characteristic. In the second experiment, the subject again showed a remarkably short period, with internal desynchronization during the last week (according to the short period during the first three weeks, with a drastically shortened activity period (Fig. 29)). Moreover, it can be concluded from table 2 that the difference in the periods between successive experiments does not depend on the interval between the experiments. The result to be derived from table 2, in general, proves that the differences between autonomous periods, obtained in the multiplicity of experiments performed under constant conditions, in fact, primarily are due to interindividual variability and only to a small degree to intraindividual variability. This result, therefore, justifies the discrimination of the periods included in figure 37, regarding personality data.

In the first step, the rectal temperature periods will be discriminated regarding sex and age of the subjects. Of the 159 subjects with autonomously running rhythms, 44 females (28% of the subjects) showed a mean period (± standard deviation) of 24.94 ± 0.56 hours and the 115 males (72% of the subjects) showed a mean period of 25.04 ± 0.45 hours. These data show that there is a weak tendency for shorter autonomous periods in females; however, this is far from statistical significance. Figure 39 shows, likewise, the age of the subjects is without influence on the period of autonomous rhythms. The (nonparametrical) coefficient of correlation getween period and age cannot be differentiated at any level of significance, from zero. On the average, the male

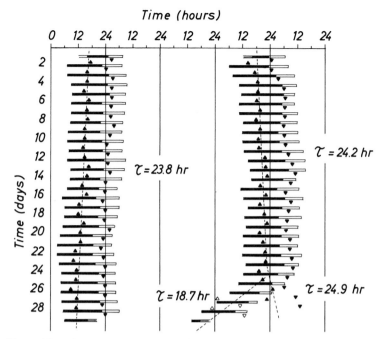

Figure 38.   Autonomous rhythms of one subject (H.S., ♀ 61y, and 62 y resp.), living under constant conditions without time cues, originating from two identical experiments performed with an interval of 1 year. Temporal courses of the rhythms of activity and rectal temperature, presented successively one period beneath the other. Indications are the same as in figure 27/I.

subjects (median age: 25.4 years old) were a little older than the female subjects (median age: 24.2 years old). Even when computed separately for the two sexes, no correlation between period and age can be found. It, therefore, can be stated, in summary, that the period of autonomously running human circadian rectal temperature rhythms does not depend on the sex or on the age of the subjects. The same result is true when only the periods of separated rectal temperature rhythms are considered (i.e., after exclusion of the interaction with activity rhythms during the state of internal desynchronization). The mean period ($\pm$ standard deviation) of the 12 females is 24.93 ± 0.17 hours and for the 26 males it is 24.87 ± 0.20 hours. The coefficient of rank correlation, between autonomous period and age, is $R = 0.01$. These figures show that the period of autonomous rectal temperature rhythms is independent of the sex and age of the subjects in

both the synchronized and desynchronized rhythm. Likewise, with other personality data, no correlations to the autonomous rectal temperature period could be found. These results are different from animal experiments where the dependency of the free running period on age was evaluated. In experiments performed with three species of rodents (Pittendrigh and Daan, 1974), the period became shorter with increasing age.

Regarding autonomous activity periods, a similar discrimination seems to be less meaningful. The reason is the occurrence of internal desynchronization in some subjects which broadened the distribution of activity periods drastically (Fig. 37). The consideration of subjects, whose rhythms stood internally synchronized (main peak in the lower histogram of figure 37), is useless since the rhythms of those subjects already were included in the consideration of rectal temperature periods. There are subjects remaining

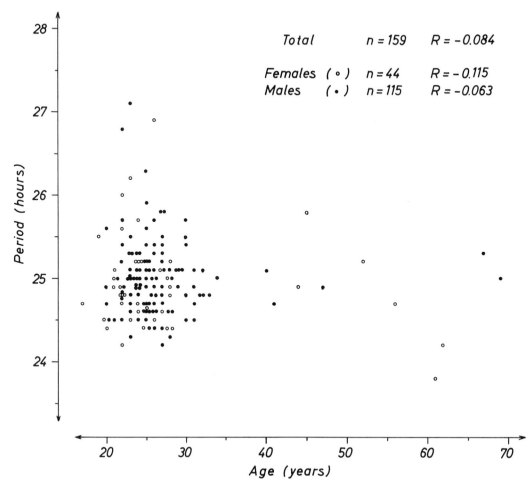

Figure 39. Autonomous rectal temperature periods of all subjects, plotted as a function of the age of the subjects (i.e., abscissa) and separated by male and female subjects. The coefficients of rank correlation (Spearman) are indicated for all subjects and separated by sex.

with internally desynchronized rhythms. Internal desynchronization with shortened activity rhythms (Fig. 28) seems to be forced by the same characteristics as internal desynchronization with lengthened activity rhythms (Fig. 27). Considering the activity periods collectively, the variability of the periods, therefore, can be expected to depend on personality data rather than the mean of the periods. In order to give a more obvious review, it seems appropriate to compare the tendency toward internal desynchronization with personality data. In the preceding chapter, the different modes of internal desynchronization and dissociation have been discussed. The frequency in

the occurrance of these different modes will be considered here depending on personality data. In order to review properly, table 3 summarizes the number of cases of the different modes observed, so far, in a sample of 151 subjects with autonomous rhythms (for each mode, it is indicated in parenthesis what figure represents an example of that specific mode). Table 3, in addition, includes a subdivision of the numbers with regard to the sex of the subjects.

Table 3 shows, for instance, that the occurrence of real internal desynchronization is more probable than of apparent internal desynchronization. It shows that in both modes, moreover, a change of the activity

Table 3.   *Frequency of Internal Rhythm Disorders*

	$\tau_{act} < \tau_{temp}$	$\tau_{act} > \tau_{temp}$	Females	Males	Totals
Number of Subjects			44 (= 100%)	115 (=100%)	159 (=100%)
Real internal desynchronization	13 (Fig. 28)	25 (Figs. 27,30)	12 (= 27%)	26 (= 23%)	38 (= 24%)
Apparent internal desynchronization	1 (Fig. 33)	11 (Fig. 32)	3 (= 7%)	9 (= 8%)	12 (= 8%)
Internal dissociation	5 (Fig. 35, right)	23 (Fig. 35, left)	7 (= 16%)	21 (= 18%)	28 (= 18%)
Initial dissociation	7 (Fig. 34, right)	[140 (Fig. 34, left)]	5	2	7

period to a lengthening one is more probable than a change to a shortening one. The same is true with internal dissociation. In all modes in table 3, except initial dissociation with an activity period which is temporarily longer than the rectal temperature period, the physiological time and the psychological time, as defined above, do not coincide during the total experiment. They differ from each other at the end of the experiment by at least 1 day. In cases of initial dissociation, as already mentioned, the mutual phase shift between different overt rhythms is, on the average, less than 90°. In all other cases, it is close to, or more than, 360°. There are, in total, 85 cases originating from 72 subjects (in 13 subjects, two different modes of internal desynchronization or dissociation occurred successively) where this discrepancy between the different courses of subjective time occurred. In other words, there are only 79 out of the 151 subjects, or 52% of the subjects, with autonomously running rhythms where the number of activity cycles during the total experiment equals the number of rectal temperature cycles. This means that in only about half of the subjects, autonomous circadian rhythms take a "normal," undisturbed course.

With regard to the sex of the subjects, table 3 shows the occurrence of internal desynchronization and dissociation is independent of the sex. With real, as well as apparent, internal desynchronization and, likewise, internal dissociation, the percentage of female and male subjects showing this type of internal rhythm disorder are nearly identical. This is true as long as the direction

of the mutual separation of the two rhythms (activity and rectal temperature) is not considered. If, however, these directions are considered separately, there is a significant influence concerning the sex of the subjects. Of the 27 female subjects who showed a rhythm disorder of a mode mentioned, with the result that they had different numbers of cycles in the overt rhythms of activity and rectal temperature during the experiment, 14 (52%) showed an activity period shorter than the rectal temperature period. Of the 58 male subjects with the same rhythm disorders, 15 (26%) showed an activity period shorter than the rectal temperature period (i.e., only half the percentage of the females). This means that, if internal desynchronization or dissociation occurs at all, these states are characterized, in females, primarily by overt activity rhythms being faster than the overt rectal temperature rhythms; in males, rather, by opposite separations (i.e., by overt activity rhythms being slower than the overt rectal temperature rhythms). The statistical probability for this difference, and even more improbable distributions, being due to chance variation is p = 0.0002 (exact Fisher-test). A subdivision in the different types of internal desynchronization and dissociation confirms this statement with regard to each single mode but, due to the lower numbers of subjects showing each single mode, not to sufficient levels of significance. Of the 12 female subjects showing real internal desynchronization, for instance, 6 (50%) had a drastically shortened activity period and of the 26 male subjects showing real internal desynchronization, only 7 (27%) had.

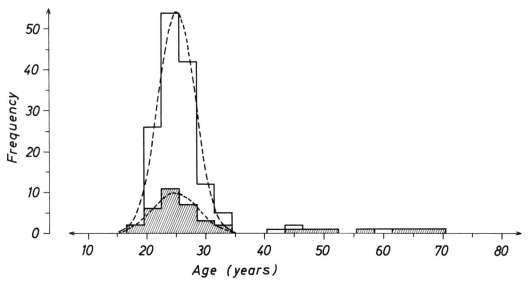

Figure 40.   Distribution of the ages of all subjects showing autonomous rhythms (open areas) and those showing real internal desynchronization (shaded areas). Dotted lines: normal distributions computed from the group of younger subjects (17 to 34 years old).

In order to determine the dependency of the tendency toward real internal desynchronization on the age of the subjects, figure 40 presents distribution of the ages of the subjects; all subjects with autonomously running rhythms, and subjects who showed real internal desynchronization. Figure 40 shows that the subjects can be subdivided into two groups, including younger subjects (between 17 and 34 years old) and older subjects. The distribution of the ages of the younger subjects nearly follows a normal distribution with 25.1 ± 3.1 years. 31 of the 141 younger subjects (22%) showed real internal desynchronization and the age distribution of these subjects again nearly follows a normal distribution with the similar parameters of 24.9 ± 3.8 years. This means that the tendency toward internal desynchronization does not depend on the age of the subjects within the younger group. This result is also true when both sexes are considered separately. Of the 35 females within this group with a mean age of 23.7 ± 2.9 years, 8 (23%), with a mean age of 23.8 ± 4.2 years, showed real internal desynchronization. Of the 106 males with a mean age of 25.6 ± 3.0 years old, 23 (22%), with a mean age of 25.4 ± 3.4 years, showed real internal desynchronization. Finally, a subdivision in both directions of internal desynchronization does not result in any detectable dependency on the age of the subjects.

There are, beside the group of the younger subjects discussed, the older subjects. Of the 10 older subjects, 7 (70%) showed real internal desynchronization. Of the three remaining older subjects who did not show internal desynchronization, one showed this state in a second experiment under equivalent conditions (Fig. 38) and another subject remained during the greatest part of the experiment, even externally synchronized (Fig. 21). In comparing the frequency in the occurrence of real internal desynchronization within the large group of the younger subjects (22%) and within the small group of older subjects (70%), this difference is far from an accidental probability ($p = 0.0026$; exact Fisher-test). Considering the wide range of ages, the tendency toward internal desynchronization depends significantly on the age of the subjects, although it is independent of age with only the younger subjects. A reasonable disentanglement of this apparent contradiction is the assumption of a threshold age (anywhere between 35 and 45 years old). The dependency of the tendency toward internal desynchronization on the age of the subjects is then not continuous but discontinuous, with a low tendency below and a high tendency above the threshold age. (After the manuscript was completed, there was a chance to test a 73-year-old female in an experiment under constant conditions. In the context discussed here, the primary result was the spontaneous occurrence of real internal desynchronization on the 5th day of the experiment.)

Within the group of younger subjects, the tendency toward internal desynchronization was shown to be independent of the sex and the age of the subjects. It is not independent of other aspects of their personalities, however. Most of the subjects were tested psychologically before and after the experiment. In the first instance, there is no systematic trend, in any respect, during the experiment. Among the many items tested, there is only one item which correlates significantly with the physiological rhythm measurements (Lund, 1974b); the tendency for neuroticism, as evaluated independently with the E.N.N.R. test (Brengelmann and Brengelmann, 1960) and with the VELA test (Fahrenberg, 1965). Both tests correlated mutually regarding the scores of neuroticism, and correlate significantly with the tendency toward internal desynchronization (Lund, 1974b). Figure 41 shows the result of the respective evaluations. The scores are significantly higher in subjects with internally desynchronized rhythms than those with internally synchronized rhythms with respect to the E.N.N.R. test ($p < 0.005$) and the VELA test ($p < 0.05$). This means that subjects with high scores of neuroticism tend to desynchronize internally rather than subjects with low scores. This correlation was tested only within the group of younger subjects (Fig. 40). Within the other group, the number of subjects is too small to make any significant statements. Of the ten older subjects, only one showed high scores of neuroticism in the tests. Most of them,

nevertheless, showed internal desynchronization. The high tendency toward internal desynchronization within this age group cannot be due to a general high tendency for neuroticism. It must be concluded, therefore, that age and neuroticism affect internal desynchronization independently of each other.

It was shown that in 52% of the subjects with autonomously running rhythms, the different rhythms measured had the same period for the whole experiment. The rhythms of these subjects can be described sufficiently under the assumption of only one circadian oscillator. The endogenous, as well as the oscillatory origin of the underlying mechanism, have been proven significantly (cf. 2.1.5). The rhythms of 16% of the

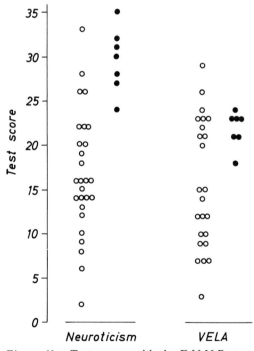

Figure 41. Test scores with the E.N.N.R. test (neuroticism; Brengelmann and Brengelmann, 1960) and VELA test (Fahrenberg, 1965), determined with subjects showing internally synchronized and desynchronized rhythms. From Lund (1974b).

subjects, who showed internal dissociation but not desynchronization, moreover, can be described under the same assumption. In these cases, the coupling between the oscillator and the different overt rhythms must be assumed to be variable. To be precise, the results of the experiments with internally synchronized rhythms, as mentioned, do not exclude the existence of more than one underlying oscillator. There are no conclusive reasons to reject the more simple hypothesis based on one oscillator only. Evidently, hypotheses based on more oscillators by no means are insufficient to describe such a system. The more complex multioscillator hypotheses, in those cases, do not have the capability to describe more details in the behavior of the circadian system than the more simple one oscillator hypothesis. Following this line of thought, some relevant features of the basic oscillator can be evaluated in experiments where the magnitude of the controlling environmental stimulus changes. As a consequence, different parameters of the autonomously running overt rhythms change their values systematically (cf. 4.1.1). Other features of the basic oscillator can be evaluated in experiments where the oscillator does not run autonomously but heteronomously (i.e., controlled by external zeitgebers of varying properties (cf. 4.1.2)). In the following, both of these courses will be followed in order to derive the basic features of the human circadian system.

Of the other subjects, at least those showing real internal desynchronization (24%) represent a circadian system that cannot be described sufficiently by the simple one oscillator hypothesis. The assumption of a multioscillator system is conclusive here. In cases where the assumption of a multioscillator hypothesis is indispensable, the features of each of the different basic oscillators can be shown to coincide with those of the single basic oscillator, as concluded from the experiments with internally synchronized rhythms mentioned earlier. The separate autonomy of the oscillators can be shown, in most experiments with internally desynchronized rhythms, by the total phase shifts

of the rhythm components against local time exceeding 12 hours (Figs. 25, 27, 30, and 36). Correspondingly, the computed 'spectral lines' are separated clearly from 24.0 hours. In all rhythm components, moreover, when considered separately, averaged periods (longitudinal) show phase angles of rectal temperature rhythms leading those of the activity rhythms, which is characteristic in autonomous rhythms. Phase angle differences between the overt rhythms cannot be determined meaningfully because they are not temporally constant. It cannot be evaluated directly whether or not the different basic processes of the multioscillator system are oscillatory or stochastic because the only competent test (i.e., the serial correlation test) cannot be applied directly. Following the multioscillator hypothesis, a separate consideration of isolated basic oscillators is impossible because each measurable overt rhythm is controlled collectively by all of the basic oscillators. The mechanism of the underlying processes, therefore, cannot be tested directly in a multioscillator system but only concluded indirectly. As long as the rhythms run internally synchronized, the oscillatory basis of the underlying processes can be proven by serial correlation tests. After separation of the rhythms in the internal desynchronization state, it is not likely that the underlying process alters from oscillatory to stochastic mechanisms.

In the great majority of experiments, the results of which suggest a multioscillatory system, the assumption of not more than two basic oscillators is sufficient. Among these cases, nearly all are included where internal desynchronization is present during only a limited section of an experiment, while the rhythms are synchronized internally during other sections. The analysis of those experiments is advantageous because they enable quantitative statements concerning the relative strengths of the different oscillators involved and, therefore, the mutual interaction between the different oscillators (cf. 4.2.3). These statements are based on the changes of the periods of the different rhythms in opposite directions when internal desynchronization occurs (Fig. 29). Other features of the interaction between different oscillators can be evaluated when, by applying corresponding zeitgebers, the oscillators become synchronized externally and separately. In the following, experiments under constant conditions and zeitgeber conditions will be considered in order to conclude the special properties of the multioscillatory origin of the circadian system.

There remain some subjects, nearly all of whom show internal desynchronization during the total experiment, whose rhythms demonstrate the cooperation of more than two oscillators in the circadian system. In single cases, possibly three (Fig. 25) or even four different oscillators (Fig. 30), which can be separated from each other, may be present. The presence of internal desynchronization during a total experiment, under conditions where other subjects do not show internal desynchronization or only during limited sections of an experiment, demonstrates a higher tendency toward internal desynchronization in these subjects. It must be concluded, therefore, that the number of basic oscillators that can be separated from each other within the circadian system, is greater the higher the tendency toward internal desynchronization becomes. It is only with regard to the very few subjects demonstrating the interaction between more than two oscillators that the two oscillator hypothesis must be extended to a multioscillator hypothesis.

The multioscillator hypothesis, though its assumption is conclusive only in a minority of subjects, is more general than the one oscillator hypothesis. It is suggested, therefore, the reader accept a multioscillator system in all subjects. Following this concept, it must be concluded that in the majority of subjects, the different oscillators run synchronously to each other so that they function outwardly as only one oscillator. Only in cases of internal desynchronization, the different oscillators become separated so that they appear obviously. In any case, it seems to be more general to describe the circadian systems of all subjects with a uni-form hypothesis rather than with different hypotheses alternating with each other. This uniform hypothesis can be only the multioscillator hypothesis.

2.4. External Modifications of Autonomous Rhythms

In the previous chapters, experiments have been discussed in detail only when the experimental conditions remained unchanged. These experiments disregard external stimuli influencing circadian rhythms. Under natural conditions, however, circadian rhythms, including human rhythms, are modified continuously by environmental stimuli. This external influence normally is manifested by a synchronization to external periodicities. This influence also can be manifested by modifications of autonomous rhythms due to changes in continuously operating external stimuli. These external modifications of autonomously running rhythms will be discussed below.

2.4.1. Influence of Light Intensity

In most animal experiments, light is the most effective external stimulus. This cannot be proven only by a synchronizing effect of light-dark cycles but also by modifying influences of the intensity of illumination on autonomous rhythms. This means that in most animals, the period and many additional parameters of these rhythms are influenced regularly by the intensity of illumination under which the circadian rhythms run autonomously. These experiments are performed in a manner where a certain light intensity is held constant for several weeks and then altered to another intensity for several other weeks.

Also, in the present investigations of human circadian rhythms, influences of the intensity of illumination have been examined (Wever, 1969a). Figure 42 shows the course of a pertinent experiment. The subject lived, during the first 10 days, under a constant

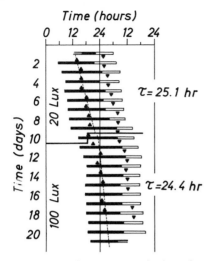

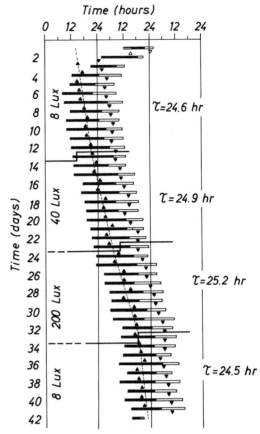

Figure 42. Autonomous rhythm of a subject (B.K., ♀ 24 y) living under constant conditions without time cues, with one alteration in the intensity of illumination. Temporal courses of the rhythms of activity and rectal temperature are presented successively, one period beneath the other. Indications are the same as in figure 16/I. From Wever (1969a).

light intensity of 22 lux. During the second 10 day section, the subject lived under a light intensity which likewise was constant but five times greater. The period of the autonomous circadian rhythm was obviously shorter during the second section, indicating an effect of the intensity of illumination on the autonomous period. If longitudinal statistics are applied, in spite of their inadmissibility because of the serial dependency, the change in the period would be guaranteed significantly. The correlation between light intensity and autonomous periods, as derived from Figure 42, is not the rule in all corresponding experiments, however. Figure 43 shows the course of another experiment, likewise performed with a young female subject in the same experimental room as the other experiment, but a few weeks later. At the beginning, internal dissociation can be observed, as discussed in Figure 34 (right). In the further course of the experiment, light intensity increased two times in 10-day intervals, as in the other experiment.

Figure 43. Autonomous rhythm of a subject (A.E., ♀ 22 y) living under constant conditions without time cues, with three alterations in the intensity of illumination. Temporal courses of the rhythms of activity and rectal temperature are presented successively, one period beneath the other. Indications are the same as in figure 27/I. From Wever (1969a).

Again, each change in the intensity of illumination is accompanied by a change in the autonomous period but with a correlation opposite to the other experiment. Each increase in the light intensity causes a lengthening in the period. At the end of the experiment, the intensity of illumination was decreased to the original value and the period likewise shortened to nearly the original value, indicating the reliability of the correlation between light intensity and period in this subject. Again, formally applied longitudinal statistics would guarantee the significance of the alteration in the period. Figure desynchronization occurs (Fig. 29). Other features of the interaction between different oscillators can be evaluated when, by applying corresponding zeitgebers, the oscillators become synchronized externally and separately. In the following, experiments under constant conditions and zeitgeber conditions will be considered in order to conclude the special properties of the multioscillatory origin of the circadian system.

There remain some subjects, nearly all of whom show internal desynchronization during the total experiment, whose rhythms demonstrate the cooperation of more than two oscillators in the circadian system. In single cases, possibly three (Fig. 25) or even four different oscillators (Fig. 30), which can be separated from each other, may be present. The presence of internal desynchronization during a total experiment, under conditions where other subjects do not show internal desynchronization or only during limited sections of an experiment, demonstrates a higher tendency toward internal desynchronization in these subjects. It must be concluded, therefore, that the number of basic oscillators that can be separated from each other within the circadian system, is greater the higher the tendency toward internal desynchronization becomes. It is only with regard to the very few subjects demonstrating the interaction between more than two oscillators that the two oscillator hypothesis must be extended to a multioscillator hypothesis.

The multioscillator hypothesis, though its assumption is conclusive only in a minority of subjects, is more general than the one oscillator hypothesis. It is suggested, therefore, the reader accept a multioscillator system in all subjects. Following this concept, it must be concluded that in the majority of subjects, the different oscillators run synchronously to each other so that they function outwardly as only one oscillator. Only in cases of internal desynchronization, the different oscillators become separated so that they appear obviously. In any case, it seems to be more general to describe the circadian systems of all subjects with a uni-

form hypothesis rather than with different hypotheses alternating with each other. This uniform hypothesis can be only the multioscillator hypothesis.

2.4. External Modifications of Autonomous Rhythms

In the previous chapters, experiments have been discussed in detail only when the experimental conditions remained unchanged. These experiments disregard external stimuli influencing circadian rhythms. Under natural conditions, however, circadian rhythms, including human rhythms, are modified continuously by environmental stimuli. This external influence normally is manifested by a synchronization to external periodicities. This influence also can be manifested by modifications of autonomous rhythms due to changes in continuously operating external stimuli. These external modifications of autonomously running rhythms will be discussed below.

2.4.1. Influence of Light Intensity

In most animal experiments, light is the most effective external stimulus. This cannot be proven only by a synchronizing effect of light-dark cycles but also by modifying influences of the intensity of illumination on autonomous rhythms. This means that in most animals, the period and many additional parameters of these rhythms are influenced regularly by the intensity of illumination under which the circadian rhythms run autonomously. These experiments are performed in a manner where a certain light intensity is held constant for several weeks and then altered to another intensity for several other weeks.

Also, in the present investigations of human circadian rhythms, influences of the intensity of illumination have been examined (Wever, 1969a). Figure 42 shows the course of a pertinent experiment. The subject lived, during the first 10 days, under a constant

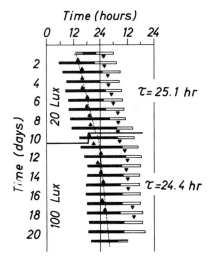

Figure 42. Autonomous rhythm of a subject (B.K., ♀ 24 y) living under constant conditions without time cues, with one alteration in the intensity of illumination. Temporal courses of the rhythms of activity and rectal temperature are presented successively, one period beneath the other. Indications are the same as in figure 16/I. From Wever (1969a).

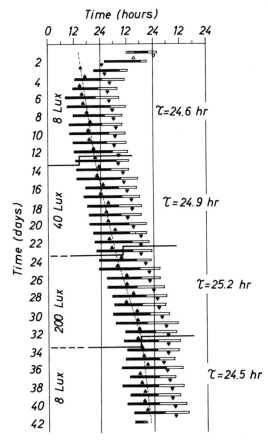

Figure 43. Autonomous rhythm of a subject (A.E., ♀ 22 y) living under constant conditions without time cues, with three alterations in the intensity of illumination. Temporal courses of the rhythms of activity and rectal temperature are presented successively, one period beneath the other. Indications are the same as in figure 27/I. From Wever (1969a).

light intensity of 22 lux. During the second 10 day section, the subject lived under a light intensity which likewise was constant but five times greater. The period of the autonomous circadian rhythm was obviously shorter during the second section, indicating an effect of the intensity of illumination on the autonomous period. If longitudinal statistics are applied, in spite of their inadmissibility because of the serial dependency, the change in the period would be guaranteed significantly. The correlation between light intensity and autonomous periods, as derived from Figure 42, is not the rule in all corresponding experiments, however. Figure 43 shows the course of another experiment, likewise performed with a young female subject in the same experimental room as the other experiment, but a few weeks later. At the beginning, internal dissociation can be observed, as discussed in Figure 34 (right). In the further course of the experiment, light intensity increased two times in 10-day intervals, as in the other experiment.

Again, each change in the intensity of illumination is accompanied by a change in the autonomous period but with a correlation opposite to the other experiment. Each increase in the light intensity causes a lengthening in the period. At the end of the experiment, the intensity of illumination was decreased to the original value and the period likewise shortened to nearly the original value, indicating the reliability of the correlation between light intensity and period in this subject. Again, formally applied longitudinal statistics would guarantee the significance of the alteration in the period. Figure

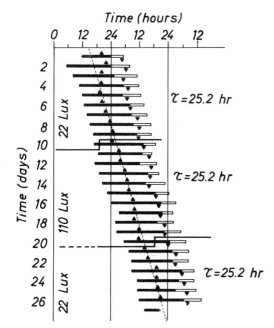

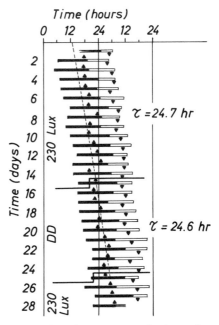

Figure 44. Autonomous rhythm of a subject (W.S., ♂ 25 y) living under constant conditions without time cues, with two alterations in the intensity of illumination. Temporal courses of the rhythms of activity and rectal temperature are presented successively, one period beneath the other. Indications are the same as in figure 16/I. From Wever (1969a).

Figure 45. Autonomous rhythm of a subject (A.A., ♂ 23 y) living under constant conditions without time cues, with two alterations in the intensity of illumination (DD = total darkness). Temporal courses of the rhythms of activity and rectal temperature are presented successively, one period beneath the other. Indications are the same as in figure 16/I. From Wever (1973e).

44 shows the course of a third experiment in this series with an increase of light intensity after 10 days and a corresponding decrease after another 10 days. In this experiment, the period remained unchanged during the experiment, in spite of the alteration in the light intensity for equal amounts as in the other experiments. This indicates independence between the autonomous period and light intensity in this subject.

It is the result of many experiments with alterations in the intensity of illumination, as shown in the three characteristic examples in figures 42 through 44, that alterations in the intensity of illumination are accompanied mostly by alterations in the autonomous period, but there is no reliable correlation between light intensity and period. It cannot be excluded from these results that a regular correlation, which is small in amount

only, is superimposed by random fluctuations and, therefore, is undetectable. Toward high light intensities, there is a limit (for technical reasons) at about 1500 lux. Toward low light intensities, however, there is no limit. Additional experiments, therefore, have been performed with decreases of the light intensity down to total darkness (Wever, 1973e). Figure 45 shows the course of such an experiment in which a subject lived initially for 2 weeks in constant bright light and afterwards for 2 weeks in total darkness. During the first part of the experiment, the subject had to learn all manipulations necessary for his subsistence and he dictated some scientific papers, which he wanted to study carefully, on magnetic tape. During the second part, during which he felt remarkably well, the subject was able to support himself perfectly (e.g., he was able

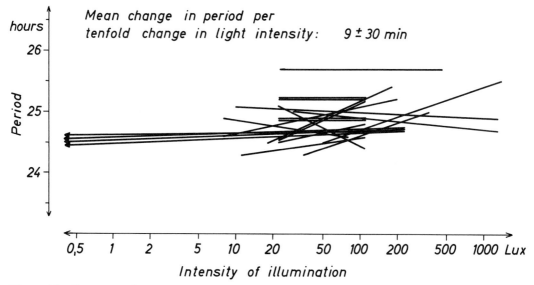

Figure 46.   Summary of all experiments with autonomous rhythms including at least one alteration in the intensity of illumination. Periods (i.e., ordinate) are plotted as a function of the intensity of illumination (i.e., abscissa). The lines combine results from different sections in individual experiments. Mean and standard deviation of the individual regressions are indicated. From Wever (1973e).

to prepare hot meals). As a result of this experiment, there was nearly no change in the period of the autonomous rhythm with the transition to total darkness. All other measurable rhythm parameters, likewise, remained unchanged. The same result has been obtained in the other three experiments with total darkness for about 2 weeks.

A summary of the results of all 20 experiments, testing the influence of light intensity on the autonomous period, is given in figure 46. The results originate from all experiments in which the intensity of illumination was changed at least once but remaining constant for intervals of at least 10 days (Figs. 42 through 45). As can be seen from this figure, the correlation between light intensity and the autonomous period is positive in some experiments, negative in others, and zero in a third group. The small positive regression, shown by the mean of all data, does not differ from zero in the statistical analysis. However, in most of the experiments the period changes with changing light intensity significantly, and in particular, it changes at the day when light intensity changes. It is, therefore, the general result

that changes in the free running period, as a consequence of changes in the intensity of illumination, are likely to occur, but the correlations between the two changing parameters are randomly distributed between positive and negative values. Every hypothesis describing the influence of light on human circadian rhythms must consider this obvious but bivalent correlation.

One possible hypothesis that could explain the apparently irregular correlation between light intensity and autonomous period, and has been discussed in the past (Lohmann, 1967), can be rejected directly from the results mentioned. This hypothesis states that the correlation (whether positive or negative) between changes in the intensity of illumination and autonomous period depends on the phase of the rhythm where the light intensity had been changed. As can be seen from figures 42 through 45, the light intensity was changed at almost the same phase of the activity rhythm in all experiments (i.e., about 3 to 6 hours after an activity onset). In contrast to the hypothesis, nevertheless, correlations between changes in light intensity and autonomous period,

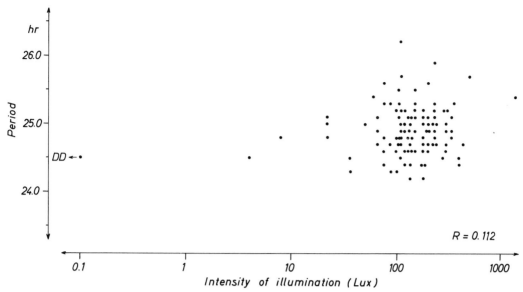

Figure 47. Summary of all experiments with autonomous rhythms, with an intensity of illumination remaining constant during the total experiment. Periods (i.e., ordinate) plotted as a function of the intensity of illumination (i.e., abscissa). The coefficient of rank correlation (Spearman) is indicated.

with both positive and negative signs, were observed.

In the greater portion of all experiments with autonomous circadian rhythm, light intensity was held constant during the total experiment. The results of those experiments, nevertheless, can be used to test the correlation between light intensity and autonomous period (Wever, 1969a, 1973e). In figure 47, the periods of the rectal temperature rhythms, obtained in 102 experiments with unchanged light intensity, are plotted against light intensity. As can be seen, only a very few points do not fit to a pure random distribution. Including all measured points, a nonparametric test of the correlation (Spearman) has to be applied. The calculation ($R = 0.112$) shows that the correlation is positive but to such a small amount that it cannot be differentiated statistically from zero, in spite of the large number of experiments included. The result of this evaluation agrees with that obtained from experiments in which the intensity of illumination had been changed at least once. This means, in summary of experiments with constant illumination, there is a weak tendency to lengthen the period of

autonomous rhythms with increasing light intensity. This tendency, however, can not be guaranteed statistically in a large number of experiments.

Apart from period length of autonomous rhythms, the tendency toward internal desynchronization (cf. 2.2.1) has been tested with regard to its dependency on the intensity of illumination. Of 105 single experiments which were performed with constant illumination, 24 (23%) showed real internal desynchronization. The light intensities in all of these experiments ranged from total darkness to 1500 Lux. In those experiments where internal desynchronization occurred, they ranged from 23 to 1500 Lux. In figure 48, a histogram of light intensities is presented. It includes the light intensities of all experiments (from experiments with more than one constant light intensity successively, each section is given separately) and shows, in a dashed subhistogram, the light intensities of those experiments (or sections) where internal desynchronization occurred. The small difference between the two median values statistically is not significant. This means that in experiments with con-

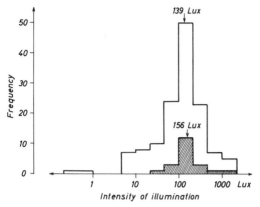

Figure 48.   Distribution of light intensities from all experiments with constant illumination (open area). From experiments with different light intensities given successively, the different sections are included separately. Hatched area: distribution of light intensities from all experiments, or sections, where real internal desynchronization occurred. The medians of the respective light intensities are indicated.

stant illumination the tendency toward internal desynchronization increases with increasing light intensity but only to such a small amount that it cannot be differentiated from zero in the statistical analysis.

In addition to the intensity of illumination, the types of illumination must be tested regarding their capacity to influence circadian rhythms (Wurtman, 1975). In most of the experiments, the experimental units were illuminated by incandescent bulbs. Only in a few experiments, especially in those using high light intensities, the illumination was based on fluorescent tubes. With both types, the light intensity could be varied continuously to zero, with all lamps in operation, by continuous changes in the mean voltage (in case of bulbs, a control transformer was used; and in case of tubes, a phase gating device was used). Depending on the intensity, the color of illumination varied considerably for incandescent bulbs but only a small amount for the fluorescent tubes.

In three experiments, the illumination had been changed from fluorescent tubes (1400 lux each) to incandescent bulbs (10, 20, and 50 lux, respectively). The results of these experiment are included in figure 46. In these experiments, the change in light intensity was combined with a drastic change in the kind of the illumination. All other experiments included in figure 46 were performed with incandescent bulbs only. In all these experiments, the change in light intensity is combined with a change in the color of the illumination. Nevertheless, there is no systematic difference, regarding the period, between experiments alternating between different types of lamps and experiments with the same type of lamps (more experiments with changing light intensity of only fluorescent tubes were performed with selfcontrolled illumination (cf. 2.4.2)). In one other experiment, an intensity of 1400 lux (fluorescent tubes) was kept constant during the total experiment. The result, which is included in figure 47, again does not deviate obviously from the results obtained with incandescent bulbs. It can be concluded, therefore, that the type of lamps constituting the illumination influences autonomously running rhythms as insignificantly as the intensity of illumination.

In summary, the result of the experiments discussed in this chapter shows light intensity significantly does not influence parameters of autonomously running circadian rhythms of man. This is true regarding the period, as well as the tendency toward internal desynchronization, and also regarding light intensities to total darkness. If the periods of the five subjects who were exposed to total darkness, at least during parts of the experiment (Figures 45, 46, and 47), are considered separately, an effect of light might be stated. They showed, during total darkness, a mean period ($\pm$ standard deviation) of 24.48 ± 0.08 hours and this mean is significantly shorter than the mean of all experiments (25.00 ± 0.50 hours; $t = 2.54$, $p < 0.01$). To be sure, the subjects who were exposed to total darkness only temporarily also showed autonomous periods shorter than the average during sections with bright light (Figure 46). Consequently, it must be considered that those subjects, who volunteer for experiments in total darkness, possibly have autonomous periods shorter than the average, independent of the actual intensity of illumination. In other words, the shortness of the periods measured in some subjects during total darkness necessarily must not be due to the absence of light; it likewise may be due to special personality data of those subjects who volunteer for this type of unusual experiment. Only further experiments will permit a decision.

In order to complete the experiments with absence of light, an experimental series with six blind subjects was undertaken (Lund, 1974a). All these subjects showed, under constant conditions without environmental time cues, clear autonomous rhythms (Fig. 98). The mean rectal temperature period ($\pm$ standard deviation) was 24.50 ± 0.42 hours. This period is significantly shorter than the mean rectal temperature period of the 147 sighted subjects (25.00 ± 0.50 hours; $t = 2.41$, $p < 0.01$). This mean period of the blind subjects coincides with the mean period of sighted subjects when living in total darkness (see above). If, instead of the rectal temperature rhythms, other vegetative rhythms of the blind subjects are taken for comparison, the difference to the sighted subjects is even greater. For instance, the autonomous rhythms of urinary cortisol excretion resulted in a mean period of 24.38 ± 0.31 hours. All autonomous rhythms measured in the blind subjects showed remarkably high reliabilities (e.g., mean reliability of rectal temperature rhythms ($82.2 \pm 7.9\%$) or mean reliability of cortisol rhythms: ($68.0 \pm 4.1\%$; Lund, 1974a)) indicating well marked autonomous rhythms. This result is of special interest since it was stated that blind subjects only have very poor circadian rhythms and, therefore, it was concluded that the perception of light is a relevant stimulus with respect to the persistence of human circadian rhythms (Hollwich and Dieckhues, 1971). Such an assumption clearly is disproven by the results mentioned. Possible reasons for the discrepancy will be discussed later (cf. 3.4).

The conclusion that parameters of autonomous rhythms do not depend on the intensity of constant illumination need not constitute a hypothesis that light is, with respect to human circadian rhythms, ineffective. From the effectiveness or ineffectiveness of a stimulus, when it is constant, it cannot be concluded to the effectiveness or ineffectiveness of the same stimulus when it is changing. In fact, there are various statements of several authors implying a clear effect of light on human circadian rhythms. These effects are, however, without exception, based on experiments performed under the influence of light-dark zeitgebers, but not under constant conditions, and, therefore, they do not contradict the results discussed in this chapter. The reports mentioned will be discussed in the context of heteronomous rhythms (cf. 3.4). Effects of changing light intensities on human circadian rhythms, conversely, can be deducted not only from heteronomous, but from autonomous rhythms as well, as will be discussed in the following.

2.4.2. Influence of Light Modality

In the experiments discussed so far, light was continuously in operation (i.e., with equal intensities during wakefulness and sleep of the subjects). On the contrary, in other experiments, the subjects were allowed to switch lights on and off at will. As a consequence, there was light during activity time and darkness during rest time. Such a light-dark cycle does not act as an entraining zeitgeber because it is itself controlled by the activity rhythm of the subject. The light-dark cycle, nevertheless, has an influence on the still free running or autonomous rhythm. Primarily, it lengthens the period (Wever, 1969a, 1973e). This can be seen in experiments where subjects lived under constant illumination during one section but under the influence of a self-controlled light-dark cycle during another section of the same experiment. An example of this type of experiment is presented in figure 49. As can be seen with the transition from constant to self-controlled illumination, the period lengthens

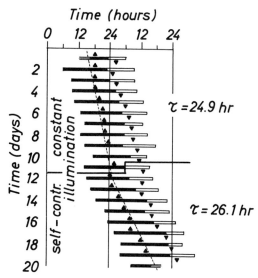

Figure 49. Autonomous rhythm of a subject (F.S., ♂ 23 y), without environmental time cues, living under constant illumination during the first section and self-controlled light-dark cycle (i.e., bright light during activity time; darkness during rest time) during the second section. Temporal courses of the rhythms of activity and rectal temperature are presented successively, one period beneath the other. Indications are the same as in figure 16/I. From Wever (1969a).

from 24.9 to 26.1 hours. A similar result has been obtained in another experiment (τ = 24.9 hours with constant, and τ = 25.5 hours with self-controlled illumination). In a third experiment of this type, internal desynchronization occurred immediately after the transition from constant to self-controlled illumination.

In order to evaluate statistically the influ-

ence of light modality, results of experiments performed under constant illumination must be compared with results of experiments with self-controlled illumination. This comparison is given in table 4. It includes all single experiments with autonomous rhythms, except the three experiments where the mode of illumination had been altered (Fig. 49). As can be seen from this table, there is a threefold effect of the mode of illumination on autonomous rhythms. Under constant illumination, the mean period is shorter, the interindividual variability of the periods around the mean is smaller, and the tendency toward internal desynchronization is smaller than under self-controlled illumination. All three differences are significant in the statistical analysis; the difference in the mean period, applying the parametric t-test as well as the nonparametric U-test. Light has been proven, consequently, to have a relevant effect on autonomous circadian rhythms of man when applied in a special mode and, therefore, the hypothesis that light is ineffective, with respect to human circadian rhythms, must be rejected.

The lengthening effect of self-controlled light conditions corresponds to similar results obtained in animal experiments (Aschoff et al., 1968). In those experiments, additionally, the correlation between light intensity and autonomous period was reversed as compared to the correlation evaluated under constant illumination. In human experiments also, the correlation between light intensity and the autonomous period

Table 4. *Effect of the Mode of Illumination*

Parameter	Single experiments with		Statistical analyses
	Constant illumination	Self-controlled illumination	
Number of subjects	103	29	
Mean period $\bar{\tau}$	24.91 hr	25.24 hr	$t = 3.10$ $p < 0.005$
Standard deviation of τ	± 0.41 hr	± 0.76 hr	$F = 3.08$ $p < 0.005$
Median of periods	24.84 hr	25.03 hr	$U/U' = 1927 / 1060$
95% confidence interval	24.78 to 24.97 hr	24.80 to 25.65 hr	$u = 2.39$ $p = 0.008$
Number of subjects with internal desynchronization	24 (= 23%)	13 (= 41%)	$p = 0.015$ (exact Fisher-test)

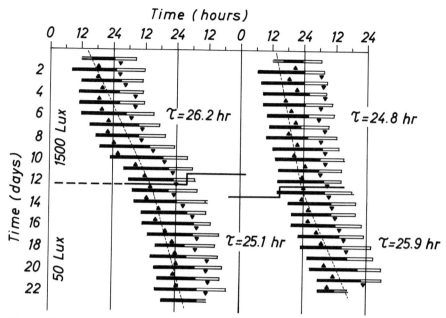

Figure 50. Autonomous rhythms of one subject (W.M., ♂ 27 y), in two different experiments, living without environmental time cues and under the influence of a self-controlled light-dark cycle (i.e., bright light during activity time; darkness during rest time), with one alteration in the intensity of illumination during the activity times in each experiment. In one experiment (left), the subject was isolated singly, while in the other experiment, performed under otherwise identical conditions, the subject was isolated collectively with another subject (right). Temporal courses of the rhythms of activity and rectal temperature are presented successively, one period beneath the other. Indications are the same as in figure 16/I. From Wever (1969a).

has been tested; not only under constant illumination but also under self-controlled illumination. The results of corresponding experiments deviate in one important point from those obtained under constant illumination; the sign of the correlation between light intensity and period depends on whether or not each subject was isolated separately, or in groups. (It must be added here that under constant illumination, positive as well as negative correlations between light intensity and period have been observed with separately isolated subjects as well as with groups of subjects, without systematic differences.) Figure 50, as one example, shows results originating from two experiments with the same subject, examined in the same experimental room under exactly the same physical conditions (self-controlled illumination, with two different light intensities) performed at an interval of sev-

eral weeks. In one experiment, however, the subject was alone (Fig. 50, left), while he was with another subject in the later experiment (Fig. 50, right). On the average, the period was longer when the subject was alone but, primarily, the correlations between light intensity and autonomous period were opposite to each other in the two experiments. The same increase in light intensity caused a lengthening of the period when the subject was alone but a shortening of the period occurred when the subject was with another subject. The other subject of this group (also a young male subject) also was examined separately under identical conditions and also showed a positive correlation between light intensity and period when he was alone, in contrast to the negative correlation in the group experiment.

The systematic difference in the results of single and group experiments can be explained by the following consideration. The system consisting of two mutually synchronized subjects can be understood as only one autonomously running oscillation. The two subjects, however, were affected by the light-dark cycle differently. The possibility of switching the light on and off was used by only one of the two subjects. In the 'morning,' the one who first decided to get up switched the lights on, and in the 'evening' the one who last went to bed switched the lights off (it need not be necessarily the same subject at both instances). The light-dark cycle lags in phase behind the activity rhythm of the subject who controls the lights and, correspondingly, it retards his rhythm. Conversely, the light-dark cycle leads the activity rhythm of the other subject and, correspondingly, it accelerates his rhythm. Since the rhythms of both subjects run synchronously, both effects neutralize each other, and the influence of the light-dark cycle, therefore, is abolished for the group as a whole. This is true with regard to the period, generally, and the influence of light intensity on the period. On the other hand, in single experiments the subject is affected by the self-controlled light-dark cycle in the manner mentioned.

As with constant illumination, with self-controlled illumination the dependency of the tendency toward internal desynchronization on light intensity, also can be tested. In 12 of the 30 experiments performed under selfcontrolled illumination, internal desynchronization occurred (Table 4). If computed in the same manner as constant illumination (Fig. 48), the median of the light intensities, taken from the corresponding sections of all experiments, is 178 Lux and the median, taken from the experiments where internal desynchronization occurred, is 206 Lux. The comparison of both of these values again may suggest a slight preference of higher intensities to produce internal desynchronization but, again, this difference is by no means significant and cannot be differentiated from a random deviation by any statistical analysis. It must be concluded, therefore, that the tendency toward internal

desynchronization with self-controlled illumination does not depend on the intensity of illumination.

Beside the intensity, the type of illumination, likewise, has been tested. From the 30 experiments with selfcontrolled illumination, 10 experiments were performed with luminescent tubes. All these experiments include at least one section with a high light intensity of 1300 to 1500 Lux. The mean period ($\pm$ standard deviation) in these sections was 25.27 ± 0.67 hours. Five of the ten experiments included, in addition, another section with lower light intensity of 30 to 50 Lux without changing the type of lamps (cf. 2.4.1.). The mean period in this section was 25.24 ± 0.38 hours. In the 20 experiments which were performed with incandescent bulbs with light intensities between 23 and 460 Lux, the mean period was 25.22 ± 0.88 hours. These results demonstrate that the period of autonomously running rhythms, when under self-controlled illumination, are independent of the type of illumination (i.e., whether the illumination is based on incandescent bulbs or fluorescent tubes).

In the experiments just discussed, the self-control mechanism was performed deliberately by the subjects themselves, with the result that the subjects were exposed to light during activity time and darkness during rest time. The light-dark cycle was delayed in relation to the activity rhythm because the subject, still in the dark, had to decide to start his activity time and then to leave the bed to reach the light switch. In the "evening" while still in bright light, he had to decide to terminate his activity time before switching off the lights. When a subject is living under constant, instead of self-controlled illumination, he subjectively experiences a similar light-dark cycle which is due to the opening and closing of the eyes. This means that even under objectively constant illumination, subjectively a self-controlled light-dark cycle is present. The influence of self-control conditions on autonomous rhythms, to be sure, is based on the delay of the environmental rhythm in comparison to the activity rhythm. The temporal delay of the subjective light-dark cycle is small in comparison to the objective light-dark cycle due to real switching on and off of the lights. The continuous presence of a self-controlled condition, though small in its effect, nevertheless, may influence human circadian rhythms even under objectively constant conditions. It may be the reason for the relatively long autonomous period of man and the shorter periods in blind subjects. It also may be the reason for the ambiguity of the correlation between the autonomous period and light intensity under constant illumination. The self-control action of light may compensate, on the average but not in each single subject, a hypothetical continuous action of light (Wever, 1969a, 1973e).

The effect of self-controlled illumination on autonomous rhythms has been confirmed frequently in animal and human experiments. The hypothesis of a self-control effect of objectively constant illumination, due to the opening and closing of the eyes, has been deduced only indirectly. However, in both cases, the basis of the self-control is a specific behavior changing the perception of light depending on the state of activity, but with a temporal delay. A rhythmic change in the sensitiveness against an external stimulus is a prerequisite for the effectiveness of this stimulus as a synchronizing zeitgeber when operating periodically. Consequences of this coincidence will be discussed later (cf. 3.5).

In summary, in the experiments performed with light as the controlling stimulus, light is effective, although only to a small amount, but does not have the capacity to affect parameters of autonomous rhythms regularly when operating continuously. It is the hypothesis that, under constant illumination, a continuous action of light intensity is more or less compensated by a self-control action. As a consequence, light is an unfit stimulus regarding the evaluation of interdependencies between different parameters of autonomous rhythms. This evaluation, however, is one of the ways to investigate general properties of the circadian system. Additionally, light is unfit in this respect

because it is perceivable consciously. This means changes in the intensity of a continuously operating illumination may affect changes in the preferred mode of activity of the subject (e.g., from reading to hearing music when the intensity decreases). And it cannot be excluded that the preferred mode of activity influences circadian rhythms indirectly.

2.4.3. Influence of Ambient Temperature

The second environmental stimulus which has to be tested, with respect to its capacity to influence autonomous rhythms, is ambient temperature. In most animal experiments, the influence of constant temperature on the autonomous period is smaller than the influence of constant light intensity. In human rhythms, even the influence of light intensity is negligible when light is continuously in operation (cf. 2.4.1). When given only in a self-control mode, light has a significant influence (cf. 2.4.2). It seems to be unlikely, therefore, that ambient temperature has the capacity to influence autonomous rhythms of man to a significant amount when it is constant. It rather is to be expected that ambient temperature has an influence when changed in a selfcontrol mode. For this reason, it appears to be useful only to test the effect of ambient temperature on autonomously running human circadian rhythms in a mode which is self-controlled by the subject (Wever, 1974b).

Figure 51 shows, as an example, the course of an experiment in which a subject lived, with constant illumination during the total experiment, under constant room temperature during the first section but the temperature was self-controlled during the second section. Self-control means the subject had decreased the setpoint of the room temperature controller by 6°C when going to bed, and he had increased the setpoint by 6°C when getting up. As the result, the autonomous period was slightly longer during the second section. Figure 52 shows another example of this series, with a reversed temporal sequence of the sections with the two different temperature modes (i.e., with a self-controlled temperature cycle (range: 6°C) during the first section and constant temperature during the second section). The autonomous period again was slightly longer during the section with the self-controlled temperature cycle and, therefore, it is unlikely that the change in period in the first experiment (Fig. 51) was simulated by a temporal trend. Since, in both experiments, the means of self-controlled temperature cycles coincided with the constant room temperatures during the other section in each case, the changes in period could not be due to differences in the levels of ambient temperature during the two sections.

In total, eight experiments were performed with constant ambient temperature during one section and self-controlled temperature during another section (with changing temporal sequence of the two sections) with equal mean temperatures during both sections. The results of these experiments are summarized in table 5. As can be seen in all experiments, the autonomous period was longer during the sections with self-controlled ambient temperature than during sections with constant temperature, without exception. The difference in the periods between the two sections is statistically significant, applying the parametric t-test as well as the nonparametric Wilcoxon-test. This result shows that the influence of a self-controlled cycle in ambient temperature coincides with a self-controlled cycle in illumination (Table 4). This result shows, in addition, that ambient temperature is not ineffective with regard to autonomous rhythms.

With light as the stimulus under self-control, not only the period was longer than under constant conditions but the interindividual variability of the periods also was larger (Table 4). With ambient temperature as the stimulus, the same result is still true, although not to a significant amount. The difference in the standard deviations between the two sections, however, suggests another interrelationship which is, in fact, significant. This is the correlation between the original period and the change in period due to the transition between the two modes of ambient temperature (Table 5). This result shows that the change in period, induced by an external stimulus, depends on the original period.

2.4.4. Influence of Natural Electromagnetic Fields

Beside the external stimuli, which can be changed arbitrarily, fixed conditions may have the capacity to influence autonomous rhythms. These conditions are the properties of the two experimental units available. The units differ visibly only in the mirror-like arrangement of the service rooms (bathroom, kitchen, and lock) relative to the living room (Fig. 10). Since the furniture within the room (except the bed) are moved frequently by the subjects themselves, there is no systematic difference in the arrangement of the furnitures between the two rooms. There is, however, an invisible difference between the units. One experimental unit is shielded against electric and magnetic fields and the other is not (cf. 1.3.1). The equipment for the shielding was built into the walls and its existence was, at least during the first years of the experiment, unknown to the subjects (Wever, 1967c). To be precise, the exterior of the units was equal only during the first five years of the running experiment. Late in 1968, one of the units (nonshielded) was equipped with a larger and more powerful air conditioning plant to perform special experiments with changing ambient temperature (cf. 2.4.3). After the exchange, the optical impression of this room was remarkably different and, therefore, it was no longer meaningful to speak of visibly identical units. If differences in the results obtained in the two different units are considered, relative to the different states of the electromagnetic shielding, it is appropriate to give emphasis on experiments performed only during the interval 1964 to 1968.

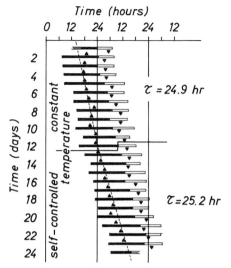

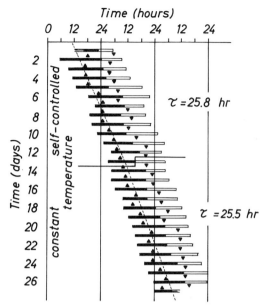

Figure 51. Autonomous rhythm of a subject (K.H., ♂ 27 y) living without environmental time cues, while under the influence of a constant ambient temperature during the first section but a self-controlled cycle of ambient temperature (i.e., warm during activity time; cold during rest time; with a range of 6°C) during the second section, and with the same average ambient temperature during both sections. Temporal courses of the rhythms of activity and rectal temperature are presented successively, one period beneath the other. Indications are the same as in figure 16/I. From Wever (1974b).

Figure 52. Autonomous rhythm of a subject (C.F., ♀ 22 y) living without environmental time cues, while under the influence of a self-controlled cycle of ambient temperature (i.e., warm during activity time; cold during rest time; with a range of 6°C) during the first section but constant ambient temperature during the second section, and with the same average ambient temperature during both sections. Temporal courses of the rhythms of activity and rectal temperature are presented successively, one period beneath the other. Indications are the same as in figure 16/I. From Wever (1974b).

Table 5.   *Effect of Ambient Temperature*

Subject	Autonomous period		
	Constant temperature	Self-controlled temperature	Difference
G.S., ♀ 23 y	24.5 hr	24.8 hr	0.3 hr
M.S., ♀ 22 y	24.6	24.8	0.2
K.H., ♂ 27 y	24.9	25.2	0.3
D.B., ♀ 21 y	24.8	25.2	0.4
W.B., ♂ 25 y	25.6	26.3	0.7
G.K., ♂ 23 y	24.8	25.3	0.5
C.F., ♀ 22 y	25.5	25.8	0.3
M.H., ♀ 17 y	24.5	24.7	0.2
Mean	24.90 hr	25.26 hr	0.36 hr
Standard dev.	±0.43 hr	±0.55 hr	± 0.17 hr

From Wever, 1974b.
Statistical analysis concerning: Difference in periods $\neq 0$ (two tailed)
t-test: $t = 6.09$, $p < 0.001$
Wilcoxon-test: $I = 0$, $p < 0.01$
Coefficients of correlation:
(1) Difference versus constant temperature: $r = 0.635$, n.s.
(2) Difference versus self-controlled temperature: $r = 0.800$, $p < 0.05$

Table 6/I. Effect of Electromagnetic Shielding

	Sample	Nonshielded room				Shielded room			
No.	Condition	No.	Mean period ± stand. dev. (hr)	Median (hr)	Int. desynchr.	No.	Mean period ± stand. dev. (hr)	Median (hr)	Int. desynchr.
	1964···1968								
1	All experiments	33	24.85 ± 0.45	24.82	4 (= 12%)	51	25.11 ± 0.59	24.98	18 (= 35%)
2	All experiments, without field sections	33	24.85 ± 0.45	24.82	4 (= 12%)	51	25.25 ± 0.91	25.02	18 (= 35%)
3	Single experiments	27	24.80 ± 0.47	24.78	3 (= 11%)	50	25.10 ± 0.59	24.97	18 (= 36%)
4	Single experiments, without field sections	27	24.80 ± 0.47	24.78	3 (= 11%)	50	25.25 ± 0.92	25.01	18 (= 36%)
5	Single experiments, without field experiments	27	24.80 ± 0.47	24.78	3 (= 11%)	37	24.97 ± 0.37	24.92	12 (= 32%)
6	Single exp., constant illumination	20	24.62 ± 0.35	24.65	1 (= 5%)	34	25.00 ± 0.41	24.95	10 (= 29%)
7	Single exp., constant ill., without field sect.	20	24.62 ± 0.35	24.65	1 (= 5%)	34	25.10 ± 0.59	24.97	10 (= 29%)
8	Single exp., constant ill., without field exp.	20	24.62 ± 0.35	24.65	1 (= 5%)	25	24.93 ± 0.32	24.92	6 (= 24%)
9	Single exp., self-controlled illumination	5	25.30 ± 0.41	25.0	1 (= 20%)	15	25.33 ± 0.84	25.1	8 (= 53%)
10	Single exp., self-contr. ill., without field sect.	5	25.30 ± 0.41	25.0	1 (= 20%)	15	25.58 ± 1.24	25.4	8 (= 53%)
11	Single exp., self-contr. ill., without field exp.	5	25.30 ± 0.41	25.0	1 (= 20%)	11	25.03 ± 0.48	24.9	6 (= 55%)
	1969···1976								
12	Single experiments	23	25.07 ± 0.47	24.99	6 (= 26%)	35	24.91 ± 0.51	24.82	11 (= 31%)
13	Single exp., constant ill.	17	24.99 ± 0.40	24.97	4 (= 24%)	32	24.94 ± 0.46	24.83	10 (= 31%)
14	Single exp., selfcontr. ill.	6	25.30 ± 0.61	25.1	2 (= 33%)	3	24.60 ± 1.06	24.2	1 (= 33%)
	1964···1976								
15	Single experiments	50	24.93 ± 0.48	24.89	9 (= 18%)	85	25.02 ± 0.56	24.90	29 (= 34%)
16	Single experiments, constant illumination	37	24.79 ± 0.41	24.77	4 (= 11%)	66	24.97 ± 0.43	24.89	20 (= 30%)
17	Single experiments, self-controlled illumination	11	25.30 ± 0.50	25.03	4 (= 36%)	18	25.21 ± 0.89	25.00	9 (= 50%)

For reference, however, it may be useful to look for additional results of later experiments.

The comparison mentioned, concerning results obtained in the two different experimental units, is given in table 6. It presents, in part I, average period values of experiments with autonomously running rhythms (periods of rectal temperature rhythms) together with the standard deviations, the median values of these periods, and the numbers of experiments resulting in internal desynchronization, for different samples of experiments and separately for each different room. Table 6 also presents, in part II, the statistical analyses concerning the differences between the two rooms, with regard to the mean period (parametric as well as nonparametric), to the interindividual standard deviations, and the tendency towards internal desynchronization. In the uppermost line of table 6, data of all experiments from the first interval of years (1964 to 1968) are given. As can be seen, the mean period is longer in the shielded than in the nonshielded room and this difference is significant when applying the parametric and the nonparametric test. Moreover, the standard deviation around the mean is larger in the shielded than in the nonshielded room and the frequency in the occurrence of real internal desynchronization is also larger in the shielded than in the nonshielded room. These two latter differences also are statistically significant. It will be shown in the next chapter (2.4.5) that, in the shielded room, some subjects were exposed to an artificial electric field which just compensates the effect of the shielding with regard to the autonomous period (i.e., during the sections where the subjects continuously are exposed to this field, the autonomous periods do not differ from those obtained in the nonshielded room). It seems to be fair, therefore, to exclude those sections from the comparison, as is done in the second line of table 6. This comparison, excluding the field sections of 13 subjects, corresponds to figures presented earlier (Wever, 1971a). Since the figures given in table 6 are based on recent reanalyses applying the strong criteria given in this paper, they deviate slightly in some details from those given earlier but, of course, not in the general result. The result is that the differences between the two rooms are marked more strongly when the

Table 6/II. *Effect of Electromagnetic Shielding. Statistical Analyses of the Differences between Nonshielded and Shielded Room*

Sample No.	Mean period		Standard deviation F-test	Internal desynchronization exact Fisher-test
	Parametric t-test	Nonparametric U-test		
1	$t = 2.16, p < 0.02$	$u = 1.76, p = 0.04$	$F = 1.72, p < 0.05$	$p = 0.012$
2	$t = 2.34, p < 0.0125$	$u = 2.16, p = 0.015$	$F = 4.09, p < 0.01$	$p = 0.012$
3	$t = 2.28, p < 0.02$	$u = 2.08, p = 0.019$	$F = 1.58$, n.s.	$p = 0.013$
4	$t = 2.37, p < 0.0125$	$u = 2.46, p = 0.007$	$F = 3.83, p < 0.01$	$p = 0.013$
5	$t = 1.62, p < 0.10$	$u = 1.88, p = 0.03$	$F = 1.88$, n.s.	$p = 0.034$
6	$t = 3.47, p < 0.001$	$u = 3.24, p = 0.0006$	$F = 1.37$, n.s.	$p = 0.027$
7	$t = 3.30, p < 0.002$	$u = 3.35, p = 0.0004$	$F = 2.84, p < 0.01$	$p = 0.027$
8	$t = 3.10, p < 0.0025$	$u = 2.83, p = 0.0023$	$F = 1.20$, n.s.	$p = 0.078$
9	$t = 0.08$, n.s.	$u = 0.17$, n.s.	$F = 4.20, p < 0.05$	$p = 0.191$
10	$t = 0.49$, n.s.	$u = 0.61$, n.s.	$F = 9.15, p < 0.01$	$p = 0.191$
11	$t = 1.08$, n.s.	$u = 1.36$, n.s.	$F = 1.37$, n.s.	$p = 0.202$
12	$t = 1.21$, n.s.		$F = 1.18$, n.s.	$p = 0.213$
13	$t = 0.38$, n.s.		$F = 1.32$, n.s.	$p = 0.227$
14	$t = 1.29$, n.s.		$F = 3.02$, n.s.	$p = 0.5$
15	$t = 0.95$, n.s.		$F = 1.36$, n.s.	$p = 0.021$
16	$t = 2.08, p < 0.025$	$u = 2.22, p = 0.013$	$F = 1.10$, n.s.	$p = 0.015$
17	$t = 0.31$, n.s.		$F = 3.17, p < 0.05$	$p = 0.236$

sections mentioned are excluded from the comparison.

It is the general result, to be discussed in chapter 2.4, that just those parameters which possibly are affected by the electromagnetic shielding (e.g., mean autonomous period and tendency toward internal desynchronization), are sensitive to other stimuli. It must be paid attention, therefore, to interferences between effects of shielding and other stimuli which may be disturbed irregularly among the two rooms. Two of these stimuli especially must be considered. The first is the number of subjects participating at an experiment (cf. 2.4.8). Since group experiments, with only one exception, were performed only in the nonshielded room, it seems appropriate, in the following, to consider only single experiments. With this restriction, the difference between the two rooms, in the number of experiments to be compared, becomes even greater. Another reason for this asymmetry is, for technical reasons, in the nonshielded room a larger portion of experiments with heteronomous rhythms were performed than in the other room (cf. 3). The second stimulus to be considered is the mode of illumination, which exerts the greatest influence on the concerned parameters (cf. 2.4.2.); experiments with two modes of illumination (constant versus self-controlled illumination), were not distributed equally among the two rooms. It seems to be appropriate, therefore, to discuss experiments with the different modes separately. Finally, the experimental series mentioned, which exposed subjects to an effective artificial electric field, included, by chance, some experiments with especially long autonomous periods (cf. 2.4.5). In order to be on the safe side, therefore, it may be appropriate to observe whether or not the exclusion of those experiments, in total, has a relevant effect on the result. In the following, several samples of all experiments will be considered in order to guarantee the result obtained from the overall comparison between the two rooms.

Table 6 shows that the differences men-tioned, between the two experimental units, are more marked than with all experiments when only single experiments are considered and are especially well marked when only experiments with constant illumination are considered. There is no relevant difference if either the field sections or the field experiments, in total (with especially long mean periods), are excluded. As a consequence, the more homogeneous a sample, the more significant are the differences between the two rooms. With self-controlled illumination the trend is similar but the small number of experiments does not guarantee the significance of the differences. There may be another reason for the missing significance, this being the mean period already is lengthened to such a degree, due to the self-control effect (compare samples 6 and 9; nonshielded room), that there is no longer a great margin for lengthening it further because of the shielding. In addition, table 6 guarantees the differences between the two modes of illumination, as given in table 4, separately for the different rooms.

While the differences in the results obtained in the two experimental units are guaranteed independently with different samples of experiments during the first interval of years (1964 to 1968), these differences could not be reproduced during the following eight years (1969 to 1976). There may be manifold reasons for this discrepancy. An obvious one is that the two rooms differed during the last interval of experiments, not only regarding the electromagnetic shielding but also in appearance (s. above). There is no way to decide independently whether or not the appearance of the room itself had any influence on autonomous rhythms. It does not seem to be meaningful, consequently, to compare, during this interval, results of the two rooms only considering differences in the electromagnetic shielding. Another reason for the apparent discrepancy between the two temporal intervals may be that, together with the alteration in the exterior of one room, psychomotor tests were introduced and were performed regularly by the subjects. As a possible result of the increased burden caused by the tests, at least in the nonshielded room and with constant illumination, the period lengthened significantly and the frequency in the occurrence of internal desynchronization increased (compare samples 6 and 13; 2.4.7). It also cannot be excluded that this significant change is due to the alteration in the appearance of the nonshielded room (s. above). Whereas the effect of the tests would concern both rooms simultaneously the latter effect would be detected only in the nonshielded room. Since the margin in the range of autonomous periods may be limited, there is no great possibility to lengthen the period further because of the shielding. With self-controlled illumination, the sample in the nonshielded room primarily includes experiments with continuous sleep recordings by EEG (4 of 6 experiments) where the period seems to be generally lengthened and the tendency towards internal desynchronization generally seems to be increased (cf. 2.4.7). Therefore, the missing differences between the results, obtained in the two different experimental units during the last interval of years (1969 to 1976), do not contradict necessarily the conclusion drawn from the significant differences during the first interval of years (1964 to 1968). At least with constant illumination, the differences mentioned are significant when all experiments, during the total time (1964 to 1976), are considered (Table 6, sample 16).

In the experiments performed in the shielded room, the subjects were protected from natural electromagnetic fields and, in most experiments, from intentionally introduced artificial fields. They, however, were exposed, as were the subjects in the nonshielded room, to the 50-Hz field generated by the technical line voltage. Since this field cannot be eliminated without major changes in equipment (e.g., air conditioning plant), care must be taken that this field is set at as equal a strength as possible among the different experiments. The main part of the technical 50-Hz field originates from the illumination, which in most experiments was based on incandescent bulbs. Only in the 15 experiments (exclusively during the first interval of years), where the illumination was based on fluorescent tubes, were higher frequencies introduced from the technical devices. It was shown earlier (cf. 2.4.1) that the type of lamps used did not influence autonomous rhythms. During the experiments with constant illumination, at least, it is guaranteed that the strength of the 50-Hz field nearly is identical in the different experiments when performed in the different units. In the experiments with self-controlled illumination, the strength of this field, indeed, is alternating (with a higher strength during activity than during rest) but, since the activity-rest ratio was, on the average, nearly identical in the two rooms, the average strength of the 50-Hz field was nearly identical in the two rooms. The differences between the two rooms, in fact, are present with self-controlled and constant illumination (Wever, 1969a). The constant influence of the technical 50-Hz field, therefore, did not affect the influence of the electromagnetic shielding against natural fields. A possible influence of the technical 50-Hz field on human circadian rhythms neither can be proven nor excluded by the results mentioned so far.

From the results in table 6, different conclusions can be drawn. The first refers to a subtle external stimulus that evidently has the capacity to affect human circadian rhythms. The total of the natural electromagnetic fields which penetrate into the nonshielded room but do not, or only to a reduced degree, penetrate into the shielded room had the ability to shorten the autonomous period, to diminish the interindividual differences in the periods, and to decrease the tendency toward internal desynchronization (Wever, 1967c). This subtle stimulus is the first which is effective but not perceivable consciously. In contrast to changes in light intensity and ambient temperature, changes in the state of this stimulus do not change the preferred mode of activity of the subjects and do not display a behavior which changes the perception of this stimulus. Therefore, electromagnetic fields, which can be taken from table 6 as being effective in the control of human circadian rhythms, may constitute a stimulus that controls these rhythms in such a regular manner, without self-control, that it allows the evaluation of interdependencies between different parameters of autonomous rhythms and, further, to the investigation of basic properties of circadian rhythmicity (Wever, 1971a). To be sure, natural fields do not constitute such a stimulus because they cannot be handled experimentally but, if natural fields are effective, it also can be assumed that artificial electromagnetic fields are effective, and these fields can be handled experimentally in a well-defined manner.

Another aspect of these studies is that they give evidence for the capacity of natural electromagnetic fields to affect the human being, in general. From this point of view, human circadian rhythms can be used as a very sensitive indicator to test biological effects of electromagnetic fields. The special sensitiveness of this indicator is, at least in part, based on its stability. The significantly measurable changes in the autonomous period, taken from table 6, are in the range of 1%; there are very few other biological parameter changes of which can be measured with such precision.

The conclusion, which may be drawn from differences in results obtained in the two experimental units to a general effect of weak electromagnetic fields, is so far reaching that it cannot be accepted without additional independent confirmations. It, in general, cannot be excluded with certainty that the differences mentioned are due to the mirror-like arrangement of the two rooms or even to any unknown difference between the two rooms. This uncertainty is supported by the comparison between the differences obtained in the two successive intervals of years (Table 6). Fortunately, there is a possibility to test the conclusion independently using artificial electromagnetic fields as the stimulus. If a definite artificial field is found to be effective, the general possibility is confirmed that weak electromagnetic fields can be effective. This special

field can be assumed to constitute the component from the wide spectrum of natural electromagnetic fields which, either alone or together with other components, is responsible for the effect of the total of the natural fields.

2.4.5. Influence of Artificial Electromagnetic Fields

A first series of experiments applying artificial fields was performed initially with DC fields as the stimulus and with field strengths about three times greater than those of the natural DC fields. Figure 53 shows the result of an experiment conducted under constant conditions in which the subject was pro-

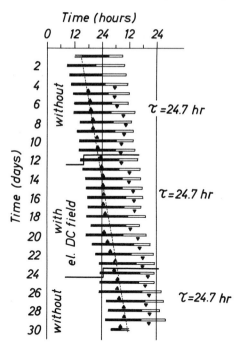

Figure 53. Autonomous rhythm of a subject (H.F., ♂ 26 y) living under constant conditions without time cues and protected from natural and artificial electromagnetic fields during the first and third sections, but under the influence of an artificial electric DC field (i.e., 300 V/m, battery operated) during the second section. Temporal courses of the rhythms of activity and rectal temperature are presented successively, one period beneath the other. Indications are the same as in figure 16/I. From Wever (1969b).

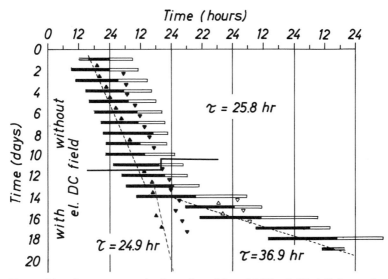

Figure 54. Autonomous rhythm of a subject (H.N., ♂ 27 y) living under constant conditions without time cues and protected from natural and artificial electromagnetic fields during the first section, but under the influence of an artificial electric DC field (i.e., 300 V/m, battery operated) during the second section. Temporal courses of the rhythms of activity and rectal temperature are presented successively, one period beneath the other. Indications are the same as in figure 27/I. From Wever (1969b).

tected from all fields during the first and the third section (with the exception of the technical 50-Hz field) but with an electric DC field continuously in operation during the second section. The homogenous field strength in the undisturbed room was 300V/m but, of course, the field was deformed by the presence of a subject and was superimposed irregularly by electric fields induced by movements of the subject. As can be seen from the figure, there is no change in the autonomous period and, in addition, no change in any other parameter when the state of the DC field alters. Figure 54 shows the result of another experiment in which the DC field was continuously in operation during the second section while the subject was protected from any field during the first section. In this experiment, internal desynchronization occurred a few days after the field had been switched on. It, of course, can not be concluded from this single result that a DC field induces internal desynchronization; but it can be stated with certainty that the DC field is not able to prevent internal

desynchronization (Wever, 1969b). In other experiments, the subjects were exposed, during one section, to a magnetic DC field (field strength: $1.5 \cdot 10^{-4}$T) while they were protected from any field during other sections. The experiments had the same result as those with the electric DC field. DC fields, either electric or magnetic, therefore, are neither able to affect the autonomous period nor to prevent internal desynchronization (Wever, 1969b). Both of these effects are characteristic for the total of the natural electromagnetic fields. If the natural electromagnetic fields are effective at all, the DC fields cannot be the relevant component. This is already unlikely, in the case of the electric DC field, because this field is distorted by the moving subject to such a degree that the original field may be negligible in comparison to the distortions.

Another series of experiments were performed with AC fields as the stimulus (Wever, 1969b). In particular, a vertical electric square wave field was applied with a frequency of 10 Hz and a field strength

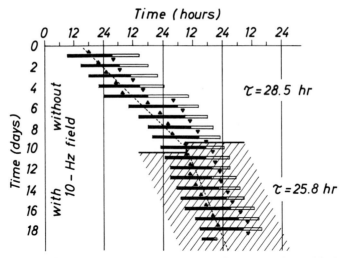

Figure 55. Autonomous rhythm of a subject (H.v.S., ♂ 23 y) living under constant conditions without time cues and protected from natural and artificial electromagnetic fields during the first section, but under the influence of an artificial electric AC field (i.e., 10 Hz square wave, 2.5 V/m) during the second section. *I.* Temporal courses of the rhythms of activity and rectal temperature, presented successively one period beneath the other. Indications are the same as in figure 16/I. Shaded area: field in operation. From Wever (1969b).

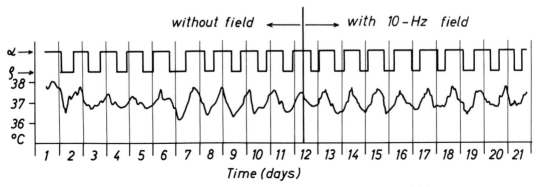

Figure 55/II. Longitudinally presented courses of the two variables.

(again measured without a subject in the room) of 2.5 V/m (total range). The result of the first experiment of this series is shown in figure 55. In this experiment, performed in the shielded room like all other experiments applying artificial fields, the subject was protected from all fields during the first section (again with the exception of the technical 50-Hz field) but continuously exposed to the 10-Hz field during the second section. According to figure 55/I, the period was shortened when the field was switched on. For com-

parison, figure 55/II shows the same original data "longitudinally" presented. This second presentation obviously shows that each section includes 9 full cycles (activity and rectal temperature) but the first section lasted longer than the second section. The result derived from the inspection of the original data (Figs. 55/I and II) is confirmed by the subsequent computer analyses. Figure 55/III presents the result of the period analyses. The spectral lines obtained in the two sections clearly are separated without

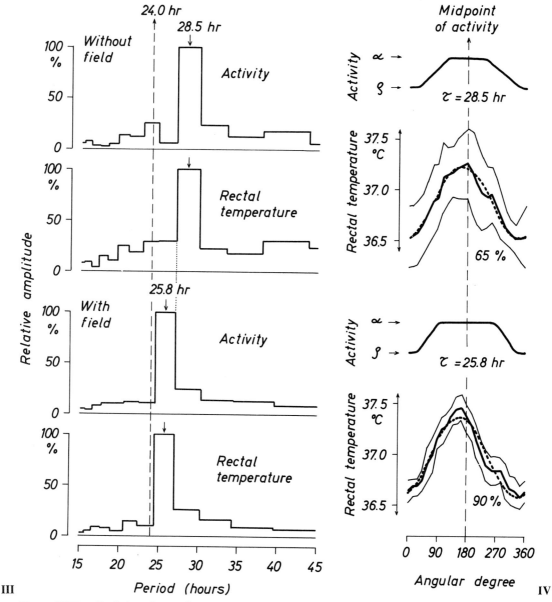

Figure 55/III. Period analyses of the two time series, presented in I and II, computed separately for the two sections, without and with the field in operation. From Wever (1973a). *IV.* Longitudinally pooled courses of the two rhythms, computed separately for the two sections, with averaging periods derived from III. Indications are the same as in figure 16/III. From Wever (1973a).

overlapping while, within each section, the two different rhythms (and all other rhythms measured but not presented) result in identical spectral lines. This indicates internally synchronized rhythms with significantly different periods during the two sections. Figure 55/IV shows the result of the longitudinal poolings, again computed separately for the two sections, and each with the relevant period determined in the preceding analyses (Fig. 55/III). In both sections, there are well marked rhythms, but the reliabilities are higher during the second section with the shorter period and, in addition, the mean value of rectal temperature is higher and the amplitude is larger during the second than during the first section. The internal phase relationship between the rhythms of activity and rectal temperature is essentially the same in both sections.

Figure 56 shows the course of another experiment of this series with reversed temporal sequence of the sections with and without the artificial field in operation. Additionally, this experiment includes a third section during which the 10-Hz field was not continuously in operation but switched on and off periodically (with a period of 23.5 hours). In this experiment, the autonomous period also was shorter when the field was continuously in operation (first section) than when not in operation (second section). In the third section, the periodically operating field seemed to entrain the subject's rhythm (suggesting a zeitgeber effect). Figure 57 shows the course of a third experiment without the field during the first and third sections and with the field continuously in operation during the second section. The comparison between the autonomous periods during the first and second sections confirms, once more, the shortening effect of the 10-Hz field. During the third section, internal desynchronization was present immediately after switching off the field. This latter result suggests a possible effect of the 10-Hz field on the mutual coupling between different rhythms. Subsequent computer analyses of the first and second sections of each of the experiments again confirmed the results. The period analyses (Figs. 56/II and 57/II) show internally synchronized rhythms with periods which are different in the two sections. The differences in period, in fact, are small and there are great overlappings in the respective spectral peaks but the differences are consistent regarding the field exposure, independent of the temporal sequence of the sections. The longitudinal poolings (Figs. 56/III and 57/III) confirm the result derived from figure 55/IV. The rectal temperature rhythms, in both experiments, are more reliable, their mean values are

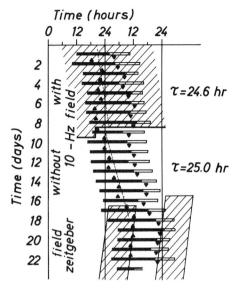

Figure 56. Rhythm of a subject (B.D., ♀ 22 y) living under constant conditions without time cues during the first and second sections, but under the influence of an artificial electric AC field (i.e., 10 Hz square wave, 2.5 V/m) during the first section, protected from natural and artificial electromagnetic fields during the second section, and under the influence of the AC field operating periodically (i.e., 11.75-hour field on and 11.75-hour field off) during the third section. *I*. Temporal courses of the rhythms of activity and rectal temperature, presented successively one period beneath the other. Indications are the same as in figure 55/I. From Wever (1970a).

higher and their amplitudes are larger during the sections with the field continuously in operation (i.e., with the shorter autonomous periods) than during the other sections without the field (i.e., with the longer periods). The suggestions of results obtained in the third section in each of the two experiments are worth considering separately and, therefore, will be subjects of special investigation.

In total, 17 experiments were performed under constant conditions, with the weak electric 10-Hz square wave field continuously in operation during one section (or even during two separated sections) of 8 to 14 days duration, and with another section (or even two separate sections), also of 8 to 14 days duration, where the subjects were protected against all fields (except the tech-

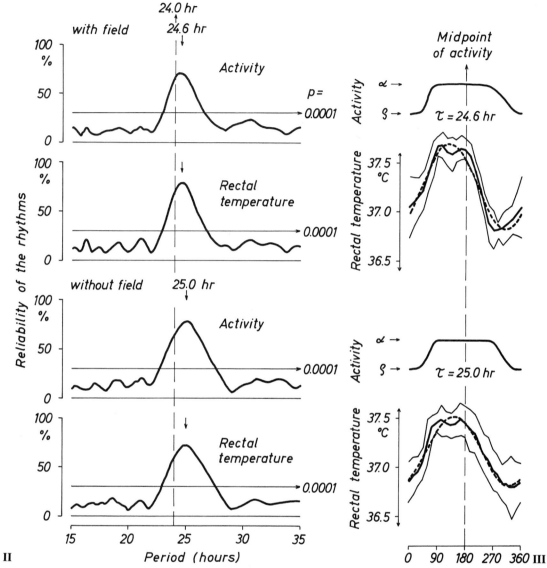

Figure 56/II.   Period analyses of the two time series, presented in I, computed separately for the first and second section, without and with the field continuously in operation. ***III.*** Longitudinally pooled courses of the two rhythms, computed separately for the first and second section, with averaging periods derived from II. Indications are the same as in figure 16/III.

nical 50-Hz field). In all these experiments, the influence of this definite artificial field could be studied with each subject as his own control. In 12 of these 17 experiments, the rhythms stood synchronized internally during at least one section, with the field, and another section, without the field continuously in operation (Figs. 55 through 57). In these 12 experiments, the influence of the artificial 10-Hz field on the autonomous pe-

riod (and on other parameters of autonomous rhythms) could be studied. In the 5 additional experiments, internal desynchronization occurred and prevented the uniform determination of autonomous periods during the different sections.

Results of the 12 experiments mentioned above are summarized, regarding the autonomous period, in the left part of figure 58. It obviously shows that the periods are consis-

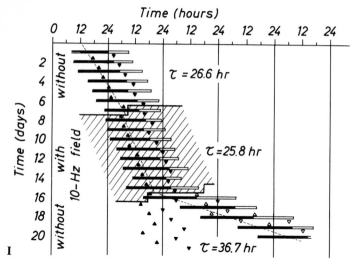

Figure 57. Autonomous rhythm of a subject (R.H., ♀ 22 y) living under constant conditions without time cues and protected from natural and artificial electromagnetic fields during the first and third section, but under the influence of an artificial electric AC field (i.e., 10 Hz square wave, 2.5 V/m) during the second section. *I.* Temporal courses of the rhythms of activity and rectal temperature, presented successively one period beneath the other. Indications are the same as in figure 55/I. From Wever (1968a).

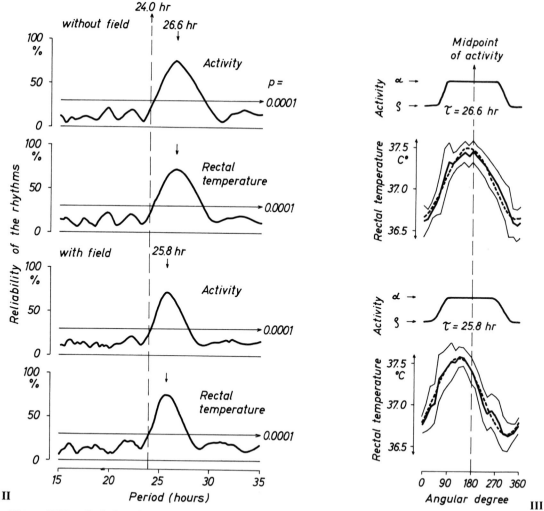

Figure 57/II. Period analyses of the two time series, presented in I, computed separately for the first and second section, with and without the field in operation. *III.* Longitudinally pooled courses of the two rhythms, computed separately for the first and second section, with averaging periods derived from II. Indications are the same as in figure 16/III.

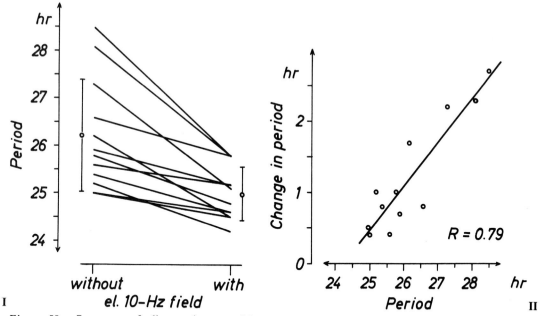

Figure 58. Summary of all experiments with autonomous rhythms, with one section under the influence of an artificial electric AC field (i.e., 10 Hz square wave, 2.5 V/m) and another without any field. *I.* Period values during the sections with and without the field continuously in operation, with lines combining results of different sections in individual experiments. Left and right: means and standard deviations of the periods within the respective sections. *II.* Amount of the effect of the field, when continuously in operation, on the period. Changes in the period, induced by the field (i.e., ordinate), plotted as a function of the period in the sections without any field (i.e., abscissa). The coefficient of rank correlation (Spearman) is indicated. From Wever (1969b).

tently shorter during the sections with the field continuously in operation than during the sections without the field. It also shows that the variability of the individual periods around a mean is smaller during the sections with the field in operation than in those without the field. In numbers, the same results are summarized in table 7, which includes details concerning the subjects and the experimental conditions. In addition, table 7 includes detailed statistical analyses of not only the total of all experiments but also subdivisions regarding the two modes of illumination (constant versus self-controlled) and regarding sex and age of the subjects. These statistical analyses have been applied to the changes in period (i.e., to the shortening effects of the 10-Hz field) because these differences in periods are independent of the interindividual variabilities of the periods. As the result, the shortening effect of the artificial electric 10-Hz square wave field, if all experiments are considered collectively, is significant at a high statistical level when

applying the parametric t-test and the nonparametric Wilcoxon-test. This effect, moreover, is significant even when the two modes of illumination and both sexes are considered separately. The period values and shortening effects are smaller with a constant than a self-controlled illumination, as with the much larger collective of all experiments (Table 4) although, due to the small number of experiments, they are only close to the limit of significance ($p < 0.1$). The period values and shortening effects, however, are nearly independent of the sex of the subjects and are not correlated to their age. Both results again correspond to results obtained with a much larger sample of subjects (cf. 2.3). It seems worth repeating that during all experiments the intensity of illumination and, of course, the mode of illumination, remained unchanged during the total experiment. The results mentioned, therefore, cannot be simulated by simultaneous changes in the illumination or the technical 50-Hz field, which is generated mainly by

Table 7. *Effect of the Artificial 10-Hz Field*

Subject	Illumination	Autonomous period		Difference
		Without 10-Hz field	With 10-Hz field	
H.v.S., ♂ 23 y	Self-control	28.5 hr	25.8 hr	2.7 hr
K.v.S., ♂ 26 y	"	25.2	24.2	1.0
M.F., ♀ 26 y	"	28.1	25.8	2.3
R.H., ♀ 22 y	"	26.6	25.8	0.8
H.R., ♂ 67 y	Constant	25.8	24.8	1.0
G.W., ♂ 26 y	"	25.6	25.2	0.4
B.D., ♂ 22 y	"	25.0	24.6	0.4
M.R., ♂ 34 y	"	25.4	24.6	0.8
M.M., ♀ 23 y	"	27.3	25.1	2.2
O.D., ♂ 22 y	"	26.2	24.5	1.7
E.P., ♀ 19 y	"	25.9	25.2	0.7
M.A., ♂ 32 y		25.0	24.5	0.5
(1) Total	(*n* = 12)	26.22 hr ± 1.18 hr	25.01 hr ± 0.56 hr	1.21 hr ± 0.81 hr
(2) Self-control only	(*n* = 4)	27.10 hr ± 1.51 hr	25.40 hr ± 0.80 hr	1.70 hr ± 0.94 hr
(3) Constant only	(*n* = 8)	25.78 hr ± 0.75 hr	24.81 hr ± 0.31 hr	0.96 hr ± 0.66 hr
(4) Females only	(*n* = 5)	26.58 hr ± 1.20 hr	25.30 hr ± 0.51 hr	1.28 hr ± 0.90 hr
(5) Males only	(*n* = 7)	25.96 hr ± 1.19 hr	24.80 hr ± 0.54 hr	1.16 hr ± 0.80 hr

Statistical analysis concerning: Difference in periods ≠ 0 (two tailed)
(1) *t*-test: $t = 5.18$, $p < 0.001$; Wilcoxon-test: $T = 0$, $p < 0.01$
(2) *t*-test: $t = 3.62$, $p < 0.05$
(3) *t*-test: $t = 4.11$, $p < 0.01$
(4) *t*-test: $t = 3.18$, $p < 0.05$
(5) *t*-test: $t = 3.84$, $p < 0.01$
Coefficient of correlation: difference in period versus age (Spearman), $R = -0.009$

the illumination. In only one of the 12 experiments, the illumination was based on fluorescent tubes; in all others on incandescent bulbs. Nothing can be stated, from these results, about a possible effect of the technical field. It can be stated with certainty, however, that such an effect, if present, does not block the significant effect of the 10-Hz field.

In figure 58/I, the lines combining the periods obtained in the different sections of each experiment are steeper the longer the period. This is due to the variability of the periods is larger for longer periods without the field than for shorter periods with the field in operation. This dependency indicates a correlation between the shortening effect of the 10-Hz field and the original period. To verify this, figure 58/II shows the differences in the periods obtained during the sections with and without the field, or the shortening

effect of the field, plotted against the original periods obtained during sections without the field in operation. As can be seen, there is a strong correlation. The computed coefficient of correlation is $r = 0.908$ (parametrically) or $R = 0.785$ (nonparametrically), respectively. It deviates significantly from zero with $p < 0.01$. In contrast to this, the other correlation, between the differences in the periods and the periods obtained during the sections with the field in operation, does not deviate significantly from zero ($r = 0.475$ or $R = 0.278$, respectively). The correlation mentioned means, in general, that the effect of the stimulus influencing the autonomous period depends on the original period and, in particular, that the shortening effect of the 10-Hz field is the stronger the longer the original period. The reversed consideration, however (i.e., the assumption of a lengthening effect with the elimination of the 10-Hz field depending on the original period measured with the field in operation), is not meaningful.

Considering the correlation included in figure 58/II, the remarkably large amount of the effect of the artificial 10-Hz field on the autonomous period, as found in the average of the experiments mentioned, becomes reduced in its meaning. This large amount is based on the fact that this series of experiments includes, by chance, some experiments with extraordinarily long periods. The average of the periods in the sections without the field (26.22 ± 1.18 hours) was much longer, and the standard deviation much larger, than the average of the periods in all experiments under comparable conditions (25.26 ± 0.85 hours) (i.e., after isolation from artificial and natural fields) (Table 6). If this latter value is taken for the starting point, the interpolation of the regression in figure 58/II results in a shortening effect of the 10-Hz field of only 0.62 hours. This means the field effect, when referred to the average of a larger sample of subjects, is expected to be only half as large as those measured averagely in the smaller sample, which included, by chance, some of the subjects with periods deviating farthest from the average. The accidental inclusion of some experiments with extraordinarily long autonomous periods in this experimental series, therefore, helped in finding the correlation between effect and original value, which possibly would not have been found with only shorter periods but may be a relevant property of the circadian system. This inclusion, however, simulates an effect that is about twice as large, on the average, as expected in a larger sample of experiments.

The natural electromagnetic fields had not only the effect of shortening the period of autonomous rhythms and diminishing the interindividual variability but, in addition, of preventing real internal desynchronization (Table 6). The question now arises whether or not the aritifical 10-Hz field also has the capability of preventing internal desynchronization. A first suggestion of this type of influence was given in figure 57. Real internal desynchronization, in fact, was ob-

served in the shielded experimental unit in 28 out of 80 subjects, where all experiments with artificial fields were performed, as long as the artificial 10-Hz field was not in operation (Table 6). This state, however, was not observed in any of the 17 subjects as long as this field was continuously in operation. Applying the exact Fisher-test, this difference statistically is significant with $p \ll 0.001$. This means the third effect of the natural electromagnetic fields (i.e., to diminish the tendency towards internal desynchronization) also has been verified with the artificial 10-Hz field (Wever, 1969b).

The summarizing inspection of all experiments has been shown to be sufficient in demonstrating the significant effect of an artificial field on the mutual coupling between different rhythms. More obvious than this collective inspection, however, is the separate inspection of single experiments. We must refer here to the 5 experiments which do not include any section with internally synchronized rhythms as long as the field was not in operation. In the experiment shown previously (Fig. 57), internal desynchronization occurred immediately after the field was switched off. This, of course, could occur by chance. Of more relevance would be an immediate terminating of internal desynchronization when the field is switched on, because a spontaneous termination of internal desynchronization seems to be a very rare exception, in contrast to a spontaneous beginning. Figure 59 gives an example that, in fact, a forced termination can occur. Internal desynchronization was present with an activity period shorter than the rectal temperature period from the beginning of the experiment. At the 17th objective day, or 21st subjective day, respectively, the artificial 10-Hz field was switched on and, on this day, the rhythm became synchronized internally. In this case, the internal resynchronization is accompanied by a lengthening of the activity period. It might be argued that this field induced lengthening is in contradiction to the stated shortening effect of the field (Table 7). The statement of a general shortening effect of the artificial 10-Hz field, however, is valid only in internally synchro-

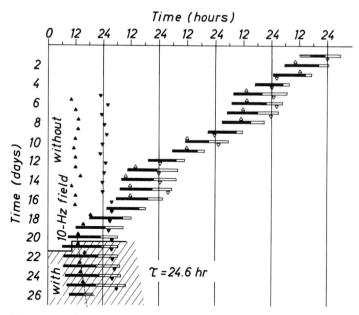

Figure 59. Autonomous rhythm of a subject (D.E., ♂ 27 y) living under constant conditions without time cues and protected from natural and artificial electromagnetic fields during the first section, but under the influence of an artificial electric AC field (i.e., 10 Hz square wave, 2.5 V/m) during the second section. Temporal courses of the rhythms of activity and rectal temperature are presented successively, one period beneath the other. Indications are the same as in figure 27/I. Shaded areas: field in operation. From Wever (1969b).

nized rhythms. It seems to be a second general effect of this field to terminate internal desynchronization. The induced internal re-synchronization is combined necessarily with changes in the periods. The direction of these changes depend on the direction of the previous internal desynchronization (i.e., whether the period of the activity rhythm was longer or shorter than the period of the rectal temperature rhythm). It is another interpretation of the same observation that the drastic lengthening of the activity period, with switching on the field, justifies the linear extrapolation of the regression between effect and original period as derived only from internally synchronized rhythms (Fig. 58/II) to periods which are much shorter than 24 hours.

In another experiment (Fig. 60), internal desynchronization again was present from the beginning of the experiment, but with an activity period longer than the rectal temper-

ature period. After the field was switched on, circa-bi-dian activity periods appeared initially (cf. 2.2.2) and circadian activity periods appeared later; indicating internal synchronization. As the experiment progressed, the artificial field was switched off and on again. When the field was in operation, the rhythms were synchronized internally with either a 1:1 or 2:1 ratio. When the field was not in operation, real internal desynchronization occurred. Another example is shown in figure 61, where real internal desynchronization again occurred from the beginning of the experiment with an activity period longer than in the other examples. After switching on the field at subjective day 10, circa-bi-dian activity periods clearly occurred, indicating internal synchronization. In this special case, the circa-bi-dian period value was closer than a circadian value to the period of the separated activity rhythm, as observed without the field, and, there-

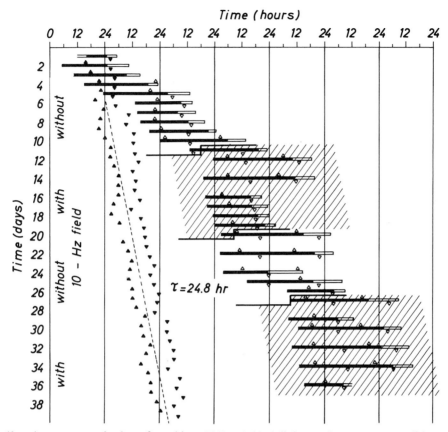

Figure 60.   Autonomous rhythm of a subject (E.R., ♂ 33 y) living under constant conditions without time cues and protected from natural and artificial electromagnetic fields during the first and third sections, but under the influence of an artificial electric AC field (i.e., 10 Hz square wave, 2.5 V/m) during the second and fourth sections. Temporal courses of the rhythms of activity and rectal temperature are presented successively, one period beneath the other. Indications are the same as in figure 59/I. From Wever (1969b).

fore, without a mutual coupling between the different rhythms. An increase in the strength of the mutual coupling must lead to circa-bi-dian rather than to circadian activity periods. After switching off the field, real internal desynchronization again occurred, not with a period between circadian and circa-bi-dian values, however, but with a period even longer than circa-bi-dian. Similar results, with temporal coincidences between switching on and off the 10-Hz field and termination and occurrence of real internal desynchronization, also have been observed in two other experiments. In summary, the frequency in these coincidences is very unlikely to occur spontaneously and, likewise, this consideration significantly

confirms the capacity of the artificial 10-Hz field to prevent internal desynchronization.

With these results, the effects of the weak artificial 10-Hz electric field are equivalent to the effects of the natural electromagnetic fields, regarding all three parameters tested (cf. 2.4.4). The electric field shortens the autonomous period, diminishes the interindividual variability, and reduces the tendency toward internal desynchronization. The results obtained in the shielded room, but under the influence of the artificial 10-Hz field (Table 7), cannot be differentiated from the results obtained in the nonshielded room (Table 6). This means that the artificial 10-Hz field only compensates the effect of the shielding. This result justifies exclusion of

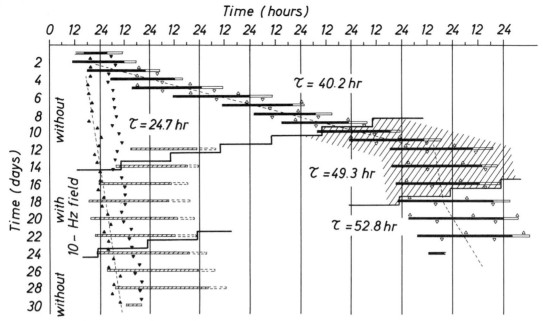

Figure 61.   Autonomous rhythm of a subject (M.B., ♂ 22 y) living under constant conditions without time cues and protected from natural and artificial electromagnetic fields during the first and third sections, but under the influence of an artificial electric AC field (i.e., 10 Hz square wave, 2.5 V/m) during the second section. Temporal courses of the rhythms of activity and rectal temperature are presented successively, one period beneath the other. Indications are the same as in figure 59/I. Shaded bars: temporally correct redrawings of corresponding full bars.

the sections with the 10-Hz field in operation from the comparison between results obtained in the shielded and nonshielded experimental unit (Table 6). A radiation with a frequency of about 10 Hz is found to be included in the natural electromagnetic fields (König, 1959; Harth, 1972, 1975) and is generated in the earth's atmosphere by resonance (Schumann, 1954). The assumption, therefore, is suggested that the 10-Hz field is at least one effective component of the great variety of frequencies included in natural fields. It can not be decided, however, whether or not additional frequencies also are effective in the control of human circadian rhythms.

With the 10-Hz electric field, an artificially applicable stimulus has been found which is effective in the control of autonomous circadian rhythms when continuously in operation, in contrast to light. This consciously perceivable stimulus was ineffective when applied continuously (cf. 2.4.1)

but effective when applied in a self-control mode. It was the hypothesis, under constant illumination, that two opposite effects neutralize each other; a continuous action and a subjective self-control action due to the opening and closing of the eyes. It is of interest to know whether or not the effect of self-controlled conditions can be demonstrated with the 10-Hz field (i.e., with a stimulus which is not perceptible consciously but effective when continuously in operation). Some experiments, therefore, have been performed where the same 10-Hz field, as applied in the other experiments, was given in a self-control mode. The field, of course, could not be switched on and off by the subjects (like light or temperature) because the subjects did not know about the field. The field, rather, was switched on automatically by the recording of activity onset and switched off automatically by the recording of termination of activity, without the knowledge and perceptibility of the subjects.

The course of one of the corresponding experiments is shown in figure 62. During the first and third sections of this experiment, the subject was protected from natural and artificial fields. During the second section, the artificial 10-Hz field was applied in a self-control mode (i.e., it was in operation only as long as the subject was active). The result of this experiment was a lengthening of the autonomous period during the second section. Although a continuously operating field shortened the period in all subjects, a field being in operation only temporarily, during the activity-time, lengthens the period. The other two experiments of this type also had the same result and, therefore, the

lengthening effect of a self-controlled field, in contrast to the shortening effect of a continuously operating field, statistically is significant with $p < 0.01$ (exact Fisher-test). These results demonstrate that the effect of self-control is not restricted to perceptible stimuli and is not restricted to those stimuli whose effects are compensated normally (e.g., light, temperature). The effect of self-controlled conditions on the autonomous period has been shown to be a general effect independent of the stimulus applied.

The results of the experiments performed with electromagnetic fields, as the controlling stimuli, have very different aspects (Wever, 1973b). The primary aspect is that they allow the evaluation of properties of human circadian rhythms more successfully than results of experiments performed with any other controlling stimulus. In the context to be discussed here, the main emphasis is given to this aspect, which applies the electromagnetic field as the only reliable tool. This aspect will be subject to further considerations (cf. 4.1.1). Another aspect of these results is that they have the capability to give significant general evidence for biological effects of electromagnetic fields (Adey and Bawin, 1977). This secondary aspect, which applies the human circadian system as an especially sensitive indicator for detecting effects of subtle stimuli, becomes of increasing practical interest (Wever, 1971a). It has been ignored widely in the past and the results obtained, so far, do not allow relevant statements. It is not clear whether the effect observed is induced directly by the electric field; or only indirectly, for example, by a magnetic field accompanying the electric field; or a change in ionization affected by the field. Moreover, it is not clear whether the applied square wave is effective due to its fundamental frequency of 10 Hz or to higher harmonics which are included in the square wave itself. Even the frequency of 10 kHz is included with a field strength of some mV/m (i.e., with a field strength comparable to the natural field with this frequency). A decision regarding this latter uncertainty is possible, in principle, by

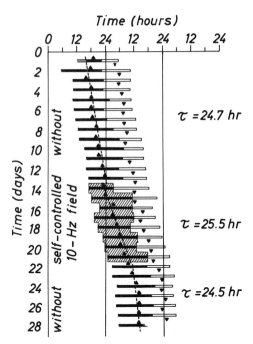

Figure 62. Autonomous rhythm of a subject (R.S., ♀ 24 y) living without environmental time cues under constant conditions and protected from natural and artificial electromagnetic fields during the first and third sections, but under the influence of a self-controlled cycle of an artificial electric AC field (i.e., 10 Hz square wave, 2.5 V/ m, in operation only during the activity time of the subject), during the second section. Temporal courses of the rhythms of activity and rectal temperature are presented successively, one period beneath the other. Indications are the same as in figure 55/I. From Wever (1968c).

applying sine waves instead of square waves of 10 Hz. Some of the preliminary experiments had results similar to those using square waves. An example of such an experiment is shown in figure 63. Some experiments, however, were not successful but did show unchanged periods, in contrast to the consistent result in all experiments using square waves. An unambiguous decision, therefore, needs more experimentation. Finally, there are no human experiments to answer the question specifically concerning the effect regarding the frequency or the field strength of the field applied. The thorough processing of this secondary aspect would need a great amount of data that cannot be obtained practically from experiments lasting not shorter than 4 weeks. Because of all these uncertainties, it must be emphasized that the term '10-Hz field,' as used in this book, is nothing but a designation for a tool, the effective component of which is still unknown. It also must be emphasized that the use of this term should not anticipate, in any way, the specific mode of action of this applied tool. There is a third, but very speculative, aspect of the present results obtained in experiments applying electromagnetic fields which may become preferential in future investigations concerning circadian rhythms; this being the circadian system is responsive to electromagnetic fields generated not only in the natural environment but also within the organism itself. This aspect may help in the search for the basic mechanism underlying circadian rhythmicity.

2.4.6. Influence of Physical Workload

To here, only effects of environmental stimuli on autonomous rhythms have been considered. There are possibly other stimuli effecting circadian rhythms which originate in the subjects themselves. Those stimuli may be connected with the special experimental conditions of strict isolation. The physical exercise performed by the subjects during an isolation experiment inside the limited experimental room, for example, can be expected to be less than during the normal life of the subjects. It also cannot be excluded that the amount of the performed workload influences the course of circadian rhytymicity. A series of experiments, therefore, has been performed to answer the question whether or not there is an influence of physical workload on the period, and other parameters, of autonomous circadian rhythms. In these experiments, the subjects had performed, during one section of the experiment lasting for about 2 weeks, a hard work-

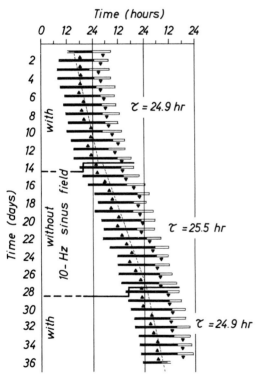

Figure 63. Autonomous rhythm of a subject (H.H., ♂ 30 y) living under constant conditions without time cues and under the influence of an artificial electric AC field (i.e., 10 Hz sine wave, 2.5 V/m) during the first and third sections, but protected from natural and artificial electromagnetic fields during the second section. Temporal courses of the rhythms of activity and rectal temperature are presented successively, one period beneath the other. Indications are the same as in figure 16/I.

load on a bicycle ergometer and were requested to behave as leisurely as possible during the other section of the same experiment, also lasting for about 2 weeks. The temporal sequence of the with and without workload sections were altered from experiment to experiment.

The temporal course of an experiment from this series is shown in figure 64. During the second section of this experiment, the subject performed, 7 times in each activity time, a workload of 100 W for 20 to 30 minutes each. The effectiveness of this hard workload could be seen in the record of the rectal temperature. Each working period resulted in an instant increase of body temperature for 0.5 to 1.0 °C. As can be seen in figure 64/I, the beginning of the working section is accompanied by a drastic retardation of the autonomous rhythms. The circadian period during the working section, in fact, is the longest autonomous period, with internally synchronized rhythms, ever seen and the alteration in the period is the greatest ever observed in a rectal temperature rhythm. This statement is confirmed by the computed period analyses (Fig. 64/II), presented separately for the sections without and with workload. In each section, only one spectral line is present in all measured rhythms but the relevant periods of the two sections are separated clearly from each other without overlapping. The longitudinal pooling of the rhythms, also computed separately for the two sections (Fig. 64/III), shows the leading phase of the rectal temperature rhythm relative to the activity rhythm, characteristic in autonomous rhythms. Figure 64/III, especially, shows that the internal phase relationship, between the two rhythms presented, is the same in both sections in spite of the different periods. This result confirms, once more, that the internal phase relationship between different autonomous rhythms is independent of the period. The reliability of the rectal temperature rhythm is not as good in the second section (with the workload) as in the first section. This difference mainly is based

on an enlarged variability of the temperature during activity but not during rest. This is due to the frequent increases in body temperature caused by the working periods. Because the intervals between successive working periods are necessarily self-selected, the working periods do not coincide in successive activity times.

In the experiment presented in figure 64, the period was much longer when performing a hard workload than without working. This interrelation, however, is not the rule in all experiments. Figure 65 shows the course of another experiment from this series, with equal temporal sequence of the sections without and with workload and equally performed workload. In this experiment, the period remained unchanged. In the seven other experiments of this series, the results are inconsistent. In all experiments, except those underlying figure 65, the period changed with the transition between the sections with and without workload, but not regularly regarding the direction, and in no other experiment as drastically as in the experiment underlying figure 64. Table 8 summarizes the results of all 9 experiments of this series. The workload was, in all experiments, the same amount described in figure 64. As can be seen from table 8, the average lengthening in the period, as a consequence of the physical workload (eliminating the interindividual variabilities), was 0.44 ± 1.35 hours. This average change surely is due to only one single experiment (Fig. 64). After elimination of this experiment, a lengthening in the period of only 0.01 ± 0.40 hours results. This means, even with a greatly increased number of corresponding experiments, a statistically significant change cannot be expected in the period.

It would, nevertheless, be hasty to conclude from these results that physical workload is ineffective regarding human circadian rhythms. This conclusion neglects the fact that in nearly all experiments the period changed on the day of the transition between the sections which were with and without a workload, though not according to a rule.

This temporal coincidence is much better than it would be with only chance variations. The effect of physical workload on the period resembles, rather, the effect of constant illumination, which had been assumed to be a net effect of two opposite actions of light (i.e., a continuous action and a self-control action due to a special behavior changing with the state of activity). A special behavior (exercising a hard workload) is the source of the effect to be expected here, and this behavior is performed only during activity time but not during rest time. It may be suggested, therefore, that the effect of physical workload on autonomously running circadian rhythms is the result of two opposite actions more or less neutralizing each other. Following this suggestion, it must be assumed the compensation mechanism was not in operation during the special experiment underlying figure 64. Future experiments will examine the correctness of this conclusion.

The effect of a physical workload is the only effect on the period of autonomous rhythms to which references from other authors are available. Webb and Agnew (1974a) have examined 14 subjects in individual isolation experiments lasting 10 to 14 days each. Seven of the subjects performed a hard physical workload on an exercise bicycle similar to that in our experiments. The other seven subjects served as controls. The authors stated an average period of 25.38 hours developed with the exercise group and 25.27 hours with the control group. As in the experiments described earlier, there is a weak tendency to lengthen the autonomous period while performing a physical workload but, again, this tendency is far from any statistical significance. Correspondingly, the authors concluded equal periods existed with and without performing the work-load but, in addition, they concluded a variability of the activity rhythms were significantly greater in the exercise group than in the control group. Figure 66 shows the courses of alternations between sleep and wakefulness of 8 of the 14 subjects (four without and four with the workload).

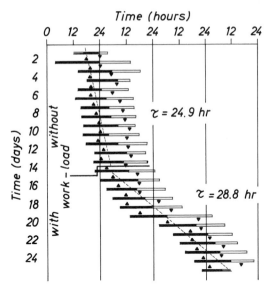

Figure 64. Autonomous rhythm of a subject (K.S., ♂ 22 y) living under constant conditions without time cues and during the second section performing a heavy workload on a bicycle ergometer (i.e., 100 W, for about 20 minutes, seven times per activity period). *I*. Temporal courses of the rhythms of activity and rectal temperature, presented successively one period beneath the other. Indications are the same as in figure 16/I.

The results obtained by Webb and Agnew (1974a) are in full agreement with the results discussed above.

2.4.7. Influence of Psychical Burden

Comparable experiments to test effects of psychical stress or extended performance tests have not been undertaken yet. Suggestions of possible effects may be deduced from the comparison between results of experiments where the subjects were not burdened by psychological or psychomotor tests and results of experiments where the subjects performed those tests. At the beginning of the experimental series, only preliminary tests in a few experiments were given the subjects by applying common types of test devices. It was the result of these studies that even multiprogramable devices could not be applied meaningful in long term experiments. Automatically operated de-

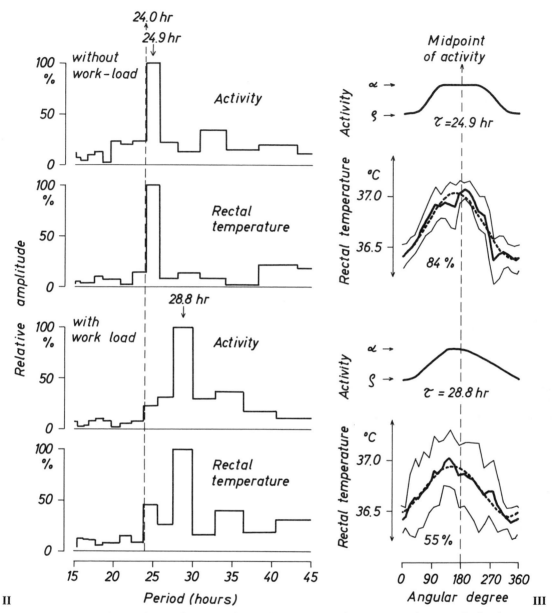

Figure 64/II.   Period analyses of the two time series, presented in I, computed separately for the two sections, without and with performing a physical workload. *III.* Longitudinally pooled courses of the two rhythms, computed separately for the two sections, with averaging periods derived from II. Indications are the same as in figure 16/III.

vices, therefore, have been developed which are controlled by random generators and do not need any cooperation with an experimenter. These automatized tests included computation speeds (Pauli-test), reaction times (multiple choice), and hand and eye coordination. During the last years, the sub-

jects had to perform, regularly in all experiments, at least one of these tests (frequently two different tests) about 6 to 10 times per 'day.'

The tests mentioned can be performed meaningful only in experiments with heteronomous rhythms. In autonomous rhythms,

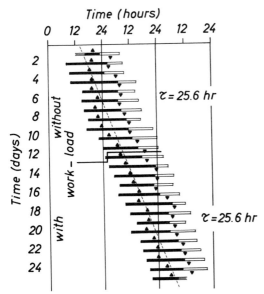

Figure 65. Autonomous rhythm of a subject (T.S., ♂ 25 y) living under constant conditions without time cues and during the second section performing a heavy workload on a bicycle ergometer (i.e., 100 W, for about 20 minutes, seven times per activity period). Temporal courses of the rhythms of activity and rectal temperature are presented successively, one period beneath the other. Indications are the same as in figure 16/I.

Table 8. *Effect of Physical Workload*

Subject	Autonomous period		
	without workload	with workload	difference
G.E., ♂ 26 y	24.5 hr	24.9 hr	0.4 hr
W.R., ♂ 28 y	24.5	24.9	0.4
K.S., ♂ 22 y	24.9	28.8	3.9
P.C., ♂ 23 y	24.6	24.4	− 0.2
K.M., ♂ 25 y	25.0	24.7	− 0.3
T.S., ♂ 25 y	25.6	25.6	0.0
T.S., ♂ 25 y	24.6	25.0	0.4
B.S., ♂ 27 y	25.5	24.8	− 0.7
H.K., ♂ 27 y	24.3	24.4	0.1
Mean (n = 9)	24.83 hr	25.27 hr	0.44 hr
Standard dev.	± 0.46 hr	± 1.37 hr	± 1.35 hr
Mean (n = 8) except Subj. K.S.	24.83 hr	24.84 hr	0.01 hr
Standard dev.	± 0.49 hr	± 0.38 hr	± 0.40 hr

Statistical analysis concerning: Difference in periods ≠ 0 (with n = 9)

  t-test: t = 0.98 n.s.
  Wilcoxon-test: T = 12 n.s.

the unavoidable 'night-gap' in the performance data prevents the determination of rhythm parameters (cf. 1.3.2). In experiments of special design, the advantages of both types of experiments (with autonomous and heteronomous rhythms) can be combined. This may be accomplished in experiments where parts of the overt rhythms are synchronized to an external zeitgeber while other overt rhythms run autonomously (cf. 3.3). In these experiments, not only the properties of performance rhythms (Fig. 86) but, also in some preliminary experiments, influences of the amount of psychical burden on circadian rhythms were evaluated (Fig. 93). Those experiments, however, have not been performed under constant conditions and, therefore, details should not be discussed in this context (cf. 3.3.2.).

Since about 1969, the performance tests mentioned were used generally in all experiments (i.e., even in experiments under constant conditions where the evaluation of parameters of performance rhythms was meaningless) (s. above). The burden to the subjects of psychical or performance tests was, on the average, higher in experiments since 1969 than in earlier experiments, independent of the type of experiment. The comparison between autonomous rhythms, measured before and after this temporal limit, was given in table 6, although originally for another purpose. For reasons to be discussed later (cf. 2.4.9), the differences between the two intervals of years (1964 to 1968 versus 1969 to 1976) can be seen only in experiments performed in one of the two experimental units available (i.e., the nonshielded room). If all single experiments are compared (Table 6, nonshielded room, samples 3 and 12), the periods are, on the average, longer during the later interval of years (1969 to 1976) than the earlier interval (1964 to 1968). The difference in the mean periods is significant when applying the parametric t-test (t = 2.03; $p < 0.025$) and the nonparametric U-test (u = 2.02; p = 0.021). Since, in the small number of experiments with self-controlled illumination, equal mean periods resulted in both intervals of years (Ta-

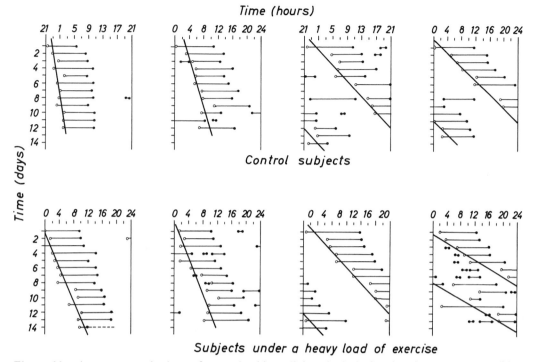

Figure 66. Autonomous rhythms of several subjects living singly isolated under constant conditions without time cues. Upper row: results from four (of seven) subjects serving as controls. Lower row: results from four (of seven) subjects performing a heavy workload. Temporal courses of the activity rhythms are presented successively, one day beneath the other. Vertical lines: sleep times of the subjects. Abscissa: local time. Ordinate: sequence of successive days. The oblique lines are regressions computed by the authors. From Webb and Agnew (1974a).

ble 6, nonshielded room, samples 9 and 14), the difference mentioned is more pronounced when experiments with only constant illumination are considered (i.e., when a more homogeneous sample is considered). Here (Table 6, nonshielded room, samples 6 and 13), the difference in the mean periods is significant at a higher level ($t = 3.00$; $p <$ 0.0025. $u = 2.62$; $p = 0.0043$). In the respective samples, the tendency towards internal desynchronization is greater during the later than the earlier interval of years, but not to a significant amount ($p = 0.12$, with all experiments, and $p = 0.11$, with constant illumination experiments only; exact Fisher-test). Considering the experiments performed in the shielded room, there are no significant differences between the successive intervals of years in any respect (Table 6).

Of course, the result just discussed (specifically, the mean period was significantly

longer and the tendency toward interval desynchronization was greater during later than earlier experiments) by no means can be attributed conclusively to psychical workload which was higher during the later than the earlier experiments. There also may be other reasons to affect such a temporal trend. The result mentioned may be only a suggestion to look more specifically for effects of psychical burdens.

There are special types of experiments where the subjects are burdened heavier than in normal experiments performed under constant conditions. These are in experiments with continuous polygraphic sleep recording. During such 4-week experiments, the isolated subject had to attach, before going to sleep, various electrodes to his head, control the contact resistances of these electrodes, and connect wires to a terminal near his bed. This total procedure lasts nearly 1 hour. The sleep itself is burdened, at least for the first time, by the unusual 'chaining up' of the isolated subjects. The continuous sleep recording by EEG is undoubtedly a stronger molestation to the subject than the unperceived sleep recording by simply measuring bed movements in the other experiments (cf. 1.3.2). Although the number of corresponding experiments is, to the present, too small to allow relevant statements, it seems obvious that the tendency toward internal desynchronization is considerably higher in these experiments than in normal experiments without EEG recording. In four out of the six EEG experiments (two out of the six have been performed after closing the tables included in this paper), internal desynchronization occured; in two from the beginning (Figure 12/13; in the other with temporarily circa-bidian activity periods) and in two experiments after 1 through 3 weeks. In the last experiments, internal dissociation occured (Figure 113), so that there was not one EEG experiment with an undisturbed rhythm as has been observed in more than half the other experiments (cf. 2.3). Moreover, the autonomous periods of the EEG experiments happened to be, on the average, longer than the average of the other experiments. These experiments again give evidence that an increasing burdening on the subjects influences human circadian rhythms in the same way as increasing the amounts of tests to be performed. The results, in fact, are significant (in the non-shielded room, 6 out of 46 singly isolated subjects without EEG record showed internal desynchronization but 4 out of 6 subjects with EEG record showed; $p = 0.002$; exact Fisher test) but may be influenced by any other factor (e.g., higher scores of neuroticism in the EEG subjects); therefore, they cannot give more than suggestions.

In summary, there are some suggestions that psychical burden on the subjects constitutes a stimulus which has the capability to influence autonomously running circadian rhythms of man. This means, in particular, a lengthening of the period and an increase in the tendency toward internal desynchroniza-

tion occurs. In contrast to effects of other stimuli discussed in this chapter, effects of 'stress' are not yet significant at a sufficient level. The main difficulty in performing experiments, with the specific objective of testing these effects quantitatively, is the impossibility of applying stressing burdens of a well defined amount. All other external stimuli discussed (including physical workload) can be measured objectively. The amount of psychical stress released by a definite stimulus (e.g., by a definite performance test), however, depends on the predisposition and the motivation of the subject. For example, a performance test of a definite amount constituted a serious molestation for one subject, according to his own statements. Another subject, who performed the same test, asked for a more extensive test in order to have sufficient psychical training. As the result, a definite change in the amount of this test would have released opposite changes in the 'stress' of the two subjects. The interindividual variability in rhythm parameters depending on changes in psychical burden, therefore, must be expected to be much greater than depending on any other stimulus.

There appears to be only one animal experiment dealing with the influence of stress on circadian rhythms. In this experiment (Stroebel, 1969), rhesus monkeys became stressed behaviorally by an experimental procedure while continuously under the influence of a 24-hour light-dark cycle. The brain temperature rhythms of the stressed animals either free-run, or showed periods of 48 hours, in spite of the persisting 24-hour light-dark cycle. These experiments were not performed under constant conditions and, therefore, are not comparable directly to the human experiments mentioned. They showed, in general, that 'stress' has the capacity to influence circadian rhythmicity.

2.4.8. Influence of Social Contacts

Finally, there is another experimental condition that may influence circadian rhythmicity; the strict isolation of subjects. In most

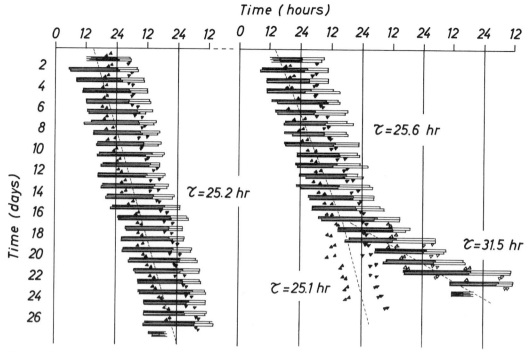

Figure 67. Autonomous rhythms of two groups of two subjects (left: W.S., ♂ 25 y, and H.O., ♂ 25 y; right: K.R., ♂ 23 y, and G.K., ♂ 23 y) living collectively under constant conditions without time cues. Temporal courses of the rhythms of activity and rectal temperature are presented successively, one period beneath the other, with the rhythms of the different subjects within one group arranged immediately one beneath the other. Indications are the same as in figure 27/I. From Wever (1975b).

experiments, subjects lived in solitary isolation and, in comparison to their normal lives, they had a lack of social contacts. It cannot be excluded that the amount of the social contacts influences the course of human circadian rhythms. The question of possible influences of such contacts on autonomous rhythms, can be answered by comparing results of experiments where subjects were isolated singly with results of group experiments where some subjects were isolated collectively. With this comparison, only experiments where the illumination was constant and not selfcontrolled can be considered. With selfcontrolled illumination, the effect of the number of subjects is superimposed by the effect of the selfcontrol which is different in individual and group experiments, as mentioned above (cf. 2.4.2).

There is generally no conspicuous difference between the results of individual and group experiments. Figure 67 shows, for example, courses of two different experiments

which were performed each with two male subjects living collectively in isolation in one experimental unit for 4 weeks under constant conditions without environmental time cues. In the experiment shown at the left side, the resulting autonomous rhythms of both subjects remained unchanged during the total experiment. The most striking result is that both subjects showed equal periods, with their activity rhythms, rectal temperature rhythms, and with all other rhythms measured. This means that the rhythms of each subject were synchronized internally and the rhythms of the two subjects were synchronized mutually. A similar result was obtained in seven more experiments with two subjects in each.

In a part of the group experiments, as in individual experiments with autonomous rhythms, internal desynchronization occurred spontaneously. This can be seen in the other example of figure 67, shown at the right side. After about 2 weeks with internally synchronized rhythms, spontaneously internal desynchronization occurred and lasted until the end of the experiment. During the first 2 weeks, the two activity rhythms and the two rectal temperature rhythms showed equal periods, indicating internal and mutual synchronization. After the occurrence of internal desynchronization, the two activity rhythms again showed equal periods, although of a much larger value. This indicates that the subjects still were synchronized with respect to their perceivable activity rhythms. It is much more remarkable that the two rectal temperature rhythms also seem to remain synchronized mutually, although these rhythms consciously were not perceivable. It can be seen in the right diagram of figure 67, during the last part of the experiment, the rectal temperature rhythms were separated from the activity rhythms but there was no systematic temporal sequence in the positions of the temperature rhythms of the two subjects. On some days, the rhythm of one subject was the leading while, on other days, the rhythm of the other subject led. This occurred without any regular sequence. It is suggested from these results that not only activity rhythms are able to synchronize with each other, but rectal temperature rhythms, although not perceivable consciously, also are capable of obtaining mutual synchronization independent of the activity rhythms. Similar results were obtained in three more group experiments, where internal desynchronization occurred. In three of these experiments, the activity period was longer than the rectal temperature period and, in one experiment, was shorter.

There was a total of twelve group experiments where two subjects lived together in isolation in the nonshielded experimental unit without environmental time cues and with constant illumination. Because of the mutual dependence of the subjects within a group, only the groups, and not the subjects, can be taken for statistical units. The results of these experiments must be compared with the results of the 37 singly isolated subjects living under identical conditions (Table 6, nonshielded room, sample 16). This comparison, together with the statistical analyses, is shown in table 9. As can be seen, the mean autonomous period is significantly longer in groups than in single experiments, as proven by applying the parametric t-test and the nonparametric U-test. The variability of the periods, moreover, is significantly smaller in groups than in single experiments (F-test) and the tendency toward internal desynchronization is greater in groups than in single experiments, but only close to the limit of significance (exact Fisher-test). In summary, it can be concluded that the mutual social contacts between the different subjects within a collectively isolated group affect autonomous circadian rhythmicity significantly. In particular, these contacts lengthen the period, diminish the interindividual variability of the periods, and tend to enlarge the frequency in the spontaneous occurrence of internal desynchronization. In the group experiment shown in figure 50, the illumination was self-controlled and the lengthening effect of the social contacts was overcompensated by the shortening effect of the self-control compensation (cf. 2.4.2).

In addition to group experiments with two subjects, there was one experiment with four subjects, isolated collectively, in the

Table 9. *Effects of Mutual Social Contacts*

Parameter	Isolation experiments with each		Statistical analyses
	one subject	two subjects	
Number of experiments	37	12	
Mean period $\bar{\tau}$	24.79 hr	25.08 hr	$t = 2.34, p < 0.0125$
Standard deviation of τ	± 0.41 hr	± 0.21 hr	$F = 3.81, p < 0.05$
Median of periods	24.77 hr	25.10 hr	$u = 2.85, p = 0.0022$
Number of experiments with internal desynchronization	4 (= 11%)	4 (= 33%)	$p = 0.072$

two experimental units, which were connected for this special experiment. This experiment was planned originally to study the social behavior within an isolated group. Emphasis in this experiment, therefore, was placed on the acquisition of psychological, instead of physiological, data (Poeppel, 1968). For instance, rectal temperature was not recorded continuously, as in all other experiments, but only during the sleep of the subjects. This experiment, nevertheless, had a remarkable result regarding physiological measurements. All four subjects were not mutually synchronized during the total experiment, regarding their activity rhythms. One subject showed, at least during the second section of the experiment, an autonomous period shorter than the autonomous periods of the other subjects. Figure 68/I shows the temporal course of the activity rhythms in this experiment. During the first section, with brighter illumination, the subject, whose activity rhythm is presented in the uppermost position, led the activity rhythms of the other subjects. During the second section, when the illumination was decreased, this subject showed an activity period which evidently was shorter than those of the other subjects. His activity rhythm seemed to be synchronized to 24.0 hours. It must be appended here that all four subjects participating in this special experiment were tested earlier in individual experiments. The subject, who seemed to be synchronized externally, was the same subject who was shown earlier to be sensitive against synchronizing social cues from the outside (Fig. 20). The other subjects showed a period of the overt activity rhythms which were longer during the second section, with dimmer illumination, than during the first section, with the brighter illumination. Since, in this experiment, the illumination was self-controlled, this result is in agreement with other results discussed earlier (Fig. 50).

Physiological data, which may help in a better understanding of the results obtained in this experiment, are available only from urine constituents. In the next step, period analyses of the rhythms of those variables, therefore, will be considered. Because the separate sections, with a constant intensity of illumination, were too short to give meaningful results, period analyses have been computed from the total experiment, regardless of the change in light intensity. Figure 68/II shows results computed from the potassium excretion and urine volume, presented separately for the four subjects in the same order, from top to bottom, as in the presentation of the activity rhythms (Fig. 68/I). Regarding the potassium excretion, all four subjects show reliable rhythms, but with different periods. The subject with the shortest activity period also shows the shortest period in potassium excretion. The other three subjects, with uniform activity periods, do not show uniform periods in the potassium excretion. Only the subject, presented in the lowermost position, shows a period coinciding in activity and potassium excretion. In the analyses of the urine volume rhythms, only two subjects show reliable rhythms, but with different periods. Period analyses from the other urine constituents (e.g., sodium, calcium) result in even more ambiguous spectra, without any reliable period. The consideration of the rhythm analyses, therefore, lead to conclusions similar to those of the overt activity rhythms. In this special experiment, the subjects, who were isolated collectively, did not show synchronous circadian rhythms. To assess this result, it must be stated that the four subjects did not know each other until the beginning of the experiment and had no strong collective interests during the experiment.

There is another series of experiments where subjects have been isolated from environmental time cues in an artificial isolation unit; seven subjects living singly and eight subjects in two groups of four (Mills et al., 1974). The experiments of this series, however, lasted only 5 to 13 days (mean ± standard deviation: 9.3 ± 2.3 days; with equal means of the solitary and group experiments). Most of the experiments did not last long enough to determine a steady state period value. Consequently, the authors stated, in most cases, different periods in the

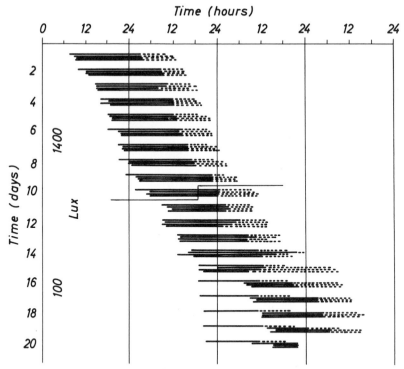

Figure 68. Autonomous rhythms of a group of four subjects (A.S., ♂ 27 y; F.M., ♂ 25 y; J.K., ♂ 23 y; and H.v.B., ♂ 28 y) living collectively under constant conditions without time cues, with one alteration in the intensity of illumination. *I.* Temporal courses of the activity rhythms, presented successively one period beneath the other, with the rhythms of the four subjects arranged immediately one beneath the other. Solid lines: activity. Dotted lines: rest. From Poeppel (1968).

rhythms of activity, body temperature, and six different urine constituents. The data available from these experiments, therefore, are not sufficient to discriminate between periods of solitary subjects and groups. Moreover, two of the seven singly isolated subjects and one of the two groups showed abnormally long activity periods, suggesting internal desynchronization. The low number of experiments and the uncertainty because of the short durations do not allow discriminations between solitary subjects and groups regarding the tendency toward internal desynchronization.

In another experiment, with a group of collectively isolated subjects (Apfelbaum and Nillus, 1967; Apfelbaum et al., 1969; Nillus, 1967), seven female subjects lived together for 14 days in a cave. The alternation between wakefulness and sleep showed

identical periods of 24.7 hours in all subjects, indicating mutual synchronization. Since there was no control experiment with subjects singly isolated under equivalent conditions, a statement about the effect of the mutual contacts on autonomous rhythms cannot be given. The same is true with an experiment of Winget (1975) where two groups of three subjects temporarily ran freely. They each showed identical periods of 24.2 hours and 25.0 hours, respectively, again indicating mutual social synchronization.

2.4.9. Summary

Summarizing the results obtained in this chapter, there are several stimuli which have the capacity to modify autonomous circa-

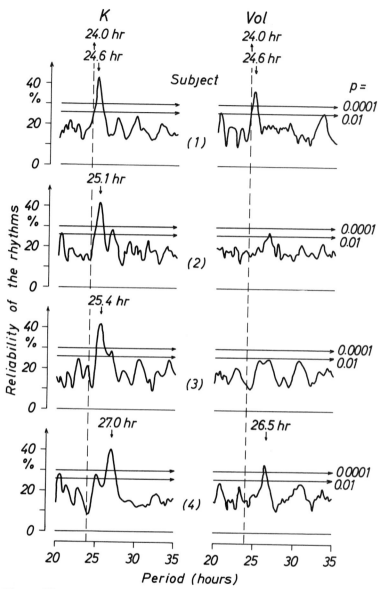

Figure 68/II.   Period analyses of the time series of potassium excretion and urine volume (i.e., mictions taken at self-selected intervals), computed for the total experiment, from data of the four different subjects.

dian rhythms of man. These stimuli are as different as light, temperature, electric AC-fields, psychical stress, and mutual social contacts. Most relevantly, all these stimuli have been shown experimentally to affect the autonomous period. In particular, with only one exception (electric AC-field), they lengthen the period. Even those stimuli with no significant effects (i.e., light intensity,

physical workload) indicate this tendency. Perhaps it is not accidental that the only external stimulus which shortens the period, when operating continuously (i.e., electric AC-field), is the only one which is not perceivable consciously. All other stimuli which, in total, lengthen the period, operate differently during activity time and rest time, either due to an artificial selfcontrol mode (i.e., light, temperature) or, though only hypothetically, a behavioral self-control (i.e., constant light) or due to an exercising which is restricted to the activity time (i.e., physical and psychical workload; social contacts). In future experiments, care must be taken to determine whether the direction of an effect released by an external stimulus depends on the quality of the stimulus or the operation mode of the stimulus (i.e., to operate with, regarding the perception of the subject, either continuous or periodic changes controlled by the activity state of the subjects). This problem is different from the problem of a periodically changing sensitiveness of a receptor as a necessary prerequisite of the synchronization by external stimuli (cf. 3.5).

The second parameter of autonomous rhythms, which is affected by the stimuli tested, is the tendency toward internal desynchronization. With all stimuli, it is a consistent result that changes in the conditions, which result in lengthened periods, simultaneously affect an increase in the tendency toward internal desynchronization. Under conditions where the autonomous periods are shortened, the frequency in the spontaneous occurrence of internal desynchronization always is diminished. Moreover, it is a consistent result, of all different types of experiments with singly isolated subjects, that changes in the conditions, which result in lengthened periods, simultaneously affect an increase in the interindividual variability of the periods. Under conditions where the autonomous periods are shortened, this variability is diminished. Only in the group experiments, where the periods are longer than in individual experiments, the variability between the groups is diminished, due to the mutual synchronization of the subjects being isolated collectively. These interdependencies between the three parameters mentioned correspond, even quantitatively, to postulations of a general oscillation model (Wever, 1971b). From this correspondence, it could be concluded that the separate consideration of the three parameters does not add to the information obtained from the consideration of only one parameter. This

conclusion, however, presupposes the adequacy of the underlying model concept and, rather, it has to be concluded reversely that the proven correspondence confirms this adequacy. The correspondence between theoretical and measured interdependencies increases the significance of the effects found experimentally, owing to the mutual confirmation of the effects shown with the separate parameters. It is characteristic, even in those cases where changes in the separate parameters cannot be guaranteed significantly (e.g., depending on the intensity of constant illumination), that the interdependencies have the same signs as in cases of significant effects.

Finally, the effect of a stimulus on the autonomous period and the other parameters has been shown to depend on the original period. This effect, in particular, is greater the longer the period. The data available are not sufficient to decide whether the relation between effect and original period is a linear one, with the consequence that the effect of a definite stimulus would be reversed when the original period is much shorter than the average and this stimulus would be ineffective with an 'optimum period'; or a nonlinear one, with the consequence that the effect of a definite stimulus is minimal with an 'optimum period' and increases in amount without changing its sign with periods increasing and decreasing from this special value. In any case, there is a special period value where the effect is minimal, or even zero. It would be of interest to know whether or not this 'optimum period' is the same with all kinds of effective stimuli. The data available, indeed, are compatible with this assumption but they are not strictly forcing this assumption. Further experiments, therefore, must be undertaken to solve this problem quantitatively.

It is an open question whether or not there exists another correlation between original period and lengthening effect of a stimulus, to the effect that the period cannot be lengthened to values beyond a certain limit. This correlation would mean a definite stimulus, which normally lengthens the period, is less effective, or even ineffective, if the original period was lengthened previously, for instance, by any other lengthening stimulus. At least the assumption of such a correlation is consistent with different experimental findings. To give examples (Table 6), electromagnetic shielding significantly lengthened the periods in experiments with constant illumination but not with self-controlled illumination where the periods previously are longer due to self-control. Furthermore, electromagnetic shielding lengthened the periods significantly during the first interval of years (1964 to 1968) but not during the second (1969 to 1976), where the periods generally were longer (possibly due to increased psychical burden). Increased psychical burden, during the second interval of years, lengthened the periods significantly in experiments which were performed in the nonshielded experimental unit but not in the shielded unit, where the periods previously were lengthened. It must be a subject of further investigations to see whether this correlation, if confirmed, is due to changing responsiveness against the stimuli, depending on period, or to a generally limited capability of the periods to exceed certain limits.

3
Heteronomous Rhythms

In all experiments discussed so far, human circadian rhythms were running autonomously (i.e., without environmental time cues). It was shown that environmental stimuli, indeed, are able to modify the rhythms, but this influencing did not break, even when effective in a self-control mode, the autonomy of the rhythms. In contrast to this, under natural conditions circadian rhythms are synchronized to the day-night cycle (i.e., to a period of exactly 24.0 hours). Two questions, therefore, arise; what is the mechanism of synchronization and what is the periodic environmental stimulus which is able to synchronize human circadian rhythms? To answer these questions, experiments must be performed where natural zeitgebers are excluded, as in experiments with autonomously running rhythms. Artificial zeitgebers then must be introduced which, in contrast to natural ones, can be manipulated experimentally regarding period, phase, and other parameters. In the first place, the question for the general effects of zeitgebers will be evaluated independently of the kind of zeitgeber that is effective.

3.1. General Effects of External Zeitgebers

3.1.1. Alterations of the Zeitgeber Period

In the first experimental series to be discussed, the period of an artificial zeitgeber has been altered. In figure 69, the course of a typical experiment is shown which was performed with a subject living in the same strict isolation from natural time cues as the other subjects with autonomous rhythms, but under the influence of an artificial "day-night" cycle of varying periods. During the first section, the zeitgeber had a period of 24.0 hours, coinciding with the natural day-night cycle. The subject (a student) was entrained, with a phase relationship about the same as during his normal life (i.e., he started his activity at about noon and terminated his activity time shortly before the end of the dark time). The subject was informed he would be exposed to an artificial day coinciding with the natural day and he was able to switch on small auxiliary lamps dur-

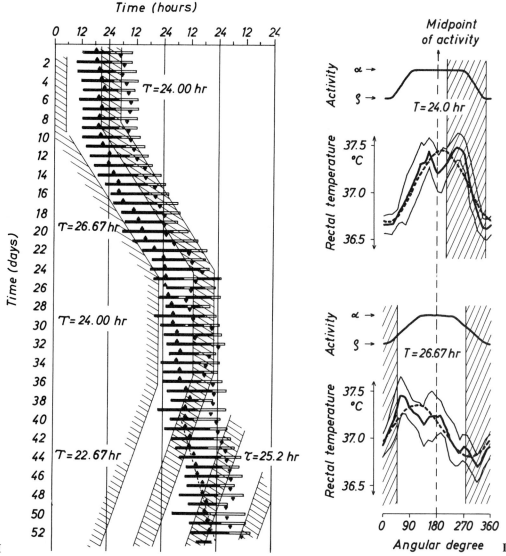

Figure 69. Rhythm of a subject (S.R., ♂ 24 y) living without environmental time cues but under the influence of an artificial zeitgeber with three alterations of the zeitgeber period. *I.* Temporal courses of the rhythms of activity and rectal temperature, presented successively one period beneath the other. Indications are the same as in figure 16/I. Shaded areas: "night time" of the zeitgeber. From Aschoff et al. (1969). *II.* Longitudinally pooled courses of the two rhythms, computed separately for the first and second sections, with an averaging period corresponding to the zeitgeber period. Indications are the same as in figure 16/III. Shaded areas: "night time" of the zeitgeber.

ing the dark-time, as in his normal life, when it became night.

After ten days, the period of the artificial zeitgeber was lengthened, without the knowledge of the subject, to 26 hours 40 minutes. The subject did not perceive this alteration but reacted to it. He, indeed, re-

mained entrained to this zeitgeber period, but with a phase relationship drastically changed. After transient periods of about 1 week duration, he started his activity around 'sun-rise' and terminated his activity shortly after 'sun-set'. Ten days after the alteration of the zeitgeber period, the subject wrote an information letter to the experimenter stating he felt very happy, possibly because of his very unusual behavior of 'getting up with the chickens', but he could not perceive any reason for this behavior. At his 25th subjective day, the zeitgeber period was realtered to 24.0 hours and this alteration was perceived well enough by the subject. The day after the alteration, he wrote another information letter stating he had perceived a very uncomfortable alteration in the experimental design, obviously resulting in absolutely abnormal conditions. Even after finishing the experiment, he could not believe that the apparently unnatural condition consisted of a 24-hour day. At subjective day 36, the zeitgeber period was once more shortened, to a value of 22 hours 40 minutes. As can be seen in figure 69/I, this period was too short to follow (i.e., it was out of the range of entrainment). The subject showed a period which must be expected under constant conditions when the rhythm runs autonomously and, therefore, it must be concluded the subject's rhythm was not synchronized to this zeitgeber period, but ran freely. It surely can be seen that the zeitgeber, during the last section, was not ineffective because the s-shaped course indicates 'relative coordination,' which is typical of a zeitgeber effect being too weak for full entrainment. The subject had not noticed, during the last section, that he was exposed to a regular light-dark cycle. He believed an irregular change in the conditions had been introduced.

In the experiment underlying figure 69, the subject's rhythms evidently were synchronized to the 24.00-hour and to 26.67-hour zeitgeber. It is not necessary, therefore, to present period analyses from the two sections. It is meaningful, however, to compare results of longitudinal pooling from these sections in order to find the mean phase relationships under the two different zeitgeber periods. Figure 69/II gives the results of this procedure, computed for the first and second section of this experiment. To eliminate the gradual transients after the alteration of the zeitgeber period, the first 3 days after this transition (day 10 to 12) are

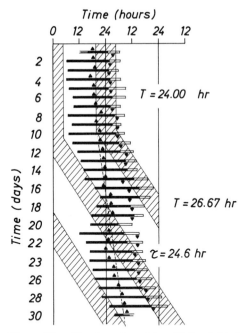

Figure 70. Rhythm of a subject (J.S., ♂ 26 y) living without environmental time cues but under the influence of an artificial zeitgeber with one alteration of the zeitgeber period. *I*. Temporal courses of the rhythms of activity and rectal temperature, presented successively one period beneath the other. Indications are the same as in figure 69/1.

not included in the computations. Figure 69/II shows that not only the external phase relationship, between the zeitgeber and the biological rhythms, changed drastically with this transition but also the internal phase relationship, between different rhythms measured in this subject. This is true not only between the rhythms of activity and rectal temperature, as presented in figure 69/II, but also between all other rhythms measured.

In general, the experiment underlying figure 69 shows that the endogenously generated rhythms can be entrained by artificial zeitgebers within a limited range of entrainment. The period of 22.67 hours is clearly below the lower limit of this range, but the upper limit cannot be detected in this special experiment. This experiment shows external and internal phase relationships depend strongly on the period, when inside the

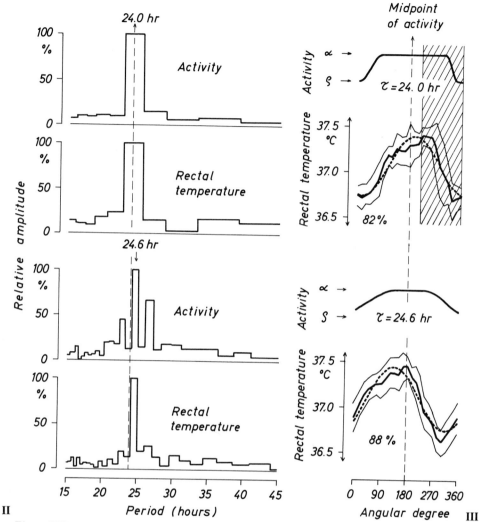

Figure 70/II. Period analyses of the two time series, presented on I, computed separately for the two sections with different zeitgeber periods. *III.* Longitudinally pooled courses of the two rhythms, computed separately for the two sections, with averaging periods derived from II. Indications are the same as in figure 69/II.

range of entrainment. However, the statements derived from this one experiment need further confirmations and, therefore, this experiment was the starting point to a series of experiments.

Figure 70 shows the temporal course of another experiment. The subject again was synchronized to the 24.00-hour zeitgeber (first section) but, in contrast to the other subject, was not synchronized to the 26.67-hour zeitgeber. During the second section, the subject showed a period, on the average,

of 24.6 hours (i.e., in the order of magnitude to be expected with autonomous rhythms). In the activity rhythm, however, this value could be observed only in the long time average due to marked "relative coordination." This means the zeitgeber period of 26.67 hours was, with this subject, just outside of the range of entrainment. The statement of the autonomy during the second section is confirmed by a period analysis, computed separately for the two sections with the different zeitgeber periods (Figure

70/II). The analyses of the first section resulted in single spectral lines with the center of gravity at 24.0 hours, this being very broad due to the short duration of this section. The analyses of the second section resulted in spectra which show spectral lines with the largest amplitude at 24.6 hours. Especially in the activity rhythm, this main peak is accompanied by smaller peaks at longer and shorter periods (the peak with the longer period at the value of the zeitgeber period), which is typical of relative coordination. The longitudinal pooling (Fig. 70/III) shows that during the first section with the 24.0-hour day, the rhythm of activity is the leading one, while during the second section, where the rhythms free run under the influence of an artificial 26.67-hour day, the rhythm of rectal temperature is the leading one.

Finally, figure 71 again shows another example of the zeitgeber experiments, with two alterations of the zeitgeber period. The rhythms clearly were synchronized to the 25.33-hour and 24.00-hour day. To the 22.67-hour day, however, only the activity rhythm seemed to be synchronized while the rectal temperature rhythm showed a deviating period of 24.8 hour (i.e., the period that must be expected with an autonomous rhythm). From this result, it must be concluded that the 22.67-hour period was within the range of entrainment of the activity rhythm, but outside this range concerning rectal temperature rhythm. The rhythms, as a consequence, were desynchronized internally. The state of internal desynchronization, in this case, did not occur spontaneously, as in all examples of this state discussed to this point (cf. 2.2.1), but was forced by the experimental conditions.

A total of 12 subjects were tested under conditions where the circadian rhythms were entrained by artificial zeitgebers of a varying period (Aschoff et al., 1969). Five of these subjects were exposed to the shortest period applied (22.67 hours). Only one of the subjects was entrained to this period with his activity rhythm, but not with other rhythms [i.e., forced internal desynchronization;

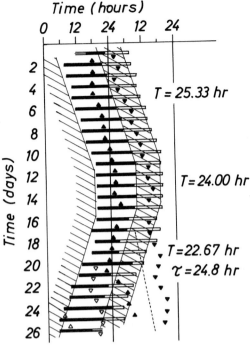

Figure 71. Rhythm of a subject (F.S. ♂ 27 y) living without environmental time cues but under the influence of an artificial zeitgeber with two alterations of the zeitgeber period. Temporal courses of the rhythms of activity and rectal temperature are presented successively, one period beneath the other. Indications are the same as in figure 69/I. From Aschoff et al. (1969).

(Fig. 71)]. The other 4 subjects showed their autonomous periods under this condition (Fig. 69). Seven of the 12 subjects were exposed to the longest of the periods applied (i.e., to a period of 26.67 hours). Three subjects were entrained fully to this period (Fig. 69). Two subjects were entrained with their activity rhythms, but not with other rhythms (i.e., forced internal desynchronization). Two subjects showed autonomous rhythms under this condition (Fig. 70). It, therefore, can be stated that entrainment, with the special kind of artificial zeitgeber applied and the special experimental conditions, ranges from about 23 to about 27 hours. These range limits of entrainment, however, are valid regarding the rhythm of rectal temperature, but the range of entrainment was found to be larger regarding the activity rhythm (Aschoff et al., 1969). The numbers mentioned show the range of entrainment is not symmetric to 24 hours, but to about 25 hours, which is the mean autonomous period of human circadian rhythms.

Six of the subjects with all overt rhythms measured, were entrained to two, or even three, different zeitgeber periods. From the results obtained in these subjects, phase relationships, depending on period, can be studied. Figure 69/II already has shown that, with lengthening the zeitgeber period, the rhythms of activity and rectal temperature shift to earlier zeitgeber phases, but for different amounts. For the average, computed from the six subjects, the phase of the activity rhythm shifts 17° and the rectal temperature rhythm shifts 38° to earlier phases of the

zeitgeber, when the period lengthens for 1 hour. The rhythm of rectal temperature, consequently, shifts, on the average, 21° to earlier phases of the activity rhythm, when the zeitgeber period lengthens for 1 hour (Wever, 1969b). The change in the phase relationships, of course, is not restricted to the rhythms of activity and rectal temperature, but is also true regarding all other rhythms measured (Wever, 1970b, 1972b). Figure 72 presents average temporal positions of acrophases of six different overt rhythms relative to the zeitgeber, plotted as a function of the zeitgeber period and computed from data of the six subjects. As can be seen in this figure, the rhythms of all variables presented shift to earlier zeitgeber

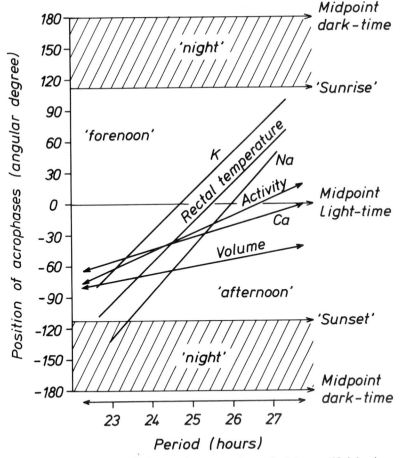

Figure 72. Summary of all experiments performed with an artificial zeitgeber of varying period. Average courses of the acrophases of six different overt rhythms relative to the zeitgeber (i.e., ordinate), plotted as functions of the period of the entraining zeitgeber (i.e., abscissa). From Wever (1972b).

phases, when the period lengthened, but with all rhythms having different slopes. This means that all rhythms shift against each other with varying zeitgeber periods. A closer inspection shows that the slopes, belonging to the different overt rhythms, do not differ irregularly, but seem to be ordered in groups. Here, the rhythms of urine volume and calcium excretion shift with similar slopes as the activity rhythm, and the rhythms of sodium and potassium excretion shift with similar slopes as the rectal temperature rhythm. The slopes of rhythms, belonging to different groups, differ from each other significantly in every case. In some cases, even the slopes within one group of rhythms differ significantly from each other (Wever, 1970b). This is the case with the rhythms of activity and urine volume and of sodium and potassium excretion ($p < 0.05$).

The rhythms of the "rectal temperature group" (Figure 72) change their external phase angle differences to the zeitgeber by an average slope of 40° per hour change in period. Since the external phase angle difference varies from one limit of the range of entrainment to the other by about 180°, independent of the size of the range of entrainment (Wever, 1965a), this slope corresponds to a range of entrainment with a size of 4.5 hours. Although the estimated linearity of the regression is only a rough approximation, this value is in good agreement with the directly measured size of the range of entrainment. With the variables of this group, the limits of the ranges of entrainment are within the range of periods presented in figure 72. The rhythms of the 'activity group' (Fig. 72) change their external phase angle differences by an average slope of only 12° per hour change in period. This value corresponds to a size of the range of entrainment of 15 hours (i.e., about 18.5 to 33.5 hours), again presupposing the linear regression is not a bad approximation. These ranges of entrainment, however, exceed the ranges of periods presented in figure 72. Considering these values, there seems to be a discrepancy. In the experiments, the range of entrainment of activity rhythms primarily does

not exceed the rectal temperature rhythm. The activity rhythm, however, is forced by not only the zeitgeber (this forcing must result in a large range of entrainment with forced internal desynchronization at zeitgeber periods between 18.5 and 23 hours and 27 and 33.5 hours) but also by the rectal temperature rhythm (cf. 4.3). This forcing must result in mutual synchronization within a large range of periods. The latter force evidently is the stronger and, therefore, forced internal desynchronization occurs only in borderline cases. If the rectal temperature rhythm is outside its range of entrainment (i.e., free running), it primarily entrains the activity rhythm, outmanoeuvring the zeitgeber effect. Only under changed experimental conditions, the large range of entrainment of the activity rhythm becomes manifest and there are large ranges of zeitgeber periods where forced internal desynchronization occurs (cf. 3.3). It must be emphasized again that all numbers mentioned are valid only with the special zeitgeber strength used. With increasing zeitgeber strength, all slopes, of course, become flatter and the ranges of entrainment enlarge. With decreasing zeitgeber strength, all slopes become steeper and the ranges of entrainment diminish (Wever, 1964b). The ratio between the two forces acting on the activity rhythm, originating from the external zeitgeber and rectal temperature rhythm, varies with the zeitgeber strength.

Inside the range of entrainment, an internal dissociation is present which manifests itself by remaining as internal phase shifts between different overt rhythms after changes in the period of an entraining zeitgeber. This internal dissociation is consistent with the multioscillator hypothesis deduced from autonomous rhythms. Following this concept, different oscillators accept equal periods, in the steady state, after the fading of the transients, during which the oscillators run temporarily with different speeds. Internal dissociation, with mutual internal phase shifts of about 180°, however, is also consistent with the more simple one oscillator hypothesis, which presupposes the coupling forces between the single oscillator and the different overt rhythms change, during the transients, by different amounts in different rhythms. Since the coupling forces, in any case, must be assumed to be different in the different overt rhythms, this presupposition always seems to be fulfilled. Experiments with heteronomous rhythms, therefore, do not enable the discrimination between one- and multioscillator hypotheses when the rhythms run synchronized internally. Only after considering the occurrence of forced internal desynchronization (Fig. 71), does the multioscillator hypothesis gain preference; as in autonomous rhythms with internally desynchronized rhythms. Following this hypothesis, the number of different slopes in the regression lines (Fig. 72) does not presuppose an equal number of different oscillators. It, rather, can be described equally well by only two, or a few, oscillators with different phase positions which contribute collectively to the different overt rhythms. The separation of the various regression slopes into two groups suggests the cooperation of only two oscillators. Within every group, one of the two oscillators is dominant. The inspection of heteronomous rhythms, under the influence of external zeitgebers of varying period, therefore, supports the same type of multioscillator hypothesis as the inspection of autonomous rhythms.

In summary, the results obtained, using artificial zeitgebers, show that human circadian rhythms can be entrained by zeitgebers, but only within limited ranges of entrainment, as typical of self-sustained oscillations. Outside this range, the rhythms run autonomously, with periods as they are accepted under constant conditions. A closer examination shows that outside this range, 'relative coordination' is present, indicated by an external phase relationship to the zeitgeber which does not vary continuously and steadily, but shows preference to fixed phases. Inside the range of entrainment, external and internal phase relationships vary, depending on the period. To be precise, there is not one range of entrainment of a

fixed size valid for all overt rhythms, but different overt rhythms can show ranges of entrainment of different sizes. Partial entrainment, therefore, can occur, due to entrainment of only part of the rhythms, while other rhythms free run autonomously with other periods (i.e., 'forced internal desynchronization').

3.1.2. Shifts of the Zeitgeber Phase

With the artificial zeitgeber, as applied in the experiments discussed so far, not only the period can be varied, but its phase also can be shifted. With these experiments, time shifts, occurring after long-distance flights over many time zones, can be simulated. Figure 73/I shows, as an example, the temporal course of such an experiment. The subject lived in an artificial 24.0-hour day, under the influence of the same zeitgeber as in the other experiments. At subjective day 8, the phase of the zeitgeber was shifted by shortening a single dark time for 6 hours, simulating an eastward flight over six time zones. The subject knew nothing about the intention of the experiment and the time shift was not announced. The subject, moreover, did not perceive any change in the experimental conditions. At subjective day 15, again the zeitgeber was shifted in the opposite direction, by lengthening a dark time for 6 hours. With this shift, a westward flight over six time zones "returning home" was simulated. The subject again did not perceive a change in the conditions. The subject, however, did react to the zeitgeber shifts as he would have reacted after real flights. Concurrent with the zeitgeber shifts, the biological rhythms also shifted. After the first 'eastward' shift, the activity rhythm shifted abruptly for about 6 hours, adopting the same phase relationship to the zeitgeber as before the shift. The rhythm of rectal temperature also advanced its phase, but more slowly. While the minimum value shifted as abruptly as the activity rhythm, the maximum value adopted its original phase relationship to the zeitgeber and activ-

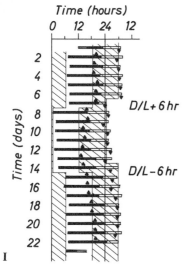

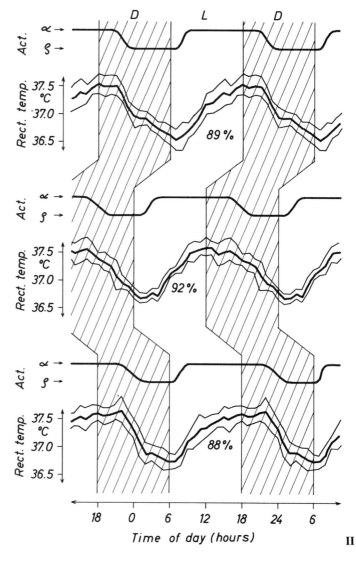

Figure 73. Rhythm of a subject (P.M., ♂ 25 y) living without environmental time cues but under the influence of an artificial 24-hour zeitgeber with two phase shifts of the zeitgeber for 6 hours. *I.* Temporal courses of the rhythms of activity and rectal temperature, presented successively one period beneath the other. Indications are the same as in figure 69/I. From Wever (1969b). *II.* Longitudinally pooled courses of the two rhythms, presented in I, computed separately for the three sections, with 24.0 hours as the averaging period. Indications are the same as in figure 69/II.

ity rhythm after about 3 days. The picture after the second, 'westward' or 'homeward', shift is similar, though generally showing a slower reaction. This lasted about 2 or 3 days before the activity rhythm reached its original phase relationship to the zeitgeber and local time. With the rhythm of rectal temperature, it was nearly 1 week before the original phase relationship was reached with regular temporal positions of maximum and minimum values.

The rhythms recorded in this experiment are pooled longitudinally and separately for the three sections (Fig. 73/II). In order to eliminate the most drastic transients, only the last 6 days of each section have been used for this procedure. The figure mainly shows both rhythms presented, and also all rhythms measured but not presented, actually shifted following the zeitgeber, with maintenance of the specific shapes of the rhythms and retention of the specific internal phase relationship between the rhythms. The simulation of a time shift, therefore, was shown to be successful. This figure also shows the high reliability of the rhythms, which is, by chance, highest when the rhythms are shifted against local time. This again confirms the correctness of the experimental conditions.

There was a total of eight experiments with phase shifts of the zeitgeber. In one of

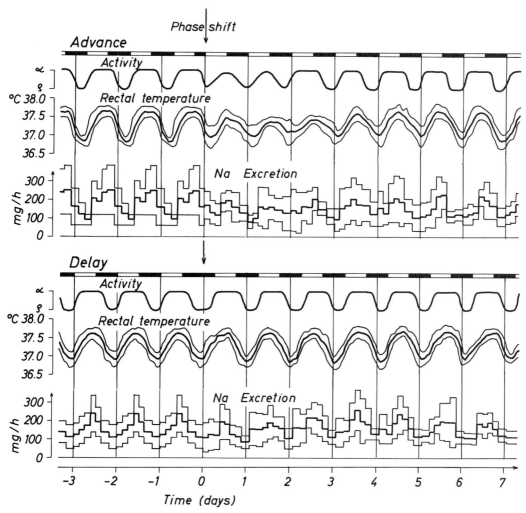

Figure 74. Summary of all experiments performed with an artificial 24-hour zeitgeber, including two phase shifts of the zeitgeber for 6 hours. Averaged courses of the rhythms of activity, rectal temperature, and sodium excretion are presented longitudinally and separately for the two zeitgeber shifts. With the rhythm of activity, the steepnesses of the transitions between activity (α) and rest (ρ) indicate the variability of this rhythm among the subjects. With the rhythms of rectal temperature and sodium excretion, the thick lines give the average courses and the thin lines give the range of the standard deviations among the subjects. Upper border in each diagram: course of the zeitgeber. "O" at the time scale (i.e., abscissa) indicates the instant when the system initially could experience the zeitgeber shift.

these experiments, there was only one 'eastward' shift. This shift was answered, by all variables measured, with an 18-hour delay instead of a 6-hour advance and the reentrainment lasting so long that the scheduled second zeitgeber shift was cancelled (Wever, 1969b). There remain seven experiments which were performed identically, with an initial 'eastward' shift, by shortening one dark time for 6 hours, and, after an interval of 8 to 15 days, a 'westward' shift

was performed, by lengthening one dark time for 6 hours. In six of the seven experiments, both shifts were answered by all overt rhythms in the same manner, as in the experiment demonstrated in figure 73. The results of these six experiments, therefore, can be pooled for further analyses. The result of the seventh experiment will be discussed separately (Fig. 77).

In figure 74, average courses of some variables are presented longitudinally and separately for the two shifts. In this type of presentation, 'zero' means the exact instant when the system could experience the zeitgeber shift. From this figure, the most obvious courses of the mean values and the amplitudes can be taken. The courses of the activity rhythms show, after the zeitgeber shifts, the ratio of activity time to rest time ('$\alpha:\rho$-ratio') is nearly unchanged. During the first 3 days after the advancing shifts, it is, on average, 95% of its original value; after the delaying shift, 92%. The course of the rectal temperature rhythm shows, during the first 3 days after the advancing shift, a conspicuous decrease in the mean value (0.09 $\pm$ 0.10°C; significant with $P < 0.05$ among the six subjects) and amplitude (down to 53 $\pm$ 10% of its original value; significant with $p <$ 0.001 among the six subjects). After the delaying zeitgeber shift, the mean value (change during the first 3 days: + 0.03 $\pm$ 0.08°C) and amplitude (relative value during the first 3 days: 100 $\pm$ 9%) remain unchanged. Fundamentally the same picture can be observed with the rhythms of sodium excretion, though with a greater interindividual variability. After the advancing zeitgeber shift, mean value (down to 86% of its original value) and amplitude (down to 48% of its original value) again are decreased. The decreases here last longer than only 3 days, in contrast to the changes with the rectal temperature rhythms. (The numbers again give average values during the first 3 days after the zeitgeber shift.) After the delaying shift, the mean value remains unchanged (decrease to 99% of its original value) while the amplitude shows a slight decrease (to 88% of its original value). In the rhythm of sodium excretion, the interindividual standard deviations are so large a statistical significance of the indicated changes cannot be guaranteed, in contrast to the data of rectal temperature. Nevertheless, in comparison to the commonly great interindividual variability of the urine constituents, the behavior of the sodium excretion, after the zeitgeber shifts, is relatively consistent and, therefore, it seems worth discussing in spite of the missed significance in the different changes.

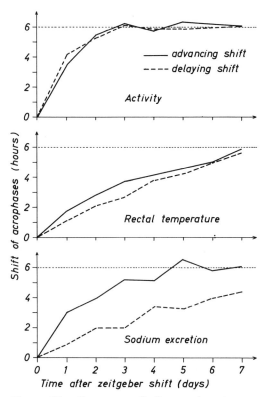

Figure 75. Summary of all experiments performed with an artificial 24-hour zeitgeber, including two phase shifts of the zeitgeber for 6 hours. The averaged duration of reentrainment to the shifted zeitgeber is presented separately for the three overt rhythms shown in Figure 74 and the two different zeitgeber shifts in opposite directions. The amount of the acrophase shift of the respective rhythm (i.e., ordinate) is plotted as a function of time following the zeitgeber shift (i.e., abscissa).

In figure 75, the courses of reentrainment are presented separately for the rhythms of the three variables. As can be seen, the activity rhythm (uppermost diagram) is reentrained fastest. This reentrainment is completed after 2 to 3 days, with a speed being independent of the shift direction. A closer inspection of the individual data shows that the termination of activity shifts faster than the activity onset in both directions. The rectal temperature rhythm (middle diagram) needs at least 1 week for full reentrainment. After 3 days, when the activity rhythms have reentrained completely, the rectal temperature rhythms were reentrained, on the average, for only half the amount of the zeitgeber shift. During the first 3 days after the zeitgeber shift, the reentrainment clearly is faster after the advancing ('eastward') shift than the delaying ('westward') shift (75 minutes per day versus 54 minutes per day). The difference in the reentrainment rates ($\pm$ standard deviation) of 21 ± 12 minutes per day deviates significantly from zero, with $p < 0.01$ (Wever, 1975c). Later, the rate of the remaining reentrainment is nearly the same in both directions, or even greater after the delaying shift, but not to a significant amount. Reentrainment for 50% of the zeitgeber shift, therefore, is reached 1 day earlier after the advancing than the delaying shift (2.2 versus 3.2 days), but reentrainment for 90% of the zeitgeber shift occurred only half a day earlier (6.4 versus 6.9 days). It is conspicuous that the direction asymmetry in the reentrainment rate is marked most strongly during those days when the amplitude is diminished after the advancing shift (Fig. 74). In the rhythm of sodium excretion (lowest diagram of figure 75), the direction asymmetry in the reentrainment is even more strongly marked than in the rhythm of rectal temperature. The duration of reentrainment is shorter than with rectal temperature rhythm after the advancing shift, but longer after the delaying shift. The direction asymmetry here is uniform during the total reentrainment; therefore, it is meaningful to give only one value. Reentrainment for 66.7% (= 4.0 hours) lasted 2.0 days after the advancing shift, but 6.0 days after the delaying shift. The difference again is significant with $p < 0.01$. It is conspicuous that the diminishing in the rhythm's amplitude lasts longer than with the rhythm of rectal temperature and is not restricted to the advancing shift. There seems, therefore, to be a correlation between the direction asymmetry in reentrainment, with a preference for advancing shift, and the diminishing of the rhythm's amplitude (Wever, 1975c).

The measured direction asymmetry in the duration of reentrainment must by no means reflect an equal direction asymmetry in the subjective discomfort after phase shifts. On the one hand, the amount of an actual reentrainment cannot be perceived consciously;

the best indication for this statement comes from the observation that nearly no subject had consciously perceived the phase shift at all. On the other hand, it can be expected that performance decrements as objectively measured after phase shifts (Klein et al., 1972) lead to subjective discomfort. Since performance is mostly closely related to body temperature, performance decrements should accompany decrements in the rectal temperature level as measured only after advancing phase shifts (see above). In fact, in those phase shift experiments where performance (computation speed) had been measured, its level was reduced after advancing but not after delaying zeitgeber shifts for 6 hours; unfortunately, these measurements had been undertaken only in a part of the relevant experiments so that statistical significance is missed. The preliminary results lead to the conclusion that the decrement in performance, and possibly also the amount of subjective discomfort, is higher after advance than after delay shifts of the zeitgeber for 6 hours each, in agreement with results of flight experiments (Klein et al., 1972). This may mean that an advance shift is, in fact, completed earlier but leads to heavier complaints than a delay shift of the same amount.

Not only changes in the amplitude during reentrainment influence the duration of reentrainment, but also the absolute value of the amplitude, measured in the steady state before the shift. This can be shown because not only the duration of reentrainment is subject to interindividual variations, but also the original amplitude. In figure 76, correlations between these two parameters are presented with the rectal temperature rhythm, displayed separately for the two shifts. For each of the six subjects, the abscissa shows the original amplitude (i.e., the average of fundamental periods, measured for 3 days preceding the shift) and the ordinate the duration of reentrainment to 66.7% of the zeitgeber shift (i.e., the time necessary for the rectal temperature rhythm to shift 4 hours). As can be seen, there are distinct positive correlations, with similar regressions for both shifts. This means the reaction of the

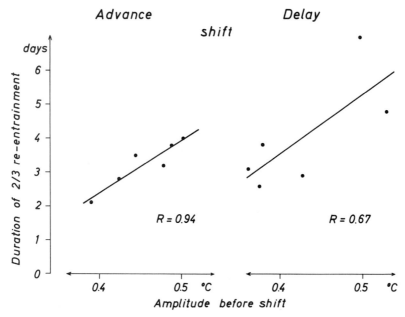

Figure 76. Summary of all experiments performed with an artificial 24-hour zeitgeber, including two phase shifts of the zeitgeber for 6 hours. The duration of reentrainment of the overt rectal temperature rhythms, to 66.7% of the zeitgeber shift (i.e. for 4 hours, ordinate), plotted as a function of the amplitude of the fundamental period during the days preceding the shift (i.e., average of 3 days each, abscissa), are presented separately for the two zeitgeber shifts in opposite directions.

rectal temperature rhythm to a 6-hour shift of the entraining zeitgeber, is faster the smaller the original amplitude. The correlation computed from the advance shift differs significantly from zero ($p < 0.02$), in spite of the small number of experiments included, but not with the delay shift. This difference is possibly caused by incomplete reentrainment after the first (advance) shift. In fact, the phases of the rectal temperature rhythms had reentrained fully in all subjects before the second (delay) shift occurred, but not the amplitude, which was reduced considerably after the advance shift and had not reached its original value during the time between the two shifts in all subjects. The (smaller) amplitude during the 3 days preceding the delay shift, therefore, did not represent the steady state amplitude, as does the (larger) amplitude during the 3 days preceding the advance shift. Figure 76 additionally demonstrates the direction asymmetry, since reentrainment, after the delaying zeitgeber shift lasts, on the average, longer than after

the advancing shift, in spite of the smaller original amplitudes (s. above).

The direction asymmetry, which has been found consistently in all experiments with two phase shifts of the zeitgeber in opposite directions, agrees with the theoretically predicted direction asymmetry (Wever, 1966a). It further agrees with results of animal experiments (Aschoff and Wever, 1963). This direction asymmetry found in simulation experiments, however, does not agree with that found in real flight experiments leading over many time zones (survey in Aschoff et al., 1975). In fact, the results of flight experiments are not as uniform as those of the simulation experiments. It is, however, the significant result for the great multiplicity of flight experiments, that the duration of reentrainment is shorter after westward than eastward flights. It even has been shown that this direction asymmetry, which is opposite to that of simulation experiments, is neither due to the temporal sequence of the flights in opposite directions nor to the actual time of day of the flight (Klein, 1973; Klein et al., 1972). The reason for this discrepancy between simulated and real flights, regarding the direction asymmetry in the reentrainment speed, remains unknown. There are many differences between the two types of experiments. One difference concerns the strengths of the zeitgeber which are the same after the simulated shifts in opposite directions (because the subjects had not perceived the shift), but possibly different in the flight experiments (e.g., social contacts are different in a strange country and at home). On the average, the zeitgeber, applied in the isolation experiments, is of a similar strength as the natural zeitgeber, as indicated by the similar reentrainment rates (compare figure 75 with table 1 in Aschoff et al., 1975). Furthermore, after flights, there may be sleep deficits which are different after flights in opposite directions, but not after the simulated shifts (s. above). Finally, the possible stress of the flight itself and the stay in another country, which may influence the reentrainment rate, is missed in the simulation experiments, where the shifts were not perceived consciously.

At the end, the difference in direction asymmetry may, in some cases, simply be a consequence of differences in the procedure of calculating the reentrainment rates. While in the simulation experiments the time base (local time) remains unchanged during the shifts, in flight experiments, the time base frequently shifts with the zeitgeber. The statement "1 day after the shift," consequently, means always 24 hours after a shift in simulation experiments, but not in all flight experiments; in some cases, 1 day after a 6 hour westward shift means 30 hours after the shift, and 1 day after a 6 hour eastward shift means 18 hours after the shift. It is evident that such discrepancies in the time bases must influence the calculations of reentrainment rate. In particular, the elimination of these discrepancies diminishes the difference between the two types of shift experiments. It must be the subject of further investigations to clarify whether or not the effects mentioned are sufficient to explain the differences between simulation and flight experiments.

In summary, sudden phase shifts of a controlling zeitgeber normally are answered by corresponding phase shifts of the biological rhythms. The circadian system, however, does not shift immediately, but with transients lasting several days, as after long distance flights over many time zones. The duration of reentrainment is different, after a definite zeitgeber shift, in the rhythms of different variables. In all cases, it is shortest with the activity rhythm. The duration of reentrainment is, with most of the overt rhythms, different after shifts of equal amounts but in opposite directions. If there is a direction asymmetry, the duration of reentrainment is shorter after advancing ('eastward') shifts than delaying ('westward') shifts. The preference of the advancing shift, regarding the duration of reentrainment, is the more remarkable since this shift always was the first. If the circadian system would not be reentrained completely after the first shift and before the second shift occurred, it must be expected, reversely, the reaction to the second ('westward') shift would be the faster one. The reason is, under this presupposition, the second shift leading back would not need reentrainment for the full shift, but only for a part. The difference in the durations of reentrainment after the two opposite shifts, therefore, cannot be due to the temporal sequence of the shifts. It, rather, must be due to the directions of the shifts, in spite of their temporal sequences applied. The degree of the direction asymmetry again is different in the rhythms of different variables. It seems to depend on the degree and the duration in the diminishing of the amplitude of the corresponding rhythm after the zeitgeber shift. As the consequence of the difference in reentrainment of different overt rhythms, internal dissociation occurred. As an additional consequence of the direction asymmetry, the amount of this dissociation is different after shifts in opposite directions. The results of these experiments again are compatible with the one- and multioscillator hypothesis, because the mutual internal phase shifts remained, in the experiments discussed so far, much less than 360°.

There is one other experiment of this type where the mutual internal phase shift, between different overt rhythms, reached 360°. The course of this experiment is shown in figure 77. After the first ("eastward") shift of the zeitgeber, the different overt rhythms shifted not only with different speeds, but also in opposite directions. The 6-hour advance of the zeitgeber was followed by the usual 6-hour advance of the activity rhythm, but by an 18-hour delay of the rectal temper-

ature rhythm. It was only after about 1 week that the original phase relationship to the zeitgeber and the different overt rhythms was reached. The second ('westward') zeitgeber shift was followed, for both rhythms, by a 6-hour delay, but the reentrainment lasted longer for the rhythm of rectal temperature than activity. At the end of the experiment, the external and internal phase relationships equalled those at the beginning. The number of cycles, during the experiment, however, was not the same in the different rhythms. It was one cycle less in the rhythm of rectal temperature than activity. The result of this special experiment, in contrast to the results of the other experiments of this series which were performed under identical experimental conditions (Fig. 73), is compatible only with the multioscillator hypothesis.

3.1.3. Entrained versus Free Running Rhythms

In the zeitgeber experiments disucssed so far, it was shown that artificial environmental periodicities have the capacity to entrain, within a limited range, human circadian rhythms. This means zeitgebers are able to alter the period and phase of circadian rhythms. There remains the question whether or not zeitgebers are able, additionally, to modify other parameters of the rhythms. In the zeitgeber experiments already discussed, the rhythm's amplitude was altered, in some cases, as a consequence of zeitgeber alterations. In those experiments, the rhythm's period, or phase, primarily were altered. It, therefore, cannot be decided whether the zeitgeber affected the amplitude directly, or only indirectly, by changes in period or phase. In order to answer this question, a series of experiments were performed with transitions between autonomous and heteronomous rhythms, but without change in the period and phase of the rhythms. In these experiments, subjects lived under constant conditions during the first section and under the influence of an

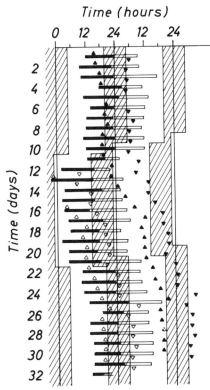

Figure 77. Rhythm of a subject (W.L., ♂ 25 y) living without environmental time cues but under the influence of an artificial 24-hour zeitgeber with two phase shifts of the zeitgeber for 6 hours. Temporal courses of the rhythms of activity and rectal temperature are presented successively, one period beneath the other. Indications are the same as in figure 69/I. White triangles: temporally correct redrawings of corresponding black triangles. From Wever (1970c).

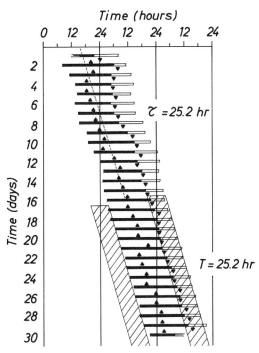

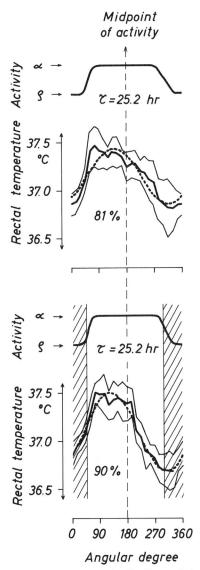

Figure 78. Rhythm of a subject (D.M., ♀ 28 y) living without environmental time cues and under constant conditions during the first section, but under the influence of an artificial zeitgeber during the second section, the period and phase of which coincided with the parameters of the autonomous rhythm determined during the first section. *I.* Temporal courses of the rhythms of activity and rectal temperature, presented successively one period beneath the other. Indications are the same as in figure 69/I.

Figure 78/II. Longitudinally pooled courses of the two rhythms, presented in I, computed separately for the two sections, without and with the zeitgeber in operation and with the same averaging period coinciding with the zeitgeber period. Indications are the same as in figure 69/II.

artificial zeitgeber during the second section; applying zeitgebers with parameters that changed neither the period nor the phase of the subject's rhythms. The effect of the transition from a free running state to entrainment, therefore, can be studied separated from changes in period or phase (Wever, 1973d).

Figure 78/I shows, for example, the course of such an experiment. During the first section, with constant conditions, the subject showed an autonomous rhythm with a period of 25.2 hours. During the second section, the artificial zeitgeber was introduced with this specific period of 25.2 hours. The phase relationship to the subject's rhythm was set in a manner, at the beginning

of the zeitgeber section, where the midpoint of light time coincided with the midpoint of activity time. The subject's rhythm, of course, was synchronized to the zeitgeber. In this case, period analyses seem meaningless for presentation because they must result in equal periods for both sections from the design of the experiment. It is of interest here to compute average periods by longitudinal poolings. Figure 78/II shows the results of these procedures, computed separately for the two sections. This figure primarily shows the amplitude of the rectal temperature rhythm is considerably larger under the influence of the zeitgeber than under constant conditions (by 45%). In contrast to the amplitude, the other rhythm parameters detected, from figure 78, remain unchanged. The internal phase relationship between the rhythms of rectal temperature and activity, and rhythms of other variables measured but not presented, is essentially the same in the two sections. The change in the amplitude, however, is enough to demonstrate that a zeitgeber is effective even when not affecting the period or phase of a circadian rhythm.

The other experiments of this series also show similar results (Wever, 1973d). The amplitude of the rectal temperature rhythm, on the average, is larger (by 50%) with the zeitgeber in operation than without it (this increase is significant with $p < 0.05$). Besides the amplitude, no other rhythm parameter shows any systematic change. In this type of experiment, it is impossible, in principle, to reverse the temporal sequence of the two sections without and with zeitgeber. It, however, has never been observed that there is a systematic temporal trend showing an increase in the amplitude, and, therefore, the change in the amplitude can be taken for a real zeitgeber effect. With this result, the effectiveness, even of artificial zeitgebers on human circadian rhythms, has been proven, independent of changes in the period and shifts in the phase.

3.2. Modalities of Effective Zeitgebers

The experiments discussed in the last chapter show the ability of human circadian rhythms to become entrained by artificial zeitgebers, which deviate in period or phase from the natural zeitgeber. The special mo-

dality of the zeitgeber having this capacity, however, were disregarded. This means, with the results discussed so far, the mode of action of effective zeitgebers can be evaluated, but not the type of periodic stimuli which are effective as zeitgebers. In the following, experiments will be discussed which deal with this problem.

3.2.1. Light-dark Zeitgebers

In most animal experiments, light-dark cycles were shown to be the most effective zeitgebers. In the human experiments discussed in the last chapter, light-dark cycles also were involved, but other periodic stimuli were administered to the subjects additionally. In the experiments performed under constant environmental conditions (cf. 2), urine samples were taken and tests performed by the subjects at self-selected intervals, which were necessarily nonequidistant. In the present experiments, an acoustic signal was introduced, at regular intervals, calling the subjects for the mictions and test sessions. The original purpose of introducing these signals was only to facilitate the analyses of the experiments, which could be done much more easily with data collection at equidistant intervals. It cannot be excluded, however, that the regular signals contribute to the zeitgeber effect. In order to discriminate between zeitgeber effects of a pure light-dark cycle and the 'enriched' zeitgeber mentioned, an additional series of experiments was performed; also with a light-dark cycle, but without the regular signals. In these experiments, the subjects themselves must select the intervals between the mictions and the test sessions, as in the constant condition experiments.

Figure 79 shows the course of a typical experiment from this series. The subject was exposed to an artificial 24.0-hour light-dark cycle, including twilight transitions, simulating the natural light-dark cycle at that time of year. The light-dark cycle concerned only the main illumination in the experimental room. The subject was able to switch on

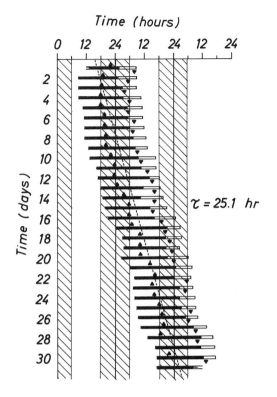

Figure 79. Rhythm of a subject (I.P., ♂ 29 y) living without environmental time cues but under the influence of an artificial light-dark zeitgeber which coincided, during the total experiment, with the natural light-dark cycle present at that time. *I.* Temporal courses of the rhythms of activity and rectal temperature, presented successively one period beneath the other. Indications are the same as in figure 16/I. Shaded areas: dark time of the zeitgeber. From Wever (1970c).

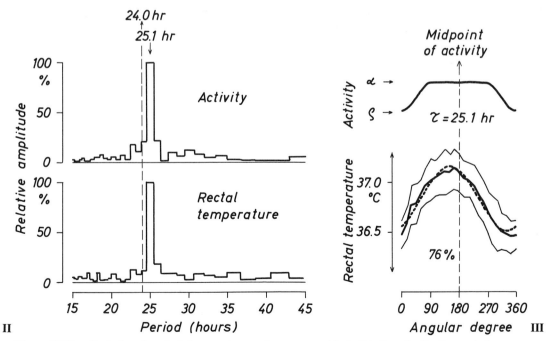

Figure 79/II. Period analyses of the two time series presented in I. *III.* Longitudinally pooled courses of the two rhythms, with an averaging period derived from II. Indications are the same as in figure 16/III.

small auxiliary lamps during the 'dark time', as in the experiments with the additional signal. The artificial light-dark change, therefore, corresponded in its meaning to the natural one where the natural sunset is also an indication to switch on artificial illumination, rather than a desire to go to bed. The subject was informed, before the experiment began, that this schedule would probably be continued during the total experiment. External time cues, other than the artificial light-dark cycle, were excluded. Figure 79/I shows that the subject was not entrained to the light-dark cycle. He showed a period of 25.1 hours, which corresponded to a free running period. After the experiment, the subject insisted he was exposed, in contrast to the announcement, to an irregular light-dark change, which was impossible to follow. He had not perceived that he shifted regularly against the light-dark change; on the average, for 1.1 hour per day. Even after showing him the records, he still could not believe the regular course of the clock, controlling the light-dark change, was accurate.

An inspection of the temporal course of the experiment (Fig. 79/I) shows the subject's rhythm shifted against local time and the artificial light-dark cycle, during the total experiment, for about 1½ days. The autonomy of the rhythm, consequently, was proven. A closer inspection of the data shows the course of the subject's rhythm was not independent, absolutely, of the light-dark cycle, but 'relative coordination' was present. When the phase relationship, between the subject's rhythm and the light-dark cycle, equalled the normal phase relationship (i.e., at the beginning of the experiment, and again at days 22 to 27), the rhythm shifted more slowly against the light-dark cycle than for the average. This phenomenon of relative coordination demonstrated that the light-dark cycle basically is not ineffective as a zeitgeber; however, the zeitgeber effect is too small to synchronize the rhythm, with an autonomous period close to 25.1 hours, to the zeitgeber period of 24.0 hours.

The computer analyses confirm these conclusions. In the period analyses (Fig. 79/II), the rhythm of activity, rectal temperature, and all other variables measured show one clear peak period, with the center of gravity at 25.1 hours. Relative coordination was so weak it was not expressed in the period analyses (cf. Fig. 70/II). The longitudinal pooling of the rhythms (Fig. 79/III) shows not only the great reliability of the rhythms, but also demonstrates the leading phase of the rectal temperature rhythm as typical of autonomous rhythms. In general, the computer analyses of this experiment, which was performed under the influence of a light-dark cycle, does not deviate in any way from analyses originating from experiments performed under constant conditions (cf. 2.1).

The experiment underlying figure 79, with autonomous rhythms, in spite of a 24.0-hour light-dark cycle, was not an isolated one. Of four additional subjects, who were also exposed to a pure light-dark zeitgeber with a period of 24.0 hours, remaining unchanged during the total experiment, one subject showed internally synchronized rhythms during the total experiment. He also showed autonomous rhythms, with a period of 24.9 hours, in spite of the 24.0-hour zeitgeber. Two more subjects were exposed to a pure 24.0-hour light-dark cycle, but with one phase shift of the zeitgeber of 6 hours, during the experiment. One final subject was exposed to the light-dark cycle, but with two zeitgeber shifts in opposite directions, following the same schedule as in the experiment underlying figure 73. The course of the last experiment is presented in figure 80. It also shows an autonomous rhythm with this subject. She is entrained to the zeitgeber as minimally as the other two subjects with only one zeitgeber shift. In total, five subjects were exposed to a 24.0-hour zeitgeber, consisting of only a light-dark cycle of the main illumination, showing rhythms remaining internally synchronized during the total experiment. Not one of these subjects had perceived the regularity of the light-dark cycle and, most importantly, not one remained

Time (hours)

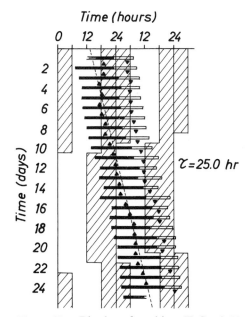

Figure 80. Rhythm of a subject (E.G., ♀ 28 y) living without environmental time cues but under the influence of an artificial light-dark zeitgeber, with two phase shifts of the zeitgeber for 6 hours. Temporal courses of the rhythms of activity and rectal temperature are presented successively, one period beneath the other. Indications are the same as in figure 79/I.

entrained to this zeitgeber. Most of these subjects, however, showed relative coordination, indicating that the zeitgeber applied was not totally ineffective, but was too weak for full entrainment (Wever, 1970c).

In general, the courses of the experiments, performed under the influence of a pure 24.0-hour light-dark zeitgeber, are very similar to those of experiments performed under constant conditions. This similarity also concerns the occurrence of internal desynchronization in some experiments. In three more experiments with the light-dark zeitgeber, this state actually occurred; in each case, after about 10 to 12 days, with internally synchronized rhythms. The course of one of these experiments is shown in figure 81. During the first 10 days, the rhythms showed, with internal synchronization, a period of 25.0 hours, in spite of the 24.0-hour light-dark zeitgeber. Internal desynchronization occurred spontaneously

and the activity rhythm showed, from this time onward, a long period of 32.6 hours. The rhythm of rectal temperature adapted to a period of 24.0 hours, which could be interpreted as being synchronized to the 24.0-hour zeitgeber. This interpretation, which precludes the assumption of an autonomous period being very close to 24.0 hours, is supported by the observation of the phase positions of the rectal temperature rhythm relative to the zeitgeber or local time (Figure 100). After the occurrence of internal desynchronization, the temperature rhythm advanced its phase, entirely in contrast to its behavior under constant conditions, until a near normal phase relationship to the natural light-dark zeitgeber was reached. This phase then remained unchanged until the end of the experiment.

The indication, concerning the periods, is supported further by the computed analyses. Figure 81/II shows the period analyses, computed for the arbitrarily separated sections A and B. In section A, there is one peak in the rhythm of activity and rectal temperature, with the center of gravity at 25.0 hours. Because of the shortness of this section, this peak is not separated significantly from 24.0 hours. The longitudinal pooling (Fig. 81/III), computed from this section, shows the leading phase of the rectal temperature rhythm, as is typical in autonomous rhythms. In section B, in the period analysis of the activity rhythm (Fig. 81/II), there is a main peak, with the center of gravity at 32.6 hours, and a small peak, with the center of gravity at 24.0 hours. A third peak, at 16.3 hours, only is due to the special shape of the rhythm as the second harmonic of the primary period. In the rhythm of rectal temperature, there is, reversely, a primary peak at 24.0 hours and a secondary peak at 32.6 hours. In this section, the rhythms can be pooled twice longitudinally, with $\tau = 24.0$ hours and $\tau = 32.6$ hours (Fig. 81/III). As in the experiments with internal desynchronization occurring under constant conditions (cf. 2.2.1), the phase relationship, between the two rhythms, is the same with the two different periods and as in the other section, with

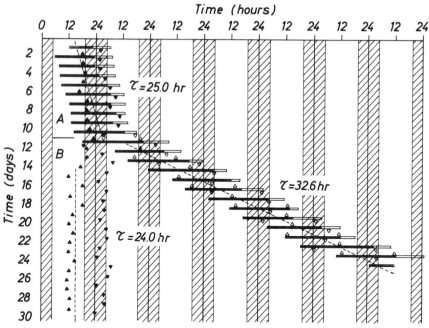

Figure 81. Rhythm of a subject (G.G., ♂ 25 y) living without environmental time cues but under the influence of an artificial light-dark zeitgeber which coincided, during the total experiment, with the natural light-dark cycle present at that time. The experiment is divided arbitrarily into two sections (A and B) for further analyses. *I.* Temporal courses of the rhythms of activity and rectal temperature, presented successively one period beneath the other. Indications are the same as in figure 79/I. White triangles: temporally correct redrawings of corresponding black triangles.

internally synchronized rhythms. In addition, with the 24.0-hour component, the external phase relationship can be determined. As can be seen in figure 81/III, the external phase relationship is similar to that measured in rhythms which are not only partially, but also fully, synchronized to a 24.0-hour zeitgeber (Fig. 100).

The computer analyses confirm that during internal desynchronization (section B) the main period of the rectal temperature rhythm is 24.0 hours; coinciding with the zeitgeber period. The same result was obtained in the two other experiments with internal desynchronization under the influence of a 24.0-hour light-dark zeitgeber. This result is compatible with the assumption that rectal temperature rhythms run autonomously with periods which are, only by chance, 24.0 hours and also is compatible with the assumption of partial synchronization of the rectal temperature rhythms only. Without exposure to a light-dark cycle, the

periods of separated rectal temperature rhythms, during internal desynchronization, follow a very small distribution (24.88 ± 0.19 hours; cf. 2.3). In all 38 cases observed, the periods are clearly longer than 24.0 hours. Based on the period distribution mentioned, it is very improbable ($p < 10^{-6}$), that in all three cases of internal desynchronization under the influence of a light-dark cycle, autonomous rectal temperature periods of 24.0 hours, or shorter, occur accidentally.

It consequently must be accepted that the rectal temperature rhythm, when desynchronized from the activity rhythm, can be synchronized to a 24.0-hour light-dark zeitgeber. The reversed case occurred in the experiment underlying figure 71. In this earlier experiment, under the influence of a zeitgeber that was shown to be stronger, only the activity rhythm was entrained, but not the rectal temperature rhythm. The hypothesis was that the range of entrainment of the activity rhythm is larger than the rectal tem-

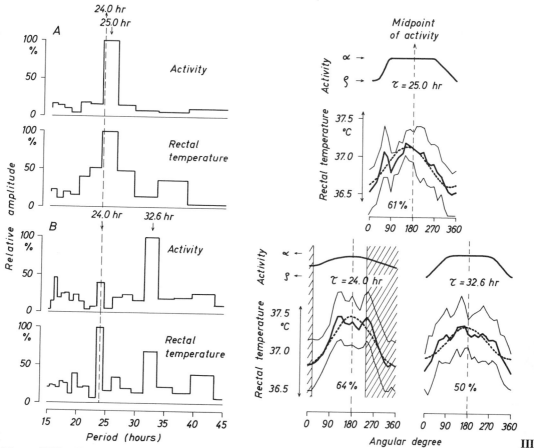

Figure 81/II.   Period analyses of the two time series, presented in I, computed separately for the two sections (A and B). *III.* Longitudinally pooled courses of the two rhythms, computed separately for the two sections (A and B), with sections A being an averaging period, derived from II, and B being two averaging periods, derived as the two most prominent peaks from II. Indications are the same as in figure 16/III. Shaded areas: dark time of the zeitgeber, with the zeitgeber period as the averaging period.

perature rhythm, so that the activity rhythm was inside, but the rectal temperature rhythm was outside, this range. The range of entrainment in the present experiment was shown to be generally small (Figs. 79 and 80). The period of the desynchronized activity rhythm, which is outside the range of entrainment, deviates from the zeitgeber period for no less than 8.6 hours. The rectal temperature period, however, must be concluded to be inside this range and, therefore, must be, without entrainment, close to 24.0 hours. In figure 81, the rhythms, as long as they run synchronized internally (section A), have a period of 25.0 hours. After the occurrence of internal desynchronization,

when the activity period becomes longer by 7.6 hours, the period of the rectal temperature rhythm must be expected to become shorter, according to the ratio 1:12, as determined in all experiments with internally synchronizing rhythms, as the average (Fig. 29), for about 0.6 hours. A natural period of about 24.4 hours, therefore, must be expected in the rectal temperature rhythm after the occurrence of internal desynchronization. This period, in fact, is close to the zeitgeber period of 24.0 hours. The range of entrainment, in this experiment, can be determined to be larger than 0.4 hours (entrainment of the separated rectal temperature rhythm in section B, with a hypothetical period of 24.4 hours), but smaller than 1.0 hour (no entrainment of the internally synchronized rhythm in section A, with a measured period of 25.0 hours). The other two experiments give similar results.

While the arguments discussed above strictly favor the assumption of partially entrained rhythms in the experiment underlying figure 81, there seems to be one argument favoring another assumption (i.e., autonomy of the rectal temperature rhythm, with a period, only by chance, very close to 24.0 hours). This argument deals with the internal phase relationship with the 24.0-hour rhythm component which shows a leading phase of the rectal temperature rhythm, in comparison to the activity rhythm; equalling the phase relationship with the other, clearly free running rhythm component and typical of autonomous rhythms (Fig. 19). The internal phase relationship, however, is applicable as a criterion indicating either autonomy or entrainment in internally synchronized rhythms only. It is not applicable to separated or desynchronized rhythm components. It is a characteristic of the multioscillator hypothesis, presented in this book that all rhythm components, as controlled by one separated oscillator, show coinciding internal phase relationships between the rhythms of activity and rectal temperature, independent of whether they run autonomous or heteronomous. This general phase relationship shows a leading phase of the rectal temperature rhythm, in comparison to the activity rhythm. Only when the different rhythm components shift against each other, following period changes of an entraining zeitgeber, the internal phase relationship between the overt rhythms changes. The constancy of the internal phase relationship within one separated or desynchronized rhythm component, therefore, does not exclude a transition from autonomous to heteronomous rhythms; as would be the case in internally synchronized rhythms.

In summary, there were eight subjects exposed to a 24.0-hour zeitgeber consisting of only a light-dark cycle of the main illumi-

nation. In five of these subjects, the rhythms were synchronized internally during the total experiment (Figs. 79 and 80) and three subjects were synchronized internally only during one section of the experiment (Fig. 81). None of the subjects were entrained, during the state of internal synchronization, to this zeitgeber. There were 16 subjects in the experiments described earlier who were exposed to a 24.0-hour zeitgeber consisting of a light-dark cycle complemented by signals at regular intervals. Eight of these subjects were in experiments with a varying zeitgeber period (cf. 3.1.1) and the other eight with shifted zeitgeber phases (cf. 3.1.2). In all 16 subjects, the rhythms were synchronized internally. All 16 subjects were clearly entrained to the 24.0-hour zeitgeber. The difference in the entrainability of rhythms, under the influence of the two zeitgeber modalities mentioned, is highly significant, with $p = 1.4 \times 10^{-6}$ (exact Fisher-test). With the pure light-dark zeitgeber, the range of entrainment was determined to be smaller than ± 1.0 hour. With the zeitgeber 'enriched' by the regular signal, the range of entrainment is about ± 2.0 hours. With this result, the question arises concerning the cause of such a remarkable difference in the strength of zeitgebers, which are apparently very similar in their modes.

3.2.2. Physical Versus Social Zeitgebers

The only difference in the two zeitgeber modalities was the additional signal, at regular intervals, which called the subjects to urine mictions and other tests in the experiments previously discussed. The signal was given acoustically, using a gong; in a 24-hour day at 3-hour intervals during light time and 4.5-hour intervals during dark time. The subjects, therefore, were given seven signals per day or period; one of which was normally during the sleep time. In artificial days of deviating durations, the intervals were changed proportionally to the period. This gong signal was originally introduced only to facilitate the analysis of the experiments. It was the distinct opinion of the experimenter that the additional signal would not influence the zeitgeber effect of an already present light-dark cycle. Nobody considered that the signals would contribute to the zeitgeber effect. Only when the gong failed to operate, shortly after the beginning of one of the experiments, the importance of the signals was discovered; the rhythm started to free run in spite of the persisting light-dark cycle. After obtaining this unexpected result, the effect of the additional signals was tested systematically. Therefore, in later experiments, tests with and without the additional gong signal were performed.

After the experiments, the subjects were examined with regard to their subjective experiences. All subjects, who were exposed to the combined zeitgeber, stated they considered the light-dark cycle was controlled automatically by a switch clock, but still perceived the gong signals as personal calls by the experimenter (i.e., social contacts). Although the subjects soon realized that the gong signals were automatically controlled by the switch clock, it was the impression that the subjects, more or less unconsciously, clung to the idea that gong signals represented social contacts, especially because of the requests transmitted by the signal. From these statements, it is suggested that the signals operated as social contacts and that this social zeitgeber is more effective than the light-dark zeitgeber. Additionally, the regular signals helped the subjects schedule their days. Some subjects numbered the signals as 'day gongs 1 to 6' and one 'night gong'. This regular temporal order also may contribute to the zeitgeber effect.

It may be argued that the strongly different capacity of the two zeitgeber modalities, with and without the additional signal, may be due to different motivations of the subjects. The motivation may depend on the instructions given to the subject. This argument can be refuted because of the accidental origin of the first experiment without the regular signals (see above). At least in this experiment, the instructions were the same as in the former experiments with the signals, because it was planned to perform this experiment in the same manner as the former experiments. Only after the technical breakdown of the gong, the subject got a letter with the instruction, because of the technical failure, to substitute the missing signals by self-selected cues of about the same frequency as the instants of mictions and test performances. In the later experiments, attention was directed to giving equal instructions in the different types of experiments.

The influence of the motivation, depending on the instructions given to the subject, was tested directly in a separate experiment. In this experiment, performed with a pure light-dark cycle (period: 25.3 hours) as the zeitgeber, the (female) subject was required to follow the zeitgeber strictly, if possible; in contrast to the instructions given for the other experiments. The temporal course of this experiment is shown in figure 82. As can be seen, the subject followed the light-dark cycle according to the instruction. The alternation between activity and rest was synchronized to the zeitgeber. A closer inspection shows that the rest times, on the average, were unusually short (6.2 ± 2.6 hours), and the subject, on some days, took naps, in contrast to her normal habit. The naps were not always positioned at the same phases of the activity time but close to the end of activity time at the beginning of the experiment, and close to the beginning of activity time at the end of the experiment. This means that the naps did not follow a 25.3-hour period, as did the 'night sleeps' according to the zeitgeber period, but followed a shorter period. On the days when the subject did not take a nap, she showed decreased amounts of activity during those instants, following a period shorter than the zeitgeber period. The subject did not perceive the shifting of the naps, relative to the period derived from the subjectively scored alternation between activity and rest. After the experiment, she insisted she always had taken naps at the same time of her subjective

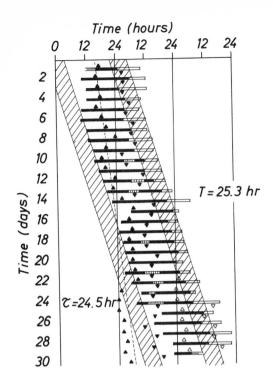

Figure 82. Rhythm of a subject (U.B., ♀ 23 y) living without environmental time cues but under the influence of an artificial light-dark zeitgeber, with strict instructions given to the subject to follow the zeitgeber. *I.* Temporal courses of the rhythms of activity and rectal temperature, presented successively one period beneath the other. Indications are the same as in figure 81/I. Hatched areas within the black bars: naps. From Wever (1975d).

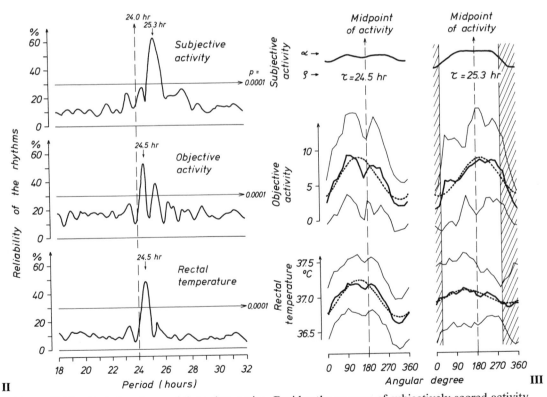

Figure 82/II. Period analyses of three time series. Besides the courses of subjectively scored activity and rectal temperature, as presented in I, the course of objectively recorded locomotor activity, from contact plates under the floor, is analyzed. *III.* Longitudinally pooled courses of the three rhythms, presented in II, with two averaging periods, derived as the two most prominent peaks from II. Indications are the same as in figure 81/III.

day. Finally, figure 82/I shows that the rectal temperature clearly followed a rhythm faster than the rhythm of the subjectively declared activity, but synchronously to the rhythm of the naps.

The computed period analyses confirm this picture, as can be seen in figure 82/II. In the time series of the subjectively declared rhythm of wakefulness and sleep, there is one clear peak at 25.3 hours (i.e., at the period of zeitgeber). This means that the rhythm obviously was entrained. The time series of the continuously recorded rectal temperature shows another clear peak, but at the shorter period of 24.5 hours. This difference in the periods may indicate forced internal desynchronization as it occurred, for example, in the zeitgeber experiment underlying figure 71, when the period was outside the range of entrainment for the rectal temperature rhythm, but inside this range for the activity rhythm. There are, however, some indications, in this experiment, that the rhythms still were synchronized internally. In the established cases of forced internal desynchronization (Fig. 71), the objectively recorded activity of the subject coincided with the subjectively declared activity, as in nearly all isolation experiments. This means that there is even a difference in the periods of the rhythms of objective activity and of rectal temperature. In the experiment underlying figure 82, however, this is not the case. The analysis of the objective activity recordings here resulted in a main period of 24.5 hours (i.e., coinciding with that of the rectal temperature rhythm), while there is a secondary peak at 25.3 hours (i.e., at the period of the zeitgeber and of the subjective activity rhythm). This twofold peak is due to the naps and reductions in activity on the days without naps, and to the 'night-sleeps' following the zeitgeber rhythm.

From these measurements in this experiment, it is improper to speak of internal desynchronization, because the period of the rectal temperature rhythm equals that of the objective activity rhythm. It can be termed as a dissociation between the activity, which was controlled by the circadian system, and another component of activity, which was forced by the subject's motivation to follow the zeitgeber rhythm. It is the outstanding result of this experiment that not even a high motivation, as can be proven by the course of the subjective activity rhythm, is able to strengthen the light-dark zeitgeber to such a degree that the range of entrainment reaches 0.8 hours (i.e., the difference between the zeitgeber period and the autonomous period of this subject). If the interpretation given above cannot be accepted, and the interpretation based on the occurrence of forced internal desynchronization is preferred, in spite of the result of the objective activity measurements, the result of this experiment also confirms the weakness of the zeitgeber effect of the pure light-dark cycle. In the experiments with the additional regular signals, the rectal temperature rhythm was synchronized, to all periods tested, within a range between 23 and 27 hours, and forced internal desynchronization occurred close to these limits only. In the experiment without the regular signals, however, forced internal desynchronization would have occurred at the period of 25.3 hours, which is close to the midpoint of the range just mentioned. The result of this experiment, therefore, confirms, in spite of the high motivation of the subject and independent of the interpretation preferred, that the zeitgeber effect of a pure light-dark cycle is small in comparison to a light-dark cycle which is completed by a signal at regular intervals calling the subjects for tests and perceived subjectively as 'social contact'.

Finally, the negligible zeitgeber effect of a light-dark cycle, in comparison to the social zeitgeber, was shown in another series of experiments. In these experiments, six subjects, in groups of two for 2 weeks, lived in a standardized environment under the influence of a strict 24-hour routine. The routine was supervised regularly by direct social contacts with experimenters. The subjects were instructed to go to bed at 23:30 and to get up at 7:30 and they received their meals at regular intervals. Every 3 hours they had

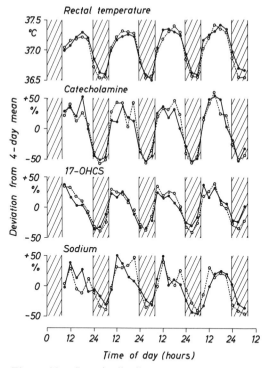

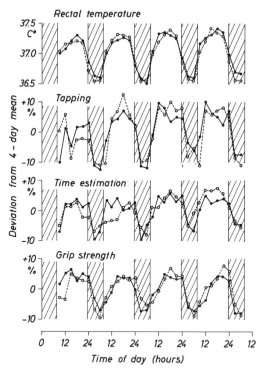

Figure 83: Longitudinally presented courses of several variables, averaged from six subjects, in groups of two, living in standardized conditions under the influence of a strict 24-hour routine performed by continuous contacts with an experimenter. From the 2 weeks of the experiment, 4 days of the first week were experimental days with a light-dark cycle, coinciding with the social routine, and 4 days of the second week were experimental days in constant total darkness. The courses of the different variables are presented separately for the section with the additional light-dark cycle (solid lines) and the second section performed under total darkness (dotted lines). *I.* Courses of some physiological variables. From top to bottom: rectal temperature, (measured continuously) and three different urine constituents (i.e., mictions taken at regular 3-hour intervals).

Figure 83/II. Courses of some psychomotor variables, measured at regular 3-hour intervals. For comparison, the course of rectal temperature is repeated from I. Data from Aschoff et al. (1971b).

to give urine samples and perform tests in the presence of an experimenter. During sleep time, the subjects were awakened for the test sessions. The two experimental weeks differed only in the mode of the illumination. The subjects, during the first week, lived under the influence of a light-dark cycle coinciding with the forced activity-rest cycle. During the second week, they lived in continuous darkness. All other con-

ditions coincided. Even the locomotor activity of the subjects was controlled for equal amounts during both weeks. The social zeitgeber, therefore, was of equal strength during both weeks, but during the first week an additional light-dark zeitgeber was present. The elimination of this additional zeitgeber, by continuous darkness, was preferred to continuous light because, in the latter case, an additional effect of a self-controlled light-dark cycle, due to opening and closing of the eyes (cf. 2.4.2) was expected.

If the additional light-dark zeitgeber has a strength comparable to the social zeitgeber, it must effect an increase in the total zeitgeber strength. This increase of strength should cause a change in the phase relationship to the zeitgeber and an increase in amplitude. The experiments showed, however, coinciding results in nearly all respects tested during both weeks, as can be seen in figure 83. Figure 83/I shows the courses of some physiological variables, and figure 83/ II shows some psychomotor variables, each presented longitudinally for the four recording days of the 2 weeks and averaged for all six subjects. As can be seen from the diagrams, and as it was tested statistically, there is no systematic difference in the results obtained during the 2 different weeks (Aschoff et al., 1971b; Giedke et al., 1974). Mean values and amplitudes, phase positions or, for instance, shapes of the rhythms are fundamentally the same with and without the additional light-dark zeitgeber, except for a significant decrease in the amplitude of Ca-excretion during the second week. The results of these experiments also confirm that the zeitgeber strength of a light-dark cycle is almost negligible in comparison to the zeitgeber strength of social contacts. The same conclusion must be drawn from another experimental series performed in a similar manner, but with continuous light (Krieger et al., 1969).

Further evidence for the importance of the ''social zeitgeber'' (Rutenfranz, 1967) comes from experiments where subjects were forced to live under unusual routines. Weitzman (1974) forced subjects to live for a 10-day period with a regular schedule alternating between 2 hours of wakefulness and 1 hour of sleep. The level of plasma cortisol remained rhythmic, with a period of 24.0 hours, and with the usual pattern. Curtis and Fogel (1971) forced subjects to live for a 14-day period with a 'random living schedule'. In this experiment, the measured circadian rhythms also remained unchanged. In both cases, the subjects had social contacts with their environment, despite their unusual living routines. It is very likely, therefore, the social contacts, in both experiments, caused the synchronization of circadian rhythmicity.

Perhaps the most convincing evidence for the social nature of the effective zeitgeber comes from an experiment performed by Klein and Wegmann (1974), who measured the rate of reentrainment after transcontinental flights over six time zones. It is well known this rate depends on the strength of the entraining zeitgeber. The control subjects, after each flight, remained continuously inside their hotel (indoor activity only), while the experimental subjects went to town every second day (in- and outdoor activity). For both groups of subjects, on every second day, several coinciding measurements were undertaken to determine circadian rhythmicity. The experimental subjects evidently had stronger social contacts with their environment than the control subjects. As the consistent result, the experimental subjects showed a shorter duration of reentrainment, or a higher reentrainment rate, than the control subjects. It, therefore, was proven that the experimental subjects, with temporary outdoor activity, were exposed to a stronger zeitgeber than the control subjects, with only indoor activity. The only difference in the zeitgebers was the increased social contact during outdoor activity. This experiment, therefore, gives clear evidence that social contacts constitute an effective zeitgeber for human circadian rhythms.

The effectiveness of social contacts as zeitgebers was firstly discovered unintentionally in experiments which should have been performed under constant conditions, but which showed, during certain sections, periods of 24.0 hours (Fig. 20). In those experiments, the measured period could be proven to be due to external synchronization. The only zeitgeber which could arrange synchronization, though unintended, was social contact with the environment. Later, the concept of 'social zeitgebers' was applied to group experiments with collectively isolated subjects. In those experiments, the different subjects normally were shown to be synchronized mutually (Fig. 67). The only stimuli, which could arrange this mutual synchronization, were the mutual social contacts between the subjects. In comparison to the zeitgeber strength of social contacts, the most obvious external zeitgeber connected with the alternation between day and night (i.e., the light-dark cycle), was shown to be weak. This statement seems contradictory to various findings concerning the effectiveness of light as a zeitgeber, even in humans. The solution of this apparent discrepancy can be discussed only after considering, systematically, the state of partial external synchronization. In the zeitgeber experiments considered so far, this state was observed only occasionally (Figs. 71 and 81). In the context to be discussed in this chapter, previously another mode of zeitgeber will be considered which leads to complete external synchronization.

3.2.3. Electric Field Zeitgebers

During the course of an experiment demonstrating the continuous action of an artificial electric 10-Hz field on autonomously running rhythms, a possible zeitgeber effect of this field was suggested (Fig. 56). In a subsequent series of special experiments, this effect was tested systematically. Figure 84 shows the course of an experiment from this series. During the first section, the subject was protected from any field, aritificial and natural, except the technical 50-Hz field. During the second section, he was exposed to a field zeitgeber with a period of 24.0 hours [i.e., the artificial electric field (10 Hz square wave, field strength 2.5 V/m), was switched on for 12.0 hours and switched off for 12.0 hours]. The illumination, and, therefore, the technical 50-Hz field, was held constant during the total experiment. As can be seen from figure 84, the subject's rhythm, which ran free during the first section, seemed to become synchronized immediately after introducing the field zeitgeber. One week later, however, the rhythm again adopted a period close to 25 hours, which may indicate an autonomous rhythm. The experiment did not last long enough to see whether or not a temporary entrainment would have occurred again later, but it positively suggests the periodically operating electric 10-Hz field can act as a zeitgeber. Such a zeitgeber, however, probably is not strong enough for full entrainment in the long run and, therefore, results in a relative coordination only. This deduction, however,

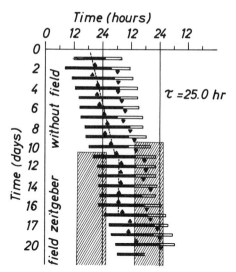

Figure 84. Rhythm of a subject (A.H., ♂ 23 y) living without environmental time cues under constant conditions and protected from natural and artificial electromagnetic fields during the first section, but under the influence of a periodically operating artificial electric AC field (i.e., 10 Hz square wave, 2.5 V/m; 12.0 hours field on, 12.0 hours field off) during the second section. Temporal courses of the rhythms of activity and rectal temperature are presented successively, one period beneath the other. Indications are the same as in figure 55/I. From Weyer (1967c).

is not conclusive for two reasons. First, the introduction of the field, though operating only temporarily, may shorten the period of a rhythm, still running autonomously, to a value which is accidentally close to 24 hours. Second, the introduction of the field may raise the sensitiveness of the rhythm, regarding a residual (usually too weak) zeitgeber, with a period of 24.0 hours. Both of these objections are unlikely, but they must be tested in subsequent experiments.

In another experiment testing the effectiveness of the field zeitgeber, the course of which is presented in figure 85, the subject again was exposed primarily to field free conditions. He showed internal dissociation, like that exemplified in figure 35 (left), with a period of the rectal temperature rhythm of 25.0 hours. After 12 days, the field zeitgeber was introduced, with a period of 23.5 hours.

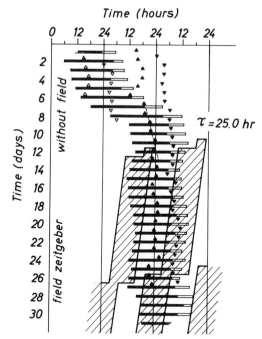

Time (hours)

τ = 25.0 hr

Time (days)

without field

field zeitgeber

Figure 85. Rhythm of a subject (H.R., ♂ 69 y) living without environmental time cues under constant conditions and protected from natural and artificial electromagnetic fields during the first section, but under the influence of a periodically operating artificial electric AC field (i.e., 10 Hz square wave, 2.5 V/m; 11.75 hours field on, 11.75 hours field off) during the second section, with a phase shift of the field zeitgeber near the end of the experiment. Temporal courses of the rhythms of activity and rectal temperature are presented successively, one period beneath the other. Indications are the same as in figure 55/I. White triangles: temporally correct redrawings of corresponding black triangles. From Wever (1969b).

This period deviates from the period of all natural zeitgebers, known or unknown, and, therefore, an entrainment cannot be due to any overlooked natural zeitgeber, but could be due only, and directly, to the artificial field zeitgeber. As figure 85 shows, the subject's rhythm seemed to become synchronized immediately after switching on the field zeitgeber. After 3 days, however, the period lengthened again, but only until another phase relationship to the zeitgeber was reached. Finally, the subject's rhythm adopted a period coinciding with that of the zeitgeber, with a phase relationship to the zeitgeber which was not only constant temporally, but also coincided with the phase relationship in the other experiment during the days of entrainment (Fig. 84). In order to test whether the coincidence with the zeitgeber period really was due to entrainment or only a chance variation in the period of an autonomously remaining rhythm, the zeitgeber phase was shifted. In case of an accidental coincidence in the periods, the zeitgeber shift is not expected to influence the subject's rhythm. Figure 85 shows, however, that the zeitgeber shift immediately was followed by a shift of the subject's rhythm. The experiment did not last long enough to reach reentrainment to the shifted zeitgeber; nevertheless, the immediate breaking off of the subject's rhythm from the zeitgeber, following the zeitgeber shift, gives additional evidence that the coincidence, between the periods of the subject's rhythm and the zeitgeber, could not be due to chance, but only to a consequence of real entrainment.

In total, 10 subjects were exposed to a field zeitgeber with periods between 23.5 and 26.0 hours for at least a section of the experiment. In all these cases, the subject's rhythms were entrained to the zeitgeber, at least for a few days, showing relative coordination (Fig. 84). Beside the temporary coincidence between the subject's period and the zeitgeber period, the main relevance for entrainment comes from the consideration of the rhythm's phases. If the coincidence in the periods would be only accidental, the external phase relationships to the zeitgeber would be distributed randomly. They, however, are concentrated significantly to a distinct phase relationship ($p < 0.01$; Fig. 100) and, therefore, entrainment is indicated. Moreover, the internal phase relationships between the rhythms of activity and rectal temperature, during the days of the possible entrainment, are significantly different from those during the days when the rhythm's periods deviate from the zeitgeber periods ($p < 0.01$; Wever, 1969b). The internal phase shifts released by the field zeitgeber further coincides exactly with internal phase shifts released by other effective external periodicities (Fig. 102). If the observed change in the period would not be based on entrainment, but on changes in the magnitude of continuously acting external stimuli, an internal phase shift would not occur (Fig. 106). With this in consideration, the effectiveness of a periodically operating weak electric square wave field, with a frequency of 10 Hz, as an entraining zeitgeber, was proven in different ways, independent of each other. The range of entrainment of this zeitgeber exceeds about ±1 hour and is larger than the other physical zeitgeber [i.e., a pure light-dark cycle (cf. 3.2.1)]. This means the field zeitgeber used is stronger than the light-dark zeitgeber, although the field zeitgeber is imperceptible consciously by the subjects. Even the possibility of applying such a zeitgeber was unknown to the subjects, while the light-dark zeitgeber is more easily perceived.

Regarding autonomous rhythms, besides the artificial 10-Hz fields, the natural electromagnetic fields were found to affect circadian rhythms (cf. 2.4.4). These natural fields include various components with different frequencies, and most are not constant temporally in intensity, but varying periodically, with periods of 24.0 hours, according to the earth's rotation. This rhythmicity concerns, for example, the component with a frequency of 10 Hz (König, 1959), which is suggested to be one of the effective components within the total of natural fields. The question arises, therefore, whether or not the daily changes in the intensity of the natural electromagnetic fields exert a zeitgeber effectiveness supporting the other natural 24-hour zeitgebers. From the experiments discussed so far, at least preliminary answers to this question can be given.

The natural electromagnetic fields penetrate into the nonshielded experimental unit to such an amount that they may cause significant effects on autonomous rhythms, as shown by the comparison of results obtained in the two different experimental units (Table 6). If the fields themselves penetrate into the room, it is obvious that their rhythmicities also penetrate. Therefore, if this rhythmicity would have any relevant zeitge-

ber effectiveness, rhythms obtained in the nonshielded room must indicate a 24-hour entrainment under intentionally constant conditions, rather than rhythms obtained in the shielded room. They at least must indicate relative coordination in several cases. In 5 of 151 experiments performed under constant conditions, the subject's rhythms remained synchronized externally to 24.0 hours against the intention of the experiment (cf. 2.1.5), either during the total experiment (Fig. 22), or only temporarily (Figs. 20 and 21). In only one experiment, an obvious zeitgeber modality (e.g., social contacts; Fig. 20) could be excluded. This means in only one of 151 experiments, an unidentified zeitgeber, with a period of 24.0 hours, was present (Fig. 21). In only this one experiment, the possibility exists that the natural electromagnetic fields exerted a zeitgeber effectiveness. This experiment, in fact, was performed in the nonshielded experimental unit. In all other experiments performed in this room, no indications for relative coordination to 24.0 hours could be detected. Not even in experiments with autonomous periods which, by chance, were very close to 24.0 hours (Fig. 24) could this be detected. Therefore, the definitely existing 24-hour variations in the intensity of the natural electromagnetic fields are normally too weak to exert a detectable zeitgeber effect on human circadian rhythms. This means that the range of entrainment of this zeitgeber cannot exceed more than a few minutes; and such a weak zeitgeber can be proven only in very rare borderline cases.

3.2.4. Summary

In summary, there are different kinds of external periodicities having the capacity to entrain human circadian rhythms as a zeitgeber. The pure physical zeitgebers are less effective than those which include a component perceived as social contacts. This means that the ranges of entrainment of the physical are smaller than those of the social zeitgebers, The effectiveness of a physical zeitgeber does not depend on its perceptibility. An imperceptible electric field zeitgeber was shown to be stronger than the easily perceptible light-dark zeitgeber. The ranges of entrainment with a definite zeitgeber, moreover, are different with different overt rhythms. As a consequence, the external phase relationships of the different overt rhythms to the zeitgeber vary differently with the zeitgeber period and, therefore, the internal phase relationship between different overt rhythms varies, depending on the zeitgeber period (Fig. 72).

It is another general result of the experiments discussed in this chapter, that all external stimuli, which are effective as zeitgebers when operating periodically, were shown earlier to influence autonomous rhythms, when operating continuously. To give an example, a pure light-dark cycle was shown to exert only a weak zeitgeber effect (cf. 3.2.1) and the intensity of constant illumination does not affect, relevantly, autonomous rhythms (cf. 2.4.1). The remarkable effectiveness of social contacts as a zeitgeber (cf. 3.2.2) coincides with a significant influence of social contacts on autonomous rhythms (cf. 2.4.8). It must be emphasized that this coincidence is not a necessity. Theoretically, other systems are as easily thinkable where effects of continuous forces on autonomous rhythms are independent of effects of periodic forces on heteronomous rhythms. Just for this reason, the experimental result mentioned is of interest, because it contributes to establishing a special model with defined properties which are not generally self-evident in rhythms or, particularly, in self-sustained rhythms.

3.3. Partial Synchronization

3.3.1. Strong Light-dark Zeitgebers

In experiments with heteronomous rhythms, as discussed so far, the applied artificial zeitgebers normally synchronized all overt rhythms (i.e., complete synchronization). In some borderline cases, only a part of the overt rhythms ran synchronously to the zeitgeber, while others free ran (i.e., partial external synchronization (Figs. 71 and 81)). This state necessarily is combined with internal desynchronization. With a special mode of zeitgeber ('strong zeitgeber'), the state of partial external synchronization, combined with forced internal desynchronization, can be induced systematically. Because of the theoretical and practical importance of this state, some experimental series, applying a strong zeitgeber, were performed.

In the preceding chapters, two zeitgebers of different strengths, using light-dark cycles, were applied. In both types, only the main illumination of the experimental room was alternated, while the subjects had the possibility to switch on small auxiliary lamps during dark time. With the stronger of the two zeitgebers, the light-dark cycle was completed by a signal, at regular intervals, calling the subjects for mictions and other tests. This zeitgeber can be strengthened once more, by also connecting the auxiliary lamps to the transformer controlling the main illumination. As a result, the subjects were not able to switch on any illumination during the scheduled dark time and, therefore, were restricted to rest when it became dark. For compensation, the dark period was limited to a quarter of the full period (i.e., to 6 hours in a 24-hour day) and the intensity of illumination during dark time was set at 0.05 lux (an intensity which allowed the subjects to recognize contours). Under the influence of this type of zeitgeber, the subjects are no longer free to select wakefulness and sleep independent of the zeitgeber but are forced to follow the zeitgeber. Subjects, indeed, were able well enough to perform activities, even during total darkness, when the darkness lasted for long periods (Figs. 45 and 83). When the darkness is limited to only a few hours, however, it acts as an inducement to rest. This "absolute light-dark cycle," in contrast to the "relative light-dark cycle" with the possibility of switching on small auxiliary lamps during dark time, was completed by gong signals at

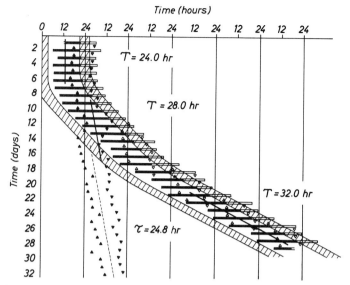

Figure 86. Rhythm of a subject (I.P., ♂ 31 y) living without environmental time cues but under the influence of a strong artificial zeitgeber (i.e., absolute light-dark cycle and regular calling signals) with two alterations of the zeitgeber period; each alteration being performed gradually and lasting 3 days. *I.* Temporal courses of the rhythms of activity, rectal temperature, and psychomotor performance, (i.e., computation speed). The two rhythms first mentioned are presented successively, one period beneath the other. The latter rhythm is indicated by the averaged temporal positions of its acrophases. Indications are the same as in figure 27/I. The thick solid lines combine the average acrophases of computation speed during each section. Shaded areas: dark time of the zeitgeber. From Wever (1973a).

regular intervals calling the subjects for mictions and test sessions, as with the zeitgeber discussed first. The subjects, therefore, awakened normally once during each sleep period. This strong zeitgeber was applied not only for periods close to 24 hours but also for more deviating periods.

Figure 86 shows the course of the first experiment of this series. The subject was exposed, during the total experiment, to the strong zeitgeber just mentioned. During the first week, the period was 24.0 hours, coinciding with the natural day-night cycle, and during this section, the subject's rhythms were entrained fully to the zeitgeber. During the following 3 days, the zeitgeber period was lengthened gradually until a period of 28.0 hours was reached. This period was maintained for 10 days. After this time, the period again was lengthened gradually, over 3 days, to a period of 32.0 hours, which was held constant until the end of the experiment. During the second and third sections of the experiment, the subject's activity

rhythm indeed was entrained to the zeitgeber, but not his rectal temperature rhythm. This rhythm showed a period of 24.8 hours, which corresponds to the average autonomous period. Forced internal desynchronization, therefore, occurred. This indicates that the range of entrainment of the rectal temperature rhythm does not cover even 28.0 hours. The range of entrainment with this strong zeitgeber, with regard to the rectal temperature rhythm, is not essentially larger than with the generally weaker zeitgeber that is based on the relative light-dark cycle. The result indicates that the range of entrainment of the activity rhythm even includes the period of 32.0 hours; the range of entrainment, with regard to this rhythm, is much larger than with the weaker zeitgeber. It is worth noting that the subject had not perceived consciously the drastic lengthening of his subjective days, as with the subjects in the constant condition experiments (cf. 2.2.1). This was true in spite of the fact that the subject, in this type of experiment,

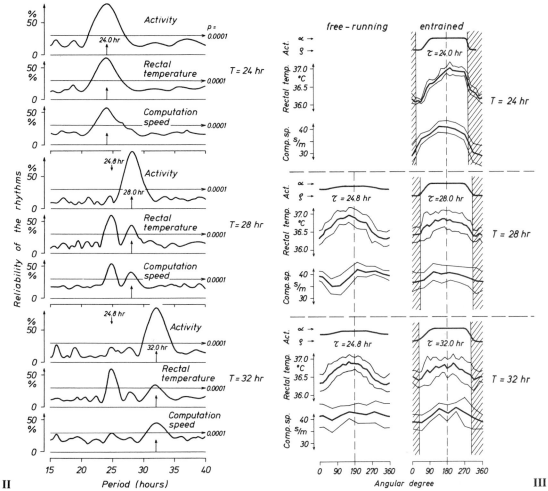

II   **III**

Figure 86/II. Period analyses of the three time series, presented in I, computed separately for the three sections with different zeitgeber periods. *III.* Longitudinally pooled courses of the three rhythms, computed separately for the three sections with different zeitgeber periods. In the first section, with the zeitgeber period as the averaging period, and in the two following sections, with the free running period which is identical in the two sections and the respective zeitgeber period as the averaging periods. Indications are the same as in figure 16/III. Shaded areas: dark time of the zeitgeber, with the zeitgeber period as the averaging period.

could not select the duration of his days spontaneously but was fixed to these days by the experimental conditions.

With the strong zeitgeber applied in the present experiments (Fig. 86), the range of entrainment of the activity rhythm is much larger than that of the rectal temperature rhythm so partial external synchronization occurs within a wide range of zeitgeber periods. This means that, with this type of experiment, internal desynchronization can

be forced easily in every subject, independent of his personality data (cf. 2.3.). This state, however, was mentioned as being of special interest, regarding the evaluation of the multioscillatory concept of the circadian system. With this type of experiment, this state can be investigated without waiting for its spontaneous occurrence. The interaction between the different oscillators, which hypothetically are involved in the multioscillator system, therefore, can be evaluated more fully in experiments with the strong zeitgeber than in those performed under constant conditions. The study of these interactions, however, is an especially suitable way to get insight into the mechanisms underlying the circadian system.

There is another advantage to the experiments performed with the strong zeitgeber, but with periods outside the range of entrainment of the vegetative rhythms, and that is the possibility of getting data from psychological rhythms. In experiments under constant conditions, there are necessarily large gaps in the acquisition of psychological data during the sleep times of the subjects, because the subjects cannot be awakened for tests without breaking the constancy of the conditions. It was discussed earlier (cf. 1.3.2) that it is meaningless to state parameters of psychological rhythms from the results of those experiments because of the regular gaps. In zeitgeber experiments it is possible to awaken the subjects in order to get psychological data ''around the clock'' without changing the intended purpose of the experiment, except with the very weak pure light-dark zeitgeber (cf. 3.2.1). Normally, in those experiments only results from entrained rhythms can be obtained. With the type of experiments presently discussed, the advantages of both types of experiments, free running and entrained rhythms, can be combined. Since a zeitgeber is present, it also is possible to get psychological or performance data at regular intervals during the sleep time of the subjects and, therefore, to state meaningful parameters of rhythms of those variables. Since the zeitgeber operates outside the ranges of entrainment of most of the rhythms, it is possible to get data from free running rhythms. Therefore, with this type of experiment (i.e., a strong zeitgeber, but operating with periods greatly deviating from 24.0 hours), data of psychological or psychomotor rhythms can be obtained meaningfully, although a part of the different overt rhythms measured free run autonomously.

In order to illustrate this possibility, in figure 86/I the course of the rhythm of the maximal computation speed (Pauli-test) is indicated by thick solid lines that combine the averaged acrophases of the rhythm of this computation speed. During the first section, the performance rhythm ran synchronously to the zeitgeber, the rhythms of activity, and rectal temperature. During the second section, with the artificial 28.0-hour day, the overt rhythm of performance showed a period of 24.8 hours, i.e., it ran synchronously to the overt rectal temperature rhythm but neither to the zeitgeber nor the overt activity rhythm). During the third section, the overt rhythm of performance, on the contrary, ran synchronously to the zeitgeber and the activity rhythm but not to the overt activity rhythm. During the third general result, the overt performance rhythm did neither run under all conditions synchronously to the overt rectal temperature rhythm, nor under all conditions synchronously to the overt activity rhythm.

The conclusions drawn from the inspection of the courses of the overt rhythms (Fig. 86/I) were confirmed by analyses computed in the usual manner. Figure 86/II shows the results of the period analyses, computed separately from the three sections with the different zeitgeber periods, and from each of the three time series presented in figure 86/I. During the first section ($T = 24.0$ hours), all three time series (i.e., activity, rectal temperature, and computation speed) show one reliable period coinciding with the zeitgeber period and indicating full entrainment of all rhythms. During the second and third section, activity also shows one reliable period coinciding with the zeitgeber period. Rectal temperature shows two reliable periods during the second and third sections. The values of the primary periods coincide among the two sections but do not coincide with the respective zeitgeber periods; the primary periods, rather, correspond to free running rhythms. This behavior indicates partial synchronization to the zeitgeber and simultaneously, internal desynchronization forced by the zeitgeber. In addition, there are secondary rectal temperature periods, each coinciding with the respective zeitgeber period. Computation speed shows, during the second section, a pattern very similar to that of rectal temperature; i. e., the primary performance period coincides with the relevant rectal temperature period but not with the activity period. The analysis of the third section results, reversely, in one reliable period coinciding with the relevant activity period, but not with the rectal temperature period. In summary, the period analyses show two rhythm components, one of which always is synchronized to the zeitgeber while the other component free runs independent of the zeitgeber, except during the first section with the 24.0-hour zeitgeber. From these results, it must be concluded that the basic oscillator controlling the rhythm component first mentioned follows the zeitgeber within a large range of entrainment, which includes all periods applied in this experiment, while the basic oscillator controlling the other rhythm component can be entrained only within a small range. The overt rhythm of the performance variable must be understood as being controlled, as with the overt rhythms of physiological variables, collectively by both underlying oscillators but with different portions during the second and third section.

This picture once more can be confirmed by the results of the longitudinal poolings (Fig. 86/III), which also have been computed separately for the three sections. In each of the sections, except in the first one, the average periods are presented twice, with the free running period (left) and the zeitgeber period (right). As can be seen, the reliability of the activity rhythm is, in all sections, much greater with the zeitgeber period than with the free running period. Contrary to this, the reliability of the rectal temperature rhythm, during the second and third section where there is a free running component, is greater with the free running than with the zeitgeber period. To be sure, in both of these sections, there are secondary rhythm components with the period of the zeitgeber. The picture is more ambiguous with the performance rhythm. During the first section where all rhythms are entrained fully both externally and internally, there is a performance rhythm of high reliability. During the second section, the performance

rhythm is reliable with both periods, but to a higher degree with the free running period. During the third section, there is a reliable performance rhythm only with the zeitgeber period. The internal phase relationships between the rhythms of activity and rectal temperature show the common picture. During the first section, with full external synchronization, the activity rhythm is the leading one and, during the other sections, the rectal temperature rhythm is the leading one with both rhythm components. The rhythm of computation speed runs in phase with the rectal temperature rhythm as long as it is synchronized to the zeitgeber. Only during the second section, where it free runs synchronously to the rectal temperature rhythm, it lags clearly behind the rectal temperature rhythm.

Results of another experiment of this series are shown in figure 87 but with the longitudinal presentation of the temporal courses (Fig. 87/I). In this experiment, the subject first was exposed for 9 days to an artificial 24.0-hour day constituted by the strong zeitgeber. He afterwards was exposed, for 21 periods (i.e., for 24.5 objective days), to a 28.0-hour day, which was known from other experiments to be too long for entrainment of the vegetative rhythms (Fig. 86). The L:D-ratio was the same, in both sections, with 18-hour light and 6-hour darkness during the first section and 21-hour light and 7-hour darkness during the second section, each calculated from one midpoint of twilight to the next. The twilight transitions lasted consistently for 40 minutes. In this example, in addition to activity, rectal temperature, and computation speed, cortisol excretion in urine is presented as representative for another type of physiological variables. Beside these four typical variables, physiological data (e.g., electrolytes in the urine) and psychological data (e.g., time estimation) were measured. The additional presentation of those variables, however, would not enlarge the understanding of the essential properties of the circadian system.

Figure 87/I shows, in its first section (24.0-hour day) clear rhythmical courses of all variables. The period analyses of this

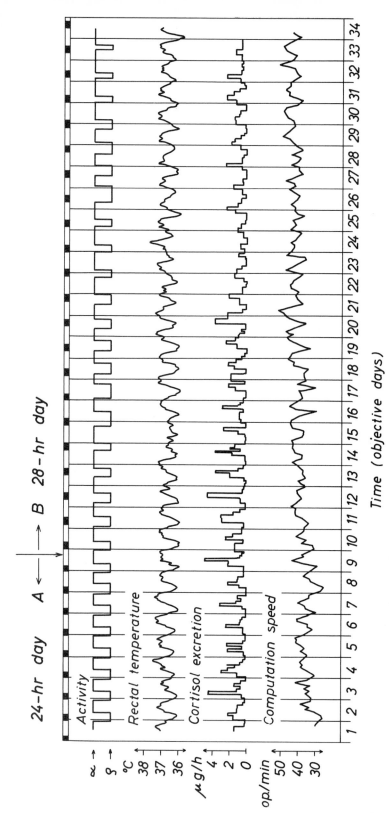

Figure 87. Rhythm of a subject (E.M., ♂ 26 y) living without environmental time cues but under the influence of a strong artificial zeitgeber with one alteration of the zeitgeber period. Presented, from top to bottom, are the rhythms of activity (i.e., alternation between activity α and rest ρ), rectal temperature (measured continuously), urinary excretion of free cortisol (i.e., mictions taken at regular intervals), and computation speed (measured after mictions with an automatic Pauli-test maschine). *I.* Longitudinally presented courses of the four variables during the total experiment.

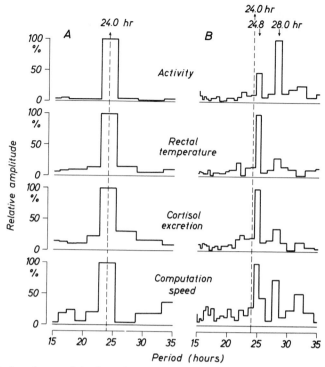

Figure 87/II. Period analyses of the four time series, presented in I, computed separately for the two sections with different zeitgeber periods (A and B).

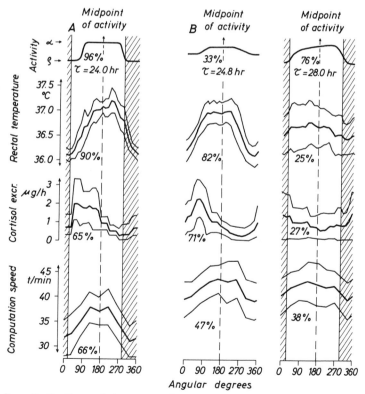

Figure 87/III. Longitudinally pooled courses of the four rhythms, computed separately for the two sections (A and B), with section A being an averaging period coinciding with the zeitgeber period and B being two averaging periods, derived from II as the two most prominent peaks; one of the periods coincides with the zeitgeber period. Indications are the same as in figure 86/III. From Wever (1975d).

165

section (Fig. 87/II), with all variables, show one 'spectral line,' with the center of gravity at 24.0 hours. These spectral lines are broad because of the shortness of this section. The longitudinal poolings (Fig. 87/III) demonstrate significantly reliable rhythms in all variables. The phase relationships between the rhythms of activity and rectal temperature correspond to those characteristic in rhythms synchronized to the natural 24-hour day [i.e., leading phase of the activity rhythm (Fig. 17)]. The phase relationship of the cortisol rhythm to the other rhythms also corresponds to the normal one. Maximal cortisol excretion occurs several hours after 'lights on' and almost simultaneously with the activity onset. With this, the urine cortisol is maximal during that part of the cycle where the body temperature increases. The performance rhythm runs nearly parallel to the rhythm of deep body temperature. It is constituted by all measured data during the full day; not only by the 'night values.' Even the slight depression in performance around noon is indicated. As the general result, all rhythms measured in this special subject were shown to correspond to normal data and, therefore, these data obtained in the 24.0-hour day can be taken for normal base line values.

In section B of this experiment (28-hour day), the activity rhythm of the subject was forced to run synchronously to the zeitgeber by the applied mode of the zeitgeber. The variability of the activity rhythm, especially that of the activity onset, however, was much greater than in section A (Fig. 87/I). In order to enable this variability the dark time was chosen to be shorter than the sleep time to be expected. In all other variables, clearly rhythmical courses are recognizable only during a few special intervals of section B (days 10 to 13, 18 to 21, and 28 to 30). If only these intervals are considered, synchronization could be concluded, as in section A, even with internal phase relationships corresponding to those observed in section A. For instance, maximal cortisol excretion occurs, during those days, shortly after "lights on" or around activity onset. Section B, how-

ever, includes other intervals of days where nearly no rhythmicity can be recognized and, especially, where internal phase relationships between the different rhythms cannot be stated meaningfully. Those 'bad' intervals (days 14/15, 23/24, and 32/33) occur between the 'good' intervals. Only the summarizing inspection of the total time series of section B, in computed analyses, can solve this apparent discrepancy. These analyses clearly demonstrate that conclusions based on the inspection of only short intervals are misleading.

In the period analyses of section B (Fig. 87/II), two peak periods generally are present. In the activity rhythm, there is, according to expectation, a primary peak at 28.0 hours, but, in addition, there is a secondary peak at 24.8 hours which is also significantly different from 24.0 hours. In all other rhythms presented, the primary period is at 24.8 hours (i.e., at a period that corresponds to an autonomous rhythm), indicating free running rhythms which are not entrained to the 28.0-hour zeitgeber or the 28.0-hour activity rhythm. In all rhythms, however, a secondary period of 28.0 hours is present, indicating another rhythm component in these rhythms runs synchronously to the zeitgeber and the activity rhythm.

More explanatory is the inspection of the longitudinal poolings of section B, which is presented with the two relevant periods of 24.8 hours and 28.0 hours (Fig. 87/III). With the 24.8-hour averaging period, the phase of the highly reliable rectal temperature rhythm leads the activity rhythm, which is characteristic in autonomously running rhythms (Fig. 17) but deviating from the phase relationship in section A. The similarly reliable cortisol rhythm has the same internal phase relationship to the rectal temperature rhythm as before, with the maximal excretion during that part of the cycle where deep body temperature increases. The rhythm of computation speed again runs parallel to the temperature rhythm. Even the noon depression is indicated. The average of the performance data is remarkably higher than in section A, due to a continuous temporal trend or 'learning effect.' This trend, in fact, enlarges the variability of the performance data, indicating once more the inadmissibility of the formally computed standard deviations for statistical purposes. It is worth noting that the reliability of the performance rhythm with this period is guaranteed even without eliminating this trend by common 'detrending' procedures. With the 28.0-hour averaging period (i.e., with the period of the zeitgeber and activity rhythm), the rhythms of rectal temperature and cortisol excretion cannot be differentiated significantly from random fluctuations. If they are still taken as being real, the cortisol rhythm especially would show a drastically differing phase relationship. The maximal cortisol excretion occurs with this rhythm component during the dark-time or sleep of the subjects and at the time of minimal body temperature, in contrast to what occurs generally in the natural day and, in particular, with this subject in the artificial 24.0-hour day and the free running rhythm component in the 28.0-hour day. Simultaneously, this experimentally determined phase relationship rejects the assumption that this component of the cortisol rhythm is nothing but a passive reaction to the light-dark cycle or the alternation between wakefulness and sleep (cf. 4.3.2). Only the performance rhythm shows a significant component with a period of 28.0 hours. The reliability of this rhythm component, however, is due to only the especially low values during dark time, the measure of which requires the subject be awakened from sleep. Excluding these 'awakening values', the remaining performance data could not be differentiated from random fluctuations. If the same data are pooled with the 24.8-hour averaging period, all average data contribute to a reliable rhythmicity. The 'awakening values' here shift continuously over the full cycle and, therefore, they contribute to all average values regularly, with the consequence they enlarge the variabilities.

Especially with the longitudinal presentation of experiments with internal desynchronization forced by a strong zeitgeber

(Fig. 87), a striking similarity to experiments with spontaneous occurrence of internal desynchronization can be recognized (Fig. 25). In both cases, there is a periodic change between intervals with well marked rhythms and badly marked rhythms which must be interpreted as beat phenomena generated by the superposition of two or several rhythm components with different periods (see Fig. 112). Both types of experiments, therefore, complement each other in evaluating the multioscillatory structure of the circadian system. In the examples of experiments with the strong zeitgeber discussed so far, there may be another similarity to autonomous rhythms with internal desynchronization. In autonomous rhythms, internal desynchronization occurred mostly spontaneously during the experiment (Figs. 27, 28, 67, and 81), but a spontaneous termination of this state has never been observed. In the strong zeitgeber experiments (Figs. 86 and 87), the rhythms ran internally synchronized during the first section and internally desynchronized until the end of the experiment. This latter behavior surely did not occur spontaneously, but was forced by the experimental design. Care must be taken, nevertheless, about whether or not a possible temporal trend, increasing the tendency toward internal desynchronization, influences this behavior. The existence of such a trend can be tested by permutating the temporal sequences of the sections with internal synchronization and desynchronization.

The course of the experiment, shown as another example (Fig. 88), differs from the examples shown earlier (Figs. 86 and 87) in two respects. First, a period shorter than 24 hours was added and, second, the 24.0-hour zeitgeber period was introduced in the middle section of the experiment. It is to be expected, therefore, to obtain not only the transition from internally synchronized to desynchronized rhythms, but also the reversed transition. Figure 88, in fact, shows that the rhythm of rectal temperature was only entrained to the 24.0-hour day, but free running in the 28.0-hour and the 20.0-hour day, while the rhythm of activity was en-

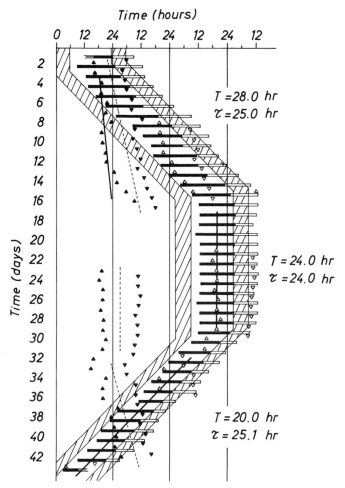

Figure 88. Rhythm of a subject (C.G., ♀ 27 y) living without environmental time cues but under the influence of a strong artificial zeitgeber with two alterations of the zeitgeber period. Temporal courses of the rhythms of activity, rectal temperature, and psychomotor performance (i.e., computation speed) are shown. The two rhythms first mentioned are presented successively, one period beneath the other. The latter rhythm is indicated by the averaged temporal positions of its acrophases. Indications are the same as in figure 86/I. From Wever (1975a).

trained to all zeitgeber periods applied. As the result, the rhythm ran synchronized internally only during the middle section with the 24.0-hour zeitgeber. After the change in the zeitgeber period from 28 to 24 hours, rectal temperature was nearly constant for several days, so no rhythmicity could be detected by any method (Fig. 118). As in figure 86, the averaged acrophases of the overt performance rhythm (i.e., computa-

tion speed) are presented by solid lines. As can be seen, this rhythm was entrained during the first section to the free running rectal temperature rhythm, but not to the zeitgeber and the activity rhythm. During the second section, all rhythms, including the performance rhythm, ran entrained fully externally and internally. During the third section, the performance rhythm was entrained to the zeitgeber and the activity rhythm, but not to

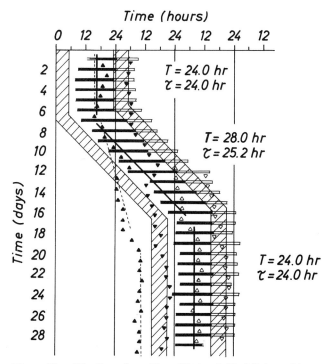

Figure 89. Rhythm of a subject (H.A., ♀ 22 y) living without environmental time cues but under the influence of a strong artificial zeitgeber with two alterations of the zeitgeber period. Temporal courses of the rhythms of activity, rectal temperature, and psychomotor performance (i.e., computation speed) are shown. The two rhythms first mentioned are presented successively, one period beneath the other. The latter rhythm is indicated by the averaged temporal positions of its acrophases. Indications are the same as in figure 86/I.

the free running rectal temperature rhythm. The result of this experiment, therefore, also confirms that the performance rhythm can follow either the activity rhythm or the rectal temperature rhythm. Similar results were obtained in four more experiments with identical sequences of the sections.

Figure 89 shows the course of an experiment with once more altered temporal sequence of the sections with different zeitgeber periods. The rhythms run internally synchronized, not during the middle section but during the first and third section (zeitgeber period 24.0 hours), and internally desynchronized during the middle section (zeitgeber period 28.0 hours). The reason for this repeatedly permutated temporal sequence is to guarantee that the results are not simu-

lated by a temporal trend, especially with regard to the performance rhythm which always is superimposed by a steady learning increase (Figs. 117 to 119). In this special experiment, the performance rhythm is synchronized to the zeitgeber and, therefore, to the activity rhythm during all sections. This means, that during the middle section, it is not synchronized to the autonomously running rectal temperature rhythm. This behavior is not a consistent rule. In another experiment of this type, on the contrary, the performance rhythm always is synchronized to the rectal temperature rhythm and, therefore, neither synchronized to the zeitgeber nor the activity rhythm during the middle section.

In other experiments of this series, the

period of the strong zeitgeber was not altered during the experiment, as in the examples shown in figures 86 to 89, but held constant during the total experiment. The reason was to evaluate the interaction between the different oscillators within internally desynchronized rhythms being undisturbed for a long time. From the results of these experiments, the period analyses of the rectal temperature rhythms are of primary interest. Figure 90 shows this type of period analyses originating from three different experiments performed immediately after each other under otherwise identical conditions where the subjects lived, during the total experiment, under the influence of a strong 28-hour, 30-hour, and 32-hour zeitgeber. With all these subjects, there were free running components of the rectal temperature rhythm, with periods that were, by

chance, very close together in all three experiments (24.7 hours). With all three subjects, there also were other rhythm components with the period of the zeitgeber, equivalent to the respective period of the overt activity rhythm. There, however, were systematic differences between the three experiments. The farther the zeitgeber period is from the free running period, the more strongly marked is the rhythm component with the freerunning period and the more weakly marked is the rhythm component with the zeitgeber period. This result was confirmed by further experiments and is in agreement with results obtained in single experiments with repeated alterations in the zeitgeber period. For instance, in the period analyses of the rectal temperature rhythm in figure 86, the entrained rhythm component is larger in reliability and amplitude when compared to the free running rhythm component in the 28-hour day than in the 32-hour day (Figs. 86/II and III). Similar results also were obtained in six more experiments with identical sequences of the sections with different zeitgeber periods. This result indicates that the ratio between the different rhythm components contributing to the overt rhythm depends systematically on the conditions (i.e., this ratio cannot be a property of the system). In other words, the different oscillators involved in the circadian multioscillator system contribute to the control of the different overt rhythms, with fractions that differ not only interindividually, but also change with the experimental condition. With regard to rectal temperature, the fractions, with which the oscillators contribute to this control, seem to vary systematically with the difference in periods between the oscillators.

The experiments forcing internal desynchronization, by a strong zeitgeber operating with a period widely deviating from 24.0 hours, were not performed only with singly isolated subjects, as discussed so far, but also with groups of collectively isolated subjects. As an example, figure 91 shows results from an experiment with four subjects living together in the two isolation units, which were connected for this experiment. During

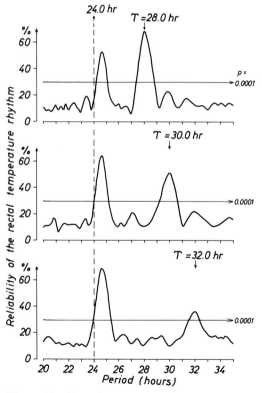

Figure 90. Rectal temperature rhythms of three subjects, in individual experiments, living without environmental time cues but under the influence of a strong artificial zeitgeber with three different zeitgeber periods. Presented are the period analyses of the rhythms.

the total experiment, they remained under the influence of an artificial 30.0-hour day generated by the strong zeitgeber (i.e., absolute light-dark cycle and regular calling signals). In this case also, it is of minor interest to analyze the activity rhythms. These rhythms, forced by the experimental condition, ran entrained collectively to the zeitgeber and, therefore, also were synchronized mutually. Of major interest, however, is the inspection of the rectal temperature rhythms of the four subjects, which ran autonomously with periods deviating from that of the activity rhythms. The lines combining the maximum and the minimum values, with different symbols characterizing the different subjects, show that the rectal temperature rhythms of the different subjects not only had equal periods, but even equal phases. There is no consistent sequence in the extreme values according to subjects but, rather, a temporal sequence changing from day to day. This indicates that the rectal temperature rhythms of the different subjects did not have, only by chance, very similar periods, but they run synchronized mutually.

The results taken from figure 91/I can be confirmed by computed analyses. Figure 91/II shows the results of period analyses. It would be of only minor interest to look for results originating from the activity rhythms. Those results coincide in all four subjects with one sharp peak at the zeitgeber period of 30.0 hours, with reliabilities between 92% and 96%. Of greater interest is the inspection of results originating from the rectal temperature rhythms. In the analyses of all four subjects, there are primary and highly reliable peaks at 24.7 hours, exactly coinciding in periods. In no subject is 24.0 hours included in the range of reliability. In all four subjects, there are secondary, but reliable, peaks at the zeitgeber period of 30.0 hours. Only in one subject (N), in addition, a reliable period of 15.0 hours is included, indicating a bimodal course of the respective 30.0-hour rhythm (cf. Fig. 91/III). In order to compare results of another physiological rhythm, from the multiplicity of rhythms measured in each subject, figure 91/II includes period analyses of potassium excretion. In contrast to the analyses of rectal temperature rhythms, they show considerable differences among the subjects. Only in two subjects (K and N), there are reliable rhythms with a period of 24.7 hours and, in only one subject (K), this is the primary period. Rhythmicities with the zeitgeber period of 30.0 hours are included reliably in all subjects. Finally, figure 91/II includes period analyses of the performance rhythms (i.e., computation speed), and there again is another picture. In one subject (N), there is no reliable rhythmicity at all and, in the other subjects, there are proportions between the periods of 24.7 hours and 30.0 hours which are different among the subjects and the proportions of the other overt rhythms in the same subjects. In summary, the contributions of the different rhythm components or the different underlying oscillators to an overt rhythm are consistent among the subjects with regard to the rectal temperature rhythm, but not to the other rhythms. As the main result, there are two different oscillators involved in the multioscillator system of every subject, and these, independent of each other, are entrained mutually among the subjects.

While the period analyses presented in figure 91/II show that those rhythm components, which run autonomously, all have the same period, another analysis shows the coincidence regarding the phases. Figure 91/III presents results of averaging procedures (longitudinal poolings) for all four subjects. The data are presented twice, with averaging periods of 24.7 hours and 30.0 hours, which are the only significant periods included in all time series (Fig. 91/II). The course of the averaged activity rhythms is presented only once for all subjects because, in this scale, the different rhythms of the four subjects would not be distinguishable. For the other variables (i.e., rectal temperature, potassium excretion, computation speed), the curves, averaged from each of the four subjects, are presented closely beneath each other to enable a comparison. As can be seen, the averaged rhythms coincide very well in their phase positions. This means

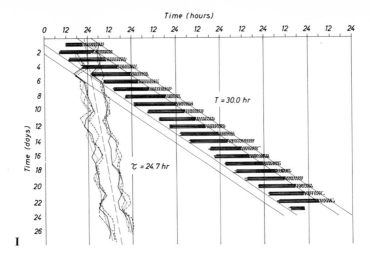

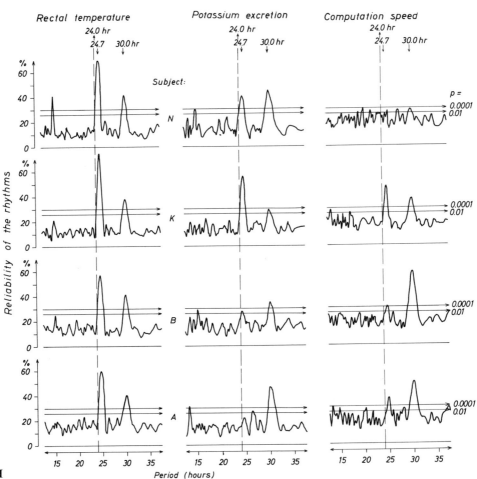

Figure 91. Rhythms of a group of four subjects (M.A., ♂ 20 y; W.B., ♂ 22 y; D.K., ♂ 22 y; and B.N., ♂ 21 y) living collectively without environmental time cues but under the influence of a strong artificial zeitgeber. *I.* Temporal courses of the rhythms of activity and rectal temperature. The activity rhythms are represented by successive lines (solid = activity; dotted = rest), one period beneath the other, with the rhythms of the different subjects arranged immediately one beneath the other. The rectal temperature rhythms are represented by lines, with different symbols characterizing the different subjects, combining the temporal positions of maximum (front group of lines) and minimum values. Framed areas: dark time of the zeitgeber. From Wever (1976a). *II.* Period analyses of the time series of rectal temperature, potassium excretion, and psychomotor performance (i.e., computation speed; mictions and tests taken at regular intervals), computed from data of the four different subjects.

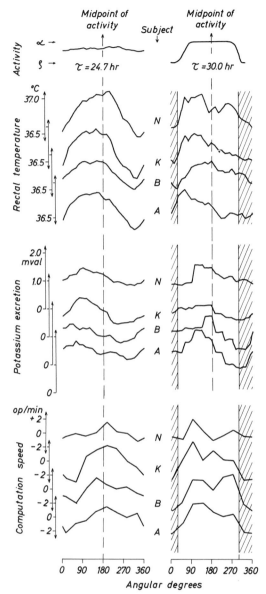

Figure 91/III. Longitudinally pooled courses of the rhythms of activity and the three rhythms, presented in II, with two averaging periods derived as the two most prominent peaks from II. The average activity cycle is presented only once in each section, since it coincides in all four subjects. The average cycles of other variables from the different subjects are arranged immediately one beneath the other. Indications are the same as in figure 86/III.

that the rhythms of the different subjects do not run only with equal periods (Fig. 91/II), but also with equal phases. In other words, the computed analyses confirm the conclusions, already drawn from figure 91/I, that

the vegetative rhythms of the four subjects are synchronized mutually. The mutual synchronization of the overt activity rhythms among the subjects is by no means remarkable. It is forced primarily by the zeitgeber condition and secondly to facilitate the companionship. It, however, is remarkable that the imperceptible rhythms of rectal temperature, which run desynchronized from the activity rhythms, are also mutually synchronized among the subjects. The only stimuli that can arrange the mutual synchronization are the mutual social contacts. With this result, an earlier suggestion, deduced from groups living collectively under constant conditions but based on intervals too short to guarantee this result (Fig. 67, right), is confirmed at a high level of reliability. The only finding, which may be comparable, is the mutual synchronization of menstrual cycles among young girls living together in a college dormitory (McClintock, 1971).

3.3.2. External Modifications of Partially Desynchronized Rhythms

In experiments with the strong zeitgeber discussed so far, the state of internal desynchronization, as forced by the special experimental design, was the main interest of discussions. For instance, it was one of the purposes of the experiments to study mutual interactions between separated oscillators in order to evaluate basic properties of the multioscillator system. In other experiments, also performed under the influence of the strong zeitgeber, the forcing of internal desynchronization was nothing but a tool; and the purpose of the experiments was to evaluate effects of environmental stimuli on vegetative rhythms that run independently of conscious activity rhythms (i.e., separated from these rhythms by internal desynchronization). Those experiments can be mentioned only in parentheses because respective experimental series are currently in progress and significant results have not been obtained yet. The approach of these experiments seems to be so promising they

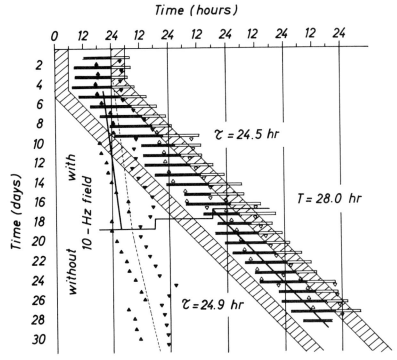

Figure 92.   Rhythm of a subject (B.K., ♀ 20 y) living without environmental time cues but under the influence of a strong artificial zeitgeber with a constant period after several initial days. The subject additionally was under the influence of a continuously operating artificial electric AC field (i.e., 10 Hz square wave, 2.5 V/m) during the first section and protected from natural and artificial electromagnetic fields during the second section. Temporal courses of the rhythms of activity, rectal temperature, and psychomotor performance (i.e., computation speed) are shown. The two rhythms first mentioned are presented successively, one period beneath the other. The latter rhythm is indicated by the averaged temporal positions of its acrophases. Indications are the same as in figure 86/I.

are worth discussion, even with only preliminary results (Wever, 1976b).

As a first example, figure 92 shows the course of an experiment where the subject was exposed to a strong 28.0-hour zeitgeber during the total experiment, except for the initial first 3 days. The result expected was that his activity rhythm would follow the forced schedule. The subject additionally was exposed continuously, during the first section of the experiment, to a weak artificial electric 10-Hz square wave field (cf. 2.4.5.). During the second section, the subject was protected from artificial, except from the technical 50-Hz field (cf. 2.4.5), and natural electromagnetic fields. The experiment was performed in the shielded experimental unit (cf. 2.4.4). The presentation at figure 92 gives the impression that the period of the rectal temperature rhythm, which,

during both sections, ran desynchronized from the activity rhythm, was shorter during the first section, with the field in operation, than during the other section. This effect of the 10-Hz field would agree with the effect of the same field on internally synchronized rhythms running under constant conditions (Table 7). The suggested change in period is close to the limit where such a change can be detected meaningfully. A greater change in period, however, cannot be expected, according to the correlation between original period and effect (Fig. 58/II). The performance rhythm included in figure 92 shows a more striking modification possibly induced by the 10-Hz field. During the first section, with the field continuously in operation, in the rhythm of computation speed (Pauli-test) only one reliable component, with a period of 24.5 hours, was present (reliability 54%)

(i.e., it ran synchronously to the rectal temperature rhythm without any detectable correlation to the activity rhythm and the zeitgeber). During the second section, the primary component of the performance rhythm had a period of 28.0 hours (reliability 54%) and a secondary component had a period of 24.9 hours (reliability 44%) (i.e., during the second section, without the field in operation, the overt performance rhythm ran synchronously to the activity rhythm and the zeitgeber, but not to the rectal temperature rhythm). If the result deduced from figure 92 can be confirmed by further experiments (to the present, there are only four experiments of this type, but with consistent results), it would mean that vegetative rhythms, when running autonomously but separated from the consciously perceptible activity rhythms by internal desynchronization, are affected by environmental stimuli in the same manner as internally synchronized rhythms; as desynchronized vegetative rhythms already were shown to be entrainable separately by external zeitgebers (Figs. 81, 91). According to the multioscillator hypothesis, this result would be a direct confirmation that every single oscillator can be excited separately by external stimuli. The result derived from figure 92 additionally would mean that the performance rhythm is affected by the 10-Hz field. In all other types of experiments performed with the artificial field (cf. 2.4.5 and 3.2.3), performance rhythms cannot be evaluated relevantly (cf. 1.3.2).

In the experiment underlying figure 92, a change in the period of desynchronized vegetative rhythms was released, which hardly can be discriminated from random fluctuations. With a special experimental design, however, it may be possible to amplify such a change in period to a considerable amount so that it can be detected clearly. This design takes advantage of the instability of a period very close to the limits of the range of entrainment (Wever, 1972a). If a rhythm operates very close to such a limit, a small change in period, which may be too small to be observable directly, may be sufficient to make the period jump from outside to inside,

or inside to outside, of the range of entrainment. As the consequence, there is a transition from externally desynchronized to synchronized vegetative rhythms or reversely, which necessarily is combined with a considerable change in the period of these rhythms. As a further consequence, if the activity rhythm is fixed in period by a strong zeitgeber, there is a simultaneous transition from internally desynchronized to synchronized rhythms or reversely. In this type of experiment, the strong zeitgeber is the tool which brings the period to the limit value desired. The experimental design will be illustrated by an experiment where the influence of psychical burden or stress is tested. It was the impression gained from experiments performed under constant conditions that, in autonomous rhythms, stress lengthens the period and increases the tendency toward internal desynchronization; these changes, however, were so small that the experimental results were not sufficient to guarantee this impression (cf. 2.4.7).

In the experiment underlying figure 93, a subject was exposed, during the total experiment, to a strong zeitgeber with a period of 22 hours 40 minutes, which was shown earlier to be very close to the lower limit of the range of entrainment of the vegetative variables (cf. 3.1.1). In addition, the subject had to perform a psychomotor test (i.e., multichoice reaction time) at regular intervals. During the first half of the experiment, the test sessions were short (3 minutes each), so the subject was not bothered by the tests. During the second half of the experiment, the test sessions were lengthened (6 to 9 minutes each), with the consequence that the subject complained about the tests without being fully aware of the reasons for his annoyance. The result of this experiment is shown in figure 93/I. The subject's rhythms were entrained fully to the zeitgeber and, therefore, internally synchronized during the first section. During the second section, only the activity rhythm was entrained to the zeitgeber, while the rectal temperature rhythm, and other vegetative rhythms, showed a typical free running period. In the computed period analyses (Fig. 93/II), the activity rhythm shows, coinciding in both sections, one clear peak corresponding to the zeitgeber. The rhythm of rectal temperature shows two peaks in every section; one corresponding to the zeitgeber (22.7 hours) and another to the free running period (24.5 hours). During the first section, however, the shorter (i.e., zeitgeber) period is dominant, indicating internal synchronization, and, during the second section, the longer (i.e., free running) period is dominant, indicating internal desynchronization. From the longitudinally averaged rhythms (Fig. 93/III) with the entrained rhythm components (22.7 hours) there results a lagging phase of the rectal temperature rhythm, which is characteristic in rhythms entrained to a short period (Fig. 72). With the free running rhythm components (24.5 hours), a rhythmicity in activity is marked by such a small amount that an internal phase relationship cannot be determined. Remarkably, during the second section, with the stronger botheration, the course of the entrained rhythm component of the rectal temperature rhythm is bimodal to an extent never seen in other experiments. During the other section, the course of this rhythm component is monomodal, as usual, like the courses of the free running components of this rhythm in both sections.

The direct effect of an increase in psychical workload on the rectal temperature rhythm must be expected to be only small. In this special experiment, the instability of the rhythm, near the lower limit of the range of entrainment, was used to amplify this small effect to a change in period of nearly 2 hours, which is detectable. It was the original interpretation that the increase in psychical workload affects a lengthening in the period, with the result that the period transgressed the limit of the range of entrainment of the zeitgeber. It is another possible interpretation that the increase in psychical workload did not affect directly the period, but the amplitude of the rectal temperature rhythm. A diminishing in amplitude also would result in a jump from inside to outside the range of entrainment, with the consequence of a drastic change in period. In this

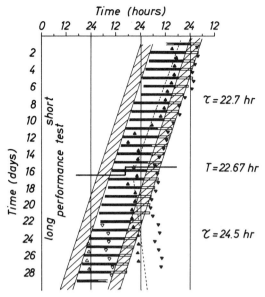

Figure 93. Rhythm of a subject (T.A., ♂ 26 y) living without environmental time cues but under the influence of a strong artificial zeitgeber with a constant period. The subject additionally had to perform a psychomotor test (i.e., multiple choice reaction time), which was of short duration during the first section but long during the second section. *I.* Temporal courses of the rhythms of activity and rectal temperature, presented successively one period beneath the other. Indications are the same as in figure 86/I.

case, the reason for the jump over the limit is not an original change in period, but a change in the position of the limit. As can be seen in figure 93/III, however, the amplitudes are larger in the second than in the first section, so the latter interpretation is rather unlikely in this special experiment. Clear discrimination between the two possible interpretations can come only from complementary experiments near the other limit of the range of entrainment. If the first interpretation is correct, increasing psychical workload must facilitate internal synchronization contrary to that suggested near the lower limit. If the second interpretation is correct, increasing psychical workload must lead to internal desynchronization near the upper limit, just as near the lower limit of the range of entrainment. In any case, the use of the instabilities close to the limits of the range of

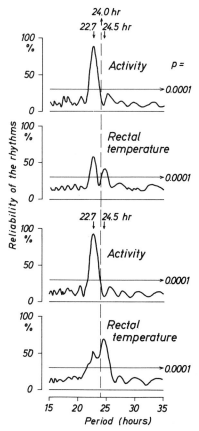

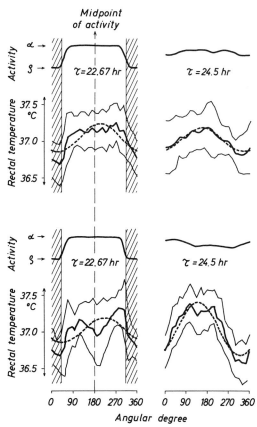

Figure 93/II. Period analyses of the two time series, presented in I, computed separately for the two sections with short and long duration performance test.

Figure 93/III. Longitudinally pooled courses of the two rhythms, computed separately for the two sections, with two averaging periods being identical in the two sections and derived as the two most prominent peaks from II. Indications are the same as in figure 86/III.

entrainment amplifies originally small affects, which may be near the limit of detection, to clearly detectable effects.

3.3.3. Experiments with Continuously Changing Zeitgeber Period

In all experiments performed with the strong zeitgeber discussed so far, the zeitgeber periods were set inside the limits of 20 and 32 hours and each zeitgeber period was held constant for at least 1 week. The main purpose of the experiments was to force internal desynchronization, in order to study interactions between different oscillators. The zeitgeber periods, therefore, must be selected so

they can be expected to be outside the smaller range of entrainment of the rectal temperature rhythm, or close to the limit of this range (Fig. 93), but inside the larger range of entrainment of the activity rhythm. From former evaluations (cf. 3.1.1), the limits of the latter range were suggested to be about 18.5 and 33.5 hours. The applied periods of the strong zeitgeber, therefore, could be expected to force internal desynchronization and make the desired investigations possible.

Another question, which also can be answered with experiments applying the strong zeitgeber, is that for evaluating the limits of the ranges of entrainment, coordinated to the different overt rhythms, more precisely. This concerns the different vegetative rhythms that were represented, in most of the experiments, by the rectal temperature rhythm, and the activity rhythm of which the limits of the range of entrainment were not transgressed, and, therefore, not demonstrated directly, in the presently discussed experiments with the strong zeitgeber. In the favored design of experiments for answering these questions, the period of the strong zeitgeber is not held constant, as in the other experiments, but continuously changing. In this type of experiment, it must be noted at which zeitgeber period the different overt rhythms break from the zeitgeber rhythm. The zeitgeber period at this instant indicates the limit of the range of entrainment of the respective rhythm. The experimental series, applying this design, is still in progress and, therefore, significant results cannot be communicated; only results of pilot studies can be used.

As an example, figure 94 shows the course of an experiment that was performed especially to detect the upper limit of the range of entrainment of the activity rhythm. In this experiment, the subject was exposed to a strong zeitgeber, of which the period was lengthened during 3 weeks, steadily and progressively, from 24.0 to 48.0 hours and then held constant at the latter value for 1 week. It was remarkable that the subject did not perceive consciously this drastic lengthening. As a primary result, the rectal temperature rhythm broke from the zeitgeber after the first week, when the zeitgeber had reached a period of 27.5 hours. It afterwards showed a free running period of 25.0 hours, independent of the zeitgeber, except for the last week (see below). Both of these findings agree with former results. They indicate a range of entrainment, coordinated to this rhythm, ranging to about 27.5 hours and a free running period coinciding with other experiments. During the last week, when the zeitgeber period was 48.0 hours, the period of the rectal temperature rhythm was 24.0 hours, indicating synchronization to a submultiple of the zeitgeber period.

Regarding the activity rhythm, the result, deduced by visual inspection from the course of the experiment (Fig. 94/I), is rather unclear. A more sophisticated consideration is necessary to see what really happened. The reason is that the subjectively stated alternation between 'day' and 'night' always followed the zeitgeber, according to the experimental design. Therefore, knowledge about activity only can come from the consideration of the objective recording (i.e., contact plates under the floor). In figure 94/II, period analyses of this activity record are presented separately for the 4 weeks of the experiment and computed with two different modes. In the left diagrams, normal period analyses are given, based on equidistantly scanned activity values. In the right diagrams, the time unit (abscissa) is not a fixed absolute value, but a fixed fraction of the zeitgeber period and, therefore, continuously increasing in length during the first 3 weeks. With this procedure, synchronization to a zeitgeber also can be detected when the zeitgeber period is changing.

The period analyses of the first week show a reliable activity period at about 25 hours (left), and an even more reliable period coinciding with the zeitgeber period (right), respectively. This result is understandable because the zeitgeber period varied only very little during this week and had a mean of about 25 hours. During the second week, there is only a small rhythm component with a fixed period. This is again 25 hours, coinciding with the period of the rectal temperature rhythm during this time (left). The right diagram indicates clear synchronization to the zeitgeber, as was the case during the first week, although the rectal temperature rhythm is no longer synchronized externally during this time. During the third week, there again is a component of the activity rhythm, with a constant period of 25 hours, which seems to be even more reliable than during the second week (left). During this week, synchronization to the zeitgeber cannot be stated (right). During the fourth week, when the zeitgeber period was held constant at 48.0 hours, there are reliable rhythm components at 48 and 24 hours, indicating external synchronization. This infor-

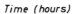

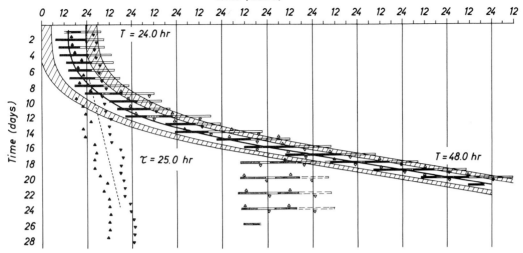

Figure 94. Rhythm of a subject (J.S., ♂ 19 y) living without environmental time cues but under the influence of a strong artificial zeitgeber, with a period steadily and progressively lengthened from 24.0 to 48.0 hours during the course of 3 weeks, and then held constant for a fourth week. *I.* Temporal courses of the rhythms of activity, rectal temperature, and psychomotor performance (i.e., computation speed). The two rhythms first mentioned are presented successively, one period beneath the other. The latter rhythm is indicated by the averaged temporal positions of its acrophases. Indications are the same as in figure 86/I. Shaded bars: temporally correct redrawings of corresponding full bars.

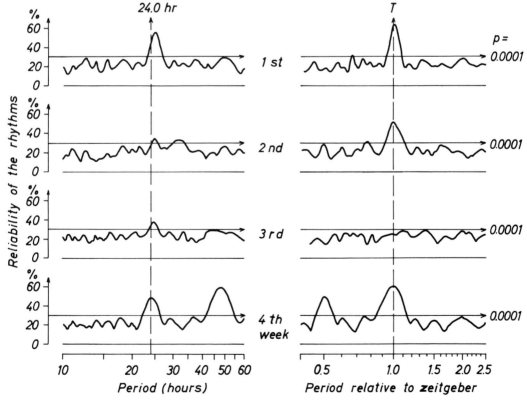

Figure 94/II. Period analyses of the objectively recorded locomotor activity from contact plates under the floor, computed separately for the 4 successive weeks of the experiment and with two different modes. Left diagrams: computed in the normal manner, with constant and equidistant scanning period presented with a logarithmic period scale (i.e., abscissa). Right diagrams: computed with the respective zeitgeber period as the scanning period (i.e., during the first 3 weeks with systematically lengthening absolute values) presented for fractions of the zeitgeber period T (i.e., abscissa).

mation consistently comes from both types of analyses (left and right diagrams).

The interpretation of this result is that the activity rhythm was synchronized to the zeitgeber during the first 2 weeks and during the last week, but not during the third week. In other words, the activity rhythm broke from the zeitgeber after the second week, when the zeitgeber reached a period of about 35 hours. It again became synchronized when the zeitgeber reached a period of 48 hours. The apparent discrepancy between the behaviors of the rhythms of the objectively measured activity and the subjectively scored alternation between 'day' and 'night' seems to be based on the naps. At the beginning, the subject did not take naps but, in the middle of the experiment, he took irregular naps on some days. At the end of the experiment, he took regular naps. To make the latter regularity obvious, the activity rhythm is redrawn in figure 94/I in a circa-bi-dian manner (shaded bars). The result mentioned is in agreement with the expectation concerning the range of entrainment of the activity rhythm, as deduced earlier (cf. 3.1.1). It further corresponds to results of all other experiments, showing internal desynchronization, that the activity rhythm includes a component that runs synchronously to the rectal temperature rhythm.

Finally, in this experiment, the rhythm of psychomotor performance (i.e., computation speed) also was measured. As can be seen in figure 94/I, it ran, on the average, synchronously to the zeitgeber during the total experiment. Only during the last week, when the zeitgeber period was 48.0 hours and the rectal temperature rhythm was synchronized to half this period, components of the performance rhythm, with periods of 24 and 48 hours, were of equal reliability (55%).

With a changing speed of the zeitgeber period, as applied in the experiment underlying figure 94, differences in the ranges of entrainment, as coordinated to the rhythms of rectal temperature and activity, in fact can be demonstrated. This speed, however, is too great to differentiate between different vegetative rhythms. In the interesting range

around 27.5 hours, the zeitgeber period increased for 1 hour per day. Other experiments, therefore, are in progress where the zeitgeber period changes very slowly, increasing from 26 to 29 hours in the course of 4 weeks. In the example shown in Figure 95, the activity rhythm is inside its range of entrainment during the entire experiment. Regarding the rectal temperature rhythm, the period of 26:50 hours is unambiguously inside the range of entrainment, but the period of 27:00 hours is just as unambiguously outside. The rhythm of urine volume remains entrained to the zeitgeber and the activity rhythm up to a period of 27:40 hours; later, it free runs in synchrony with the rectal temperature rhythm. In conclusion, the different overt rhythms alternate from the entrained to the free-running oscillator at different period values and are, therefore, temporarily separated from each other. This example illustrates that with "fractional desynchronization" the ranges of entrainment of different overt rhythms can be determined precisely and separately, independent of each other and of activity. The end of this temporal fractioning is the testing of functional interdependencies in operation modes of different physiological and psychological variables.

Finally, it must be considered that in experiments of the type shown in figures 94 and 95, the increase in the zeitgeber period crept into an originally synchronized system. It is still an open question whether or not the ranges of entrainment will be the same size if the rhythms originally are free running. Theoretically, it is a fundamental property of self-sustained oscillations, due to the nonlinearities, that it must be differentiated between an always larger "range of holding" and an always smaller "range of catching" a rhythm (Wever, 1962). In the experiments discussed so far, only the "range of holding" can be determined. It would be of interest, however, to perform, additionally, experiments starting with a zeitgeber period outside the range of entrainment and then changing the period to values closer to the free running period.

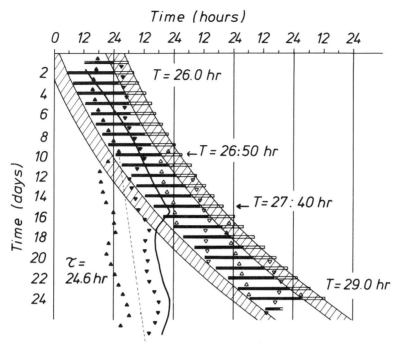

Figure 95. Rhythm of a subject (H.F., ♂ 22 y) living without environmental time cues but under the influence of a strong artificial zeitgeber, with a period of 26.0 hours during the first 5 days and then steadily and uniformly lengthened to 29.0 hours. Temporal courses of the rhythms of activity, rectal temperature, and urine volume. The two rhythms first mentioned are presented successively, one period beneath the other. The latter rhythm is indicated by the temporal positions of its acrophases. Indications are the same as in figure 27/I. The solid line combines the acrophases of the urine volume rhythm. Shaded areas: dark time of the zeitgeber.

3.3.4. Review of Partially Synchronized Rhythms

Before summarizing the experiments with the strong zeitgeber, showing partial external synchronization combined with internal desynchronization, and then drawing conclusions, the state of the activity rhythm must be considered once more. Under the influence of weaker zeitgebers (cf. 3.1 and 3.2), the activity rhythm, in fact, behaves oscillatorily, like the other overt rhythms. It, nevertheless, might be argued that the activity really is not entrained (i.e., phase controlled) under the influence of the strong zeitgeber, but passively phase set (i.e., not influenced oscillatorily). The reason would be that the strong external force annihilates the internal drive. Since the state of internal

desynchronization, as forced by the strong zeitgeber, was proposed especially to study interactions between different oscillators, this assumption would be a serious objection. However, there are several arguments strongly suggesting also the oscillatory origin of the activity rhythm when entrained by the strong zeitgeber and, therefore, justifying the conclusions to be drawn.

The first argument is the limitation of the range of entrainment of the activity rhythm, as suggested in figure 94. If this result can be confirmed significantly by further experiments, it gives the strongest evidence for the oscillatory origin of the activity rhythm. An only passively driven rhythm would run synchronously to every zeitgeber period. The second argument is the change in the external phase relationship between the activity rhythm and a strong zeitgeber depending on the zeitgeber period. An only passively driven rhythm would hold a fixed phase relationship with all periods. Under the influence of the strong zeitgeber, however, there is normally a systematic change in the external phase relationship with the zeitgeber period, as can be seen especially in figures 86 and 120. The dependency of the phase relationship between the activity rhythm and zeitgeber, as found with a strong zeitgeber, corresponds to that found with other zeitgebers (Fig. 72), and as postulated from oscillation laws under the presupposition of an oscillatorily generated rhythm.

Other evidence for the oscillatory origin of the activity rhythm comes from experiments where the activity rhythm first was entrained to the strong zeitgeber and then left in constant conditions. If the activity rhythm is entrained oscillatorily, the transition into the free running state must be expected to continue the phase of the entrained rhythm and, therefore, to last several days where transients are present. If the activity rhythm is passively driven by the zeitgeber, it must shift immediately to the steady free running state. The difference between the two possible kinds of transition would be obvious especially if, at the instant of the transition, the different rhythms run counterphased during the course of internal desynchronization. Figure 96 shows the course of an experiment where such a transition can be observed. The subject was first exposed to a strong 30.0-hour zeitgeber and then left in constant total darkness. At the end of the zeitgeber section, the rhythms of activity and rectal temperature, just by chance, ran counterphased. The temperature maximum fell into rest time and the temperature minimum fell into activity time. As can be seen in figure 96, the activity rhythm did not jump immediately after the zeitgeber was cut off

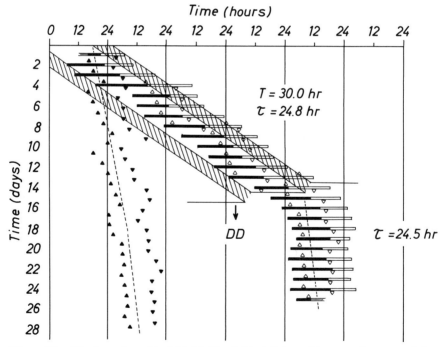

Figure 96.   Rhythm of a subject (A.McK., ♂ 24 y) living without environmental time cues and under the influence of a strong artificial zeitgeber with a constant period during the first section, but exposed to constant total darkness during the second section. Temporal courses of the rhythm of activity and rectal temperatures are presented successively, one period beneath the other. Indications are the same as in figure 27/I. Shaded areas: dark time of the zeitgeber.

in the "right" phase position relative to the more or less persisting rectal temperature rhythm, but shifted gradually, during several days and continuing its previous course, in the steady state phase position, indicating transient behavior. This rhythm pattern gives strong evidence to the oscillatory origin of the activity rhythm (i.e., the phase of the alternation between wakefulness and sleep was not set only passively by the zeitgeber but, due to endogenous rhythmicity, entrained to the zeitgeber). This example is one of only two experiments of this type performed; however, the consistency in the results, especially the agreement with other evidences, justifies the rejection of the assumption the activity rhythm under the influence of a strong zeitgeber is passively phase set instead of oscillatorily phase controlled.

To the present, 34 subjects in 30 experiments were exposed to the strong zeitgeber, consisting of an absolute light-dark cycle completed by regular signals calling the subjects for urine mictions and test sessions; with periods between 20 and 32 hours persisting for at least 1 week. In these experiments, without exception, the overt activity rhythms were entrained to the zeitgeber. This is true with regard to the subjectively scored alternation between 'day' and 'night' and the objectively recorded activity. On the other hand, none of the five subjects exposed to a 20-hour zeitgeber was entrained with his rectal temperature rhythm to this period (Fig. 88); and in none of the 23 experiments with a strong zeitgeber, with periods of 28, 30, and 32 hours, was the subject entrained with his rectal temperature rhythm to the zeitgeber (Figs. 86 to 89, 91, 92, and 96). Only to a strong zeitgeber with periods of 24.0 hours (17 experiments) and $25\frac{1}{3}$ hours (1 experiment) was rectal temperature rhythms entrained for all subjects. To strong zeitgebers with a period of $22\frac{2}{3}$ hours (six experiments), were rectal temperature rhythms either not entrained (three subjects) or entrained only during parts of the experiment (three subjects) (Fig. 93). In most of the experiments, the zeitgeber applied was

the only relevant experimental condition. In eight experiments, in addition, the magnitude of a continuously operating external stimulus was changed (Figs. 92 and 93). The results regarding these additional stimuli, however, are not enough to allow significant statements.

In all experiments where internal desynchronization was forced by the zeitgeber, (with zeitgeber periods outside the range of entrainment of the rectal temperature rhythm), i.e., with rectal temperature rhythms which free ran in spite of the presence of the zeitgeber, the overt rectal temperature rhythms showed periods very close to those periods that were measured in desynchronized rectal temperature rhythms under constant conditions (Fig. 29; Chap. 2.3). On the average ($\pm$ standard deviation) a period of 24.78 ± 0.13 hours resulted. This average period cannot be discriminated from the period of the lunar day (24.83 hours), just as little as the rectal temperature period during spontaneously occurring internal desynchronization (cf. 2.3). Only after having closer knowledge of the mode of zeitgeber action, can it be decided whether this coincidence is only accidental and the desynchronized rectal temperature rhythms really are free running, or this coincidence is due to entrainment of desynchronized rectal temperature rhythms to the lunar day (cf. 3.5).

With regard to the activity rhythm, significant results are not available yet. To the present, the results of only two pilot studies are in agreement with former indirect evaluations (cf. 3.1.1). They indicate an upper limit of the range of entrainment of the activity rhythm of close to 35 hours (Fig. 94). This result means that forced internal desynchronization occurs, with certainty, with zeitgeber periods between 28 and 32 hours and, very likely in the opposite range, between 19 and 22 hours. During this state, the different overt rhythms show different periods. It, however, must be kept in mind, with a closer inspection, that different rhythm components, which are included simultaneously in all overt rhythms, show different periods. In a more precise expression, it must be stated that the rhythm component that is normally dominant in the overt rectal temperature rhythm, shows a smaller range of entrainment, and another rhythm component that is normally dominant in the overt activity rhythm, shows a larger range of entrainment. This correlation, however, is not general. At least in one case, the dominant component of the rectal temperature rhythm was synchronized to the strong zeitgeber, with a period of 28.0 hours, while the free running component, with a period of 24.7 hours, was smaller in amplitude and reliability (Fig. 90, uppermost diagram).

The experiments discussed in this chapter, which were performed under the influence of a strong artificial zeitgeber outside the range of entrainment of the vegetative rhythms, center the present investigations. They, in particular, seem to enlarge our knowledge of the multioscillatory structure of the human circadian system in an effective manner. The main reason is the possibility of forcing the state of internal desynchronization in every subject, independent of his personality data. And this state occurs in a very regular manner: just the oscillator that shows a large inter- and intraindividual variability (i.e., the 'activity oscillator'; Figs. 29 and 37) is fixed, with respect to its period, by the experimental conditions; and only the oscillator that is remarkably stable (i.e., the 'rectal temperature oscillator'; Figs. 29 and 37) runs autonomously. Only these experiments, moreover, enable a meaningful evaluations of properties of psychical and performance rhythms in the free running state. Under constant conditions, these rhythms cannot be detected (cf. 1.3.2). It is another aspect of the present investigations that those experiments showing only partial synchronization to an external zeitgeber are of increasing practical interest.

3.4. General Effectiveness of Light-Dark Zeitgebers

It was concluded from the zeitgeber experiments discussed up to this point that a light-dark cycle is a weak zeitgeber in comparison with social contacts. A relative light-dark cycle had been shown to have a range of entrainment of about ± 0.5 hours. This is, for the most part, too small to entrain human circadian rhythms even at a period of 24 hours. Only after completing the experiments by having a regular signal that summoned the subjects for tests and mictions (considered by most subjects to be a social contact from the experimenter) was the zeitgeber strength sufficient to result in a range of entrainment of about ± 2 hours. An absolute light-dark cycle had been shown to be a much stronger zeitgeber than a relative light-dark cycle when also completed by the regular signals. It must be concluded from this comparison that an absolute light-dark cycle without the signals exerts just as well a stronger zeitgeber effectiveness as a pure relative light-dark cycle (of course, at lower levels than with the signals), although corresponding experiments have not yet been performed. However, in all these cases the limits between physical and social effects are hard to define. On the one hand, an absolute light-dark cycle affects the behavior of the subjects much more than a relative and may, therefore, frequently be perceived as a social stimulus; on the other hand, the regular signals were originally of the same physical nature as the light-dark cycle, and their social nature existed only in the imagination of the subjects. In general, a clear definition of what is, in this context, a "social contact" operating as a zeitgeber cannot, at the present, be given. Nevertheless, several different types of experiments indicate that the most effective zeitgeber in human circadian rhythms of man is related in any way to "social contacts", but great efforts have to be undertaken in the future to elucidate the special meaning of this term more unambiguously. However, before arriving at further conclusions, results of other authors dealing with this topic should be reviewed.

The first investigators who performed comparable experiments were Lewis and Lobban (1957). The authors exposed 12 subjects in Spitsbergen, under constant natural illumination, to artificial days of 21 and 27 hours duration, using manipulated watches. The living routines of the subjects followed the course of the watches. As the result, some of the overt rhythms 'adapted' to the course of the living routine, whereas other overt rhythms, especially potassium excretion in urine, persisted with a period of 24 hours. 'Dissociation' of the rhythms, therefore, occurred. It is not clear from the measurements whether the 'persisting' rhythms really persisted synchronized to a 24-hour zeitgeber (e.g., the course of the sun relative to landmarks), or they free ran with periods slightly deviating from 24.0 hours. Later, similar experiments (Simpson and Lobban, 1967), also performed in Spitsbergen with an artificial 21-hours day, gave clearer results. Rhythms of some urine constituents again were measured. The authors concluded that 'adaptation' to the changed living routine was very slow in some rhythms (e.g., 17-OHCS and potassium) but more rapid in others (e.g., sodium, chloride, and water). A later reanalysis of the data (Simpson et al., 1970) resulted in two major clusters of periods around 21.0 and 24.2 hours, indicating two rhythm components, one of which was synchronized to the living routine. Computations of acrophases of the slower rhythm component, computed arbitrarily with a period of 24.0 hours, suggested a steady phase shift against local time indicating a period slightly longer than 24.0 hours and, therefore, a free run of this rhythm component. In summary, these experiments showed, for the first time, that a forced living routine, which can be called a 'social zeitgeber' but which was not accompanied by any physical periodicity in the environment, had the capacity to entrain at least one component of the circadian rhythms of the subjects. The state of the other component, which either ran freely or entrained to any one of the physical periodicities present in the environment, could not be determined clearly. In any case, forced internal desynchronization was present, in the meaning defined in this book, and was forced by a social zeitgeber.

Experiments closest in their design to the experiment discussed here were performed by Orth et al. (1967). These authors forced subjects to sleep-wake cycles of 12, 19, and 33 hours duration. After adhering strictly to the particular sleep-wake schedule for 4 to 42 days, blood samples were taken at hourly intervals for 1 to 3 days, and the plasma 17-OHCS concentration was determined. The authors state that "normal subjects lose, in these conditions, their 24-hour 17-OHCS cycles and establish new cycles which appear to be synchronized with their new sleep-wake schedules". This result would be in contradiction to the results of the experiments discussed in this chapter, which clearly show ranges of entrainment for the vegetative rhythms not exceeding a few hours. However, Orth et al. (1967) measured the subjects only during short intervals several days after transferring them into the changed conditions. It was emphasized in the context of figure 87 that the inspection of only short intervals may lead to misleading interpretations. Also from figure 87, the inspection of only those intervals where the rhythms are shown clearly and which included the majority of days, a synchronization to the 28-hour day would have been concluded. It is obvious here that the inspection of the total time series leads to another result; there is no synchronization to the 28-hour day, or even better, there is only synchronization of a small secondary rhythm component. It, therefore, is not conclusive, from the results presented by Orth et al. (1967) that, in their experiments, the rhythms were synchronized to periods widely deviating from 24 hours as long as this conclusion is not confirmed by long term analyses.

More recently, comparable experiments were performed by Webb and Agnew (1975). The authors forced 14 subjects to activity and sleep cycles between 9 and 36 hours for 6 to 14 days. As the result, all subjects followed their sleep habits with the imposed cycles. The purpose of these experiments was to determine sleep latency depending on cycle length. Variables other than sleep were not stated. Applying the results of other experiments, the presence of forced internal desynchronization also must be expected in the experiments of Webb and Agnew (1975), with cycles sufficiently deviating from 24 hours. Direct evidence, with regard to this state, however, cannot be taken from these experiments.

In experiments performed by Meddis (1968), subjects were exposed to an artificial 48-hour day without sufficiently excluding natural time cues. As the result, the experiments were not successful, but showed normal rhythms with periods of 24.0 hours. Furthermore, Jouvet et al. (1974) claimed to have synchronized a subject, living in a cave without environmental time cues, to a 48-hour zeitgeber. The fact is, after the subject had spontaneously reached a circa-bi-dian activity rhythm with about 34 hours of wakefulness and about 15 hours of sleep (cf. 2.2.4), illumination was switched on by the subject after awakening, but switched off externally after 34.0 hour. The duration of activity time, therefore, was controlled externally, but not the duration of sleep. Consequently, the period also was not controlled externally. As the further consequence, the condition did not correspond to a zeitgeber condition in the generally accepted definition, but rather to a self-control condition. Finally, the term ''synchronization'' is not adequate. As the result of the condition really applied, the period deviated clearly from 48.0 hours, as can be seen in the records presented by Jouvet et al. (1974).

In summary, there are a few evidences from other authors stating forced internal desynchronization was observed in human subjects. There also are evidences for the zeitgeber effectiveness of social contacts. There seems to be only one comparable finding in animals. Szafarczyk et al. (1974) exposed rats to artificial days of 24, 36, and 48 hours durations. While the activity rhythms always followed the forced schedule, there were indications that plasma 17-OHCS exhibited shorter rhythms, with periods of 27.5 hours in the 36-hour day and 30.0 hours in the 48-hour day. Since the latter analyses are based on 17-OHCS determinations covering only short intervals (i.e., 24 hours in the 24-hour day, 144 hours in the 36-hour day, and 48 hours in the 48-hour day), a significant statement of exact period values hardly can be given.

There are other experimental series, specifically dealing with the influence of light on circadian rhythmicity of man, performed in the 24-hour day. Orth and Island (1969) exposed three groups, of three subjects each, to identical sleep routines but different lighting conditions. After an adaptation period of 10 to 14 days, blood was sampled at hourly intervals during 2 to 3 days for plasma 17-hydroxycorticosteroid determinations. The results of this experimental series are redrawn in figure 97. As can be seen, all three experimental groups show remarkably similar courses of the 17-OHCS concentration, in spite of the very different lighting conditions. For instance, the highest concentration is always around 9 hours in the morning, with a sharp subsequent decrease, independent of whether there was light (group I), transition from darkness to light (group II), or darkness (group III). There is always a secondary peak concentration around 19 hours, even in group II, where there was no change in illumination. (Group II consisted of the same three subjects as group I.) From only the comparison of the three experimental groups, it is unjustified to infer a considerable effect on plasma 17-OHCS caused by illumination. The authors compare every experimental group separately with a control group and, in fact, claim considerable differences. The peak concentration was delayed, relative to termination of sleep, in the experimental groups, and the secondary peak was present only in the experimental groups, but not in the control group. Both of these effects are stated as being due to the shifted lighting conditions. The control group, however, was not tested with the experimental groups mentioned, but at another time and with another experimental series (Orth et al., 1967). It, therefore, does not seem to be a guarantee that the activity habit of the subjects, which was essentially the same in

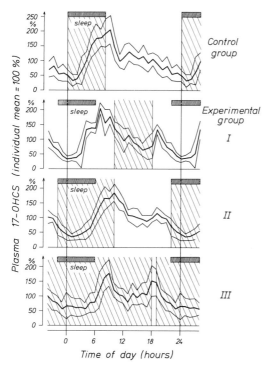

Figure 97. Rhythms of plasma 17-OHCS in four groups of subjects (i.e., control group: 8 studies of 6 subjects; experimental groups: 3 subjects each), measured at hourly intervals. In the experimental groups, the sleep times coincided, but the lighting regimes were different. The blood samples were taken after an adaptation period of 10 to 14 days in the respective condition. The thick curves indicate the means of all subjects, within the respective group, averaged over 2 to 3 sampling days. The thin lines indicate the ranges of standard deviations, computed from the different subjects and the successive sampling days. After Orth and Island (1969).

the three experimental groups, was also the same in the control group (e.g., sleep times did not coincide). As the consequence, it seems appropriate to compare the experimental groups mutually, rather than separately with the control group. The comparison first mentioned shows a direct effect of light on 17-OHCS as stated by the authors, but an effect that is small in comparison to the effect of the time of day or sleep habit. The results of Orth and Island (1969), therefore, support, rather than contradict, the findings discussed in this paper; that light exhibits only a poor zeitgeber effectiveness in comparison to social contacts (cf. 3.2.2).

Hildebrandt and Lowes (1972) exposed 5 subjects to a transition from 8 hours previously present darkness to light (500 lux), six different times of day. They stated, in all cases, considerable effects on vegetative variables (e.g., a drop in the number of eosinophiles or an increase in urine cortisol and in pulse rate) followed the illumination. In addition, they stated varying effects of the illumination, depending on time of day. Since such a phase depending effectiveness is the prerequisite of zeitgeber effectiveness (cf. 3.5), the authors conclude that light must act as a potential zeitgeber. If a zeitgeber effect of light cannot be found in a special experiment, the applied experimental conditions should have suspended the natural phase dependency of illumination effects. Against the conclusions of the authors, it can be argued that the subjects "did sleep mostly during darkness but were always awake during the following light time" (Hildebrandt and Lowes, 1972). It is impossible to decide, from these experiments, whether the measured effects really are due to illumination or the awakening of the subjects, where the degree of the change in the state of activity following illumination may depend on time of day. Moreover, the phase dependency of effects of a special stimulus, as a necessary prerequisite of zeitgeber effectiveness of this stimulus, concerns only phase shifting effects of the stimulus. These effects, however, have not been tested. The findings of Hildebrandt and Lowes (1972), therefore, are consistent enough with the assumption that light-dark cycles are only weak zeitgebers.

In addition, there are various papers stating a dominant role of light on vegetative functions, like the number of eosinophiles or concentration of plasma corticosteroids (Appel, 1938; Appel and Hansen, 1952; Radnot et al., 1960; Sharp, 1960a, 1960b). All of these papers, however, do not state a zeitgeber effect of light controlling the circadian system, but rather a direct effect on the variables measured. The stated result, therefore, is of interest in itself, but not relevant in the context to be discussed here. There are some findings in blind subjects which need attention, since they state considerable effects, because of the absence of light perception, on circadian rhythms. In some papers (e.g., Migeon et al., 1956), rhythms, very similar to those in sighted subjects, were described. In other papers (e.g., Hollwich and Dieckhues, 1971), the absence of any rhythmicity in some vegetative variables was stated. In the majority of papers (Appel and Hansen, 1952; Bodenheimer et al., 1973; Lobban and Tedre, 1964, 1967; Krieger and Glick, 1971; Krieger and Rizzo, 1971; Orth and Island, 1969; Remler, 1948), marked rhythms with unusual phase relationship to the 24-hour day were found. Finally, there are some indications (D'Allesandro et al., 1974; Orth and Island, 1969) that circadian rhythms in blind subjects may tend to free-run in the normal 24-hour day. Because of the discrepancies in the existing results, an experimental series with totally blind subjects was performed. This series included not only a section with synchronization to the 24-hour day under standardized conditions, but also included a section with free running rhythms under constant conditions, because only the combined inspection of rhythms under both conditions leads to co-

gent conclusions about properties of circadian rhythms (Lund, 1974a). Results of the sections with free running rhythms already have been mentioned (cf. 2.4.1).

Figure 98 presents, longitudinally, the course of an experiment of this series. It shows, apart from the sleep-wake cycle, the courses of rectal temperature and urinary excretion of free cortisol. The totally blind subject lived for 7 days socially synchronized to the experimeter with a strict regular 24.0-hour schedule. He afterwards lived in isolation without time cues, and the only contacts consisted of an exchange of magnetic tapes with messages, once per period. As can be seen from this figure, the rhythms look essentially like those of sighted subjects, with respect to the amplitudes and mean values. The same is true in all other blind subjects examined in this series. On the average, there are no significant differences between rhythms of blind and sighted subjects, with respect to amplitude and mean value. There is a difference to rhythms of sighted subjects, however, and that is with regard to the interindividual variability of external phase relationships to an entraining zeitgeber. This variability is considerably larger in blind than sighted subjects. Since

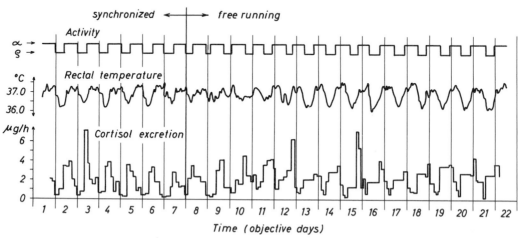

Figure 98.   Rhythm of a blind subject (P.T., ♂ 27 y, totally blind since 16 years), living socially synchronized by regular contacts with an experimenter for 1 week, and without environmental time cues for 2 weeks. Presented longitudinally are the rhythms of activity (i.e., alternation between wakefulness α and rest ρ), rectal temperature (measured continuously), and urinary excretion of free cortisol (i.e., mictions taken at regular intervals during the first section, and at self-selected intervals during the second section). From Lund (1974a).

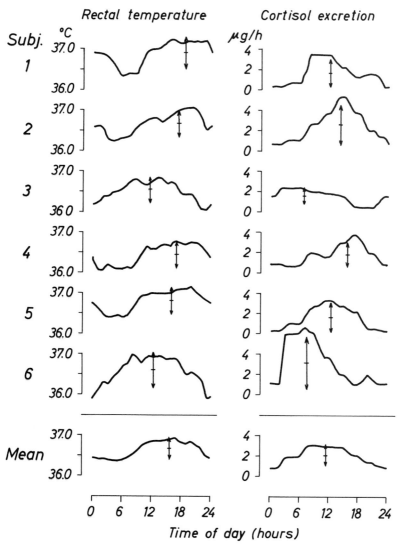

Figure 99. Daily courses of the rhythms of rectal temperature and urinary excretion of free cortisol, measured in six blind subjects during social entrainment to the 24-hour day and averaged over 6 successive days (first section of Fig. 98). Mean value and amplitude of the fundamental periods are presented at the position of the respective acrophase. The upper six diagrams, in every column, are computed from individual data of the six subjects. The lowest diagrams are computed from data averaged from the six subjects. Data from Lund (1974a).

this large variability may have caused discrepancies between statements of different authors, it will be treated in more detail.

Figure 99 shows individual courses of rectal temperature and cortisol excretion of the six blind subjects averaged over 6 days of the first section, with socially entrained rhythms. In every diagram, the mean value, amplitude, and acrophase of the fundamental period are indicated. As obviously can be seen, the acrophases show considerable interindividual variability. At the bottom, courses of the rhythms, as averaged from the six individual courses, are presented. The parameters of the fundamental period again are indicated. It is evident that the mean values (i.e., 36.68 ± 0.19°C in rectal temperature, and 2.08 ± 0.68 μg/h in cortisol excretion) and acrophases (e.g., 15.7 ± 3.0 hours CET in rectal temperature and 11.6 ± 3.7 hours CET in cortisol excretion), as averaged from the parameters of the individual rhythms (± standard deviations), are identical with the parameters of the averaged rhythms. This identity, however, is not true with regard to amplitude. In the rectal temperature rhythms, the mean of the individual amplitudes is 0.37 ± 0.06°C, but the amplitude of the average rhythm is only 0.27°C (= 73%). This difference would be significant even in the statistical analysis with $p < 0.01$ if it would not be only an artefact of the averaging procedure. In the cortisol rhythms, the individual amplitudes have a mean of 1.62 ± 0.63 μg/h, but the amplitude of the average rhythm is only 1.08 μg/h (= 67% of the mean of the individual amplitudes). This flattening of the average rhythms, due to the averaging procedure, is much less in sighted subjects since there is a much smaller interindividual variability in the phases. In six sighted subjects, living under a 24.0-hour routine (Fig. 83), the mean acrophase (± standard deviation) of the rectal temperature rhythms is at 18.3 ± 1.2 hours CET and, as a consequence of the small variability, the range of oscillation of the averaged rhythms (0.75°C) is nearly as large (= 93%) as the mean of the individual ranges (0.81 ± 0.18°C; Aschoff et al., 1974a; Wisser et al., 1973). The same is true in cortisol, which was determined, using the same method, in nine sighted subjects for comparison (Sieber, 1976). In cortisol excretion, the mean acrophase is at 10.9 ± 1.8 hours CET and, as a consequence of the small variability, the amplitude of the average rhythm (1.58 μg/h) is nearly as large (= 90%) as the mean of the individual amplitudes (1.76 ± 1.11 μg/h). Simultaneously, these numbers show that there is nearly no difference in the individual amplitudes of blind and sighted subjects.

In the comparison between blind and sighted subjects, with regard to the acrophase of rectal temperature rhythms, the advance in blind, compared with sighted subjects ($t = 1.97$), and the increase in variability in blind, compared with sighted subjects ($F = 6.25$), is significant statistically ($p < 0.05$ each). The earlier phase in the blind subjects could be due to either stronger zeitgeber effectiveness or shorter autonomous periods in the blind subjects (cf. 3.1.1). In fact, autonomous periods in blind subjects were shown to be significantly shorter than in sighted subjects (cf. 2.4.1). The second reason, therefore, is very likely but, in addition, the first reason may contribute. The increase in variability in the blind subjects could be due to weaker zeitgeber effectiveness. In this case, the increase in the interindividual variability must be accompanied by an increase in the intraindividual variability of the rhythms also (Wever, 1971b). This, however, is not the case. The intraindividual variability of a rhythm can be expressed in its reliability; the reliability of rectal temperature rhythms in blind subjects was especially high (on the average, 88.2 ± 5.5%; Lund, 1974a). There are numerous experiments in sighted subjects that include a section of sufficiently long duration with a 24.0-hour zeitgeber comparable to that applied for the blind subjects (Figs. 14, 69, 70, 73, and 86 to 89). In a sample of twelve subjects living under the influence of a corresponding 24.0-hour zeitgeber, the mean reliability of the rectal temperature rhythm (± standard deviation) was 86.6 ± 4.5%. It cannot be guaranteed statistically that the reliability is greater in blind than in sighted subjects, but these numbers clearly reject the assumption that rectal temperature rhythms in blind subjects are more variable than those in sighted subjects. As the consequence, it must be concluded that blind subjects are, in the 24-hour day, under the influence of a zeitgeber that, definitely, is not weaker than the zeitgeber that is effective in sighted subjects. This zeitgeber further seems to have great interindividual differences in its properties. Since only social zeitgebers can be effective in blind subjects, the quality of social contacts is not the same in different blind subjects. Finally, this means that social contacts, operating separately, can have a zeitgeber effectiveness that, definitely, is not weaker than the effectiveness of the combined zeitgebers entraining sighted subjects.

In summary, there are several findings that show an effectiveness of light on circadian rhythms of man. All these findings additionally show that the zeitgeber effectiveness of light-dark cycles is small in comparison to that of social contacts. This especially means that light-dark zeitgebers are effective within only small ranges of entrainment. In animals, where the light-dark zeitgeber is normally dominant, only some evidence for social entrainment are known. Gwinner (1966) has shown that species-specific song cycles, from a tape recorder, can sychronize circadian rhythm of birds within a small range. Rohles and Osbaldiston (1969) have shown social entrainment in rhesus monkeys.

3.5. General Mode of Zeitgeber Action

It is the summarized result of the experiments, discussed in chapters 3.1 to 3.3, that human circadian rhythms can be synchronized by artificial zeitgebers, with periods varying within a limited range of entrainment and any phase relationship to local time. Artificial zeitgebers can be tested only after the subjects are isolated from all natural time cues of the environment and all information related to local time. In other words, the necessary prerequisite for the demonstration of an artificial zeitgeber, which deviates from the natural zeitgeber, is a condition under which circadian rhythms would free run autonomously, unless the artificial zeitgeber is introduced.

After establishing some features of special artificial zeitgebers, it generally is possible to draw conclusions concerning the mode of action of zeitgebers. In this context, the question arises whether an effective zeitgeber primarily controls the phase or the frequency of a rhythm. Phase control, which includes the control of the overt frequency

indirectly, causes, with defined periods of the rhythm and the zeitgeber, a distinct phase relationship between the rhythm and that zeitgeber. It further causes, with changing periods, a distinct correlation between the ratio of the periods and the mutual phase relationship. Finally, under phase control, the mutual phase relationship regularly depends on the strength of the zeitgeber. Frequency control also causes a coincidence in the periods of the rhythm and the zeitgeber, but with an indefinite mutual phase relationship. The coincidence necessarily must be sloppy because of the inevitable slip and, therefore, the mutual phase relationship between rhythm and zeitgeber cannot be even temporally constant. Changes in period and strength of the zeitgeber, moreover, do not affect the mutual phase relationship in any way. As the consequence of the missing regularity in the phase angle differences, these values must be expected, with frequency control, to be randomly distributed among different subjects.

In human circadian rhythms, as in animal rhythms, phase control is realized. Evidence for this type of control comes primarily from the determination of phase relationships between human rhythms and zeitgebers. Since the periods of autonomous rectal temperature rhythms change very little around a general mean (cf. 2.3), these rhythms will be used for the following analyses. A zeitgeber of a given period should synchronize the rectal temperature rhythms with a definite phase, if phase control is present. Figure 100 shows that this is, in fact, the case for two very different zeitgeber modes. In the left diagram, the phase positions of rectal temperature acrophases are presented as derived from all experiments where subjects were exposed to a 24.0-hour zeitgeber consisting of a relative light-dark cycle and a regular calling signal (cf. 3.1). In the right diagram, phase positions are presented as derived from all experiments where subjects stood synchronized under the influence of a periodically operating electric 10-Hz field, with periods between 23.5 and 24.0 hours (cf. 3.2.3). Because of the small number of

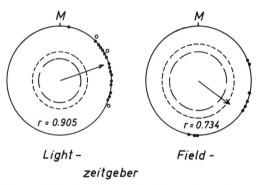

M   M

r = 0.905   r = 0.734

Light -   Field -
            zeitgeber

Figure 100. Angular distributions of acrophases of rectal temperature rhythms, relative to artificial zeitgebers. Left: light-dark zeitgeber of medium strength (i.e., relative light-dark cycle and regular calling signals) with a period of 24.0 hours. Right: field zeitgeber (i.e., artificial electric AC field, 10 Hz square wave, 2.5 V/m; operating periodically) with periods between 23.5 and 24.0 hours. Each dot represents an acrophase obtained, on the average, from one experiment. Open circles in the left diagram: acrophases of desynchronized rectal temperature rhythms under the influence of the pure light-dark zeitgeber (Fig. 81). M = zeitgeber reference: midpoint of light time (left) or midpoint of field time (right), respectively. Inner circles: probability references with regard to the mean vector (arrow). Innermost (widely hatched) circle: $p = 0.05$. Medium (narrowly hatched) circle: $p = 0.01$. The mean vector is indicated by the arrow.

subjects, the two adjoining periods are combined. In both cases, the obtained distributions of phase relationships differ from random distributions at a high level of significance. The mean of the phase relationship, moreover, varies with the zeitgeber mode. The combined light zeitgeber was shown to be stronger than the field zeitgeber (cf. 3.2), because its range of entrainment is about twice as large as that of the field zeitgeber. If both zeitgebers generally operate with identical phases, the acrophases of the rectal temperature rhythms must be closer to the zeitgeber acrophase with the stronger zeitgeber (Wever, 1964b); and this is, in fact, the case. Moreover, the phase distribution, under the influence of the stronger zeitgeber, can be seen to be more concentrated, which again is in agreement with theoretical necessities of a phase control mechanism. In fig-

ure 100, circular presentations are given to allow comparisons with other phase distributions, although the narrowness of the distributions also would allow linear presentations.

In the phase distribution derived from experiments with the light zeitgeber, the results of those three experiments are presented, but not included in the statistical calculations, where only the separated rectal temperature rhythms ran synchronized to the zeitgeber, while the activity rhythms free ran with other periods (Fig. 81). As the result, rectal temperature rhythms have almost the same phase relationship to the zeitgeber, when separated by internal desynchronization, as when internally synchronized.

Second evidence for phase control, in contrast to frequency control, comes from the detection of the correlation between the period and phase relationship to the zeitgeber. In many animal species, the variability of the autonomous periods is large enough to detect a correlation between the autonomous period and the phase relationship between the animal's rhythm and a zeitgeber of a fixed period (Aschoff and Wever, 1962c, 1966). In man, the variability of the autonomous rectal temperature periods is generally so small that the opposite method only is practicable (i.e., to detect the correlation between the varying period of the zeitgeber and the external phase relationship with nearly fixed autonomous periods). Only in the comparison between blind and sighted subjects, is there a significant difference in the autonomous periods (cf. 2.4.1), and also a significant difference in the phase relationship to the 24-hour day (cf. 3.4), confirming the phase control mode. The correlations between the zeitgeber period and external phase relationships already were shown in figure 72. This figure showed significant correlations regarding all different overt rhythms. This result again is consistent with phase control, but not with frequency control, as the mode of zeitgeber action. This result was deduced only from experiments with the light zeitgeber, since the subjects were entrained only to this zeitgeber with different zeitgeber periods, as long as the rhythms ran synchronized internally. With the field zeitgeber (Fig. 100, right diagram), one subject was tested with a zeitgeber period deviating from that applied in all other experiments (26.0 hours instead of 23.5 or 24.0 hours) (Wever, 1969b). This subject showed an external phase relationship that was very different from those shown in figure 100 (i.e., +144° instead of −126°, which was the mean of the nine other subjects).

It had been shown, with two quite different zeitgebers, that the mode of zeitgeber action is phase control and not frequency control; with the easily perceptible light zeitgeber and the subtle field zeitgeber, which cannot be perceived consciously. The biological meaning of circadian rhythmicity demands phase control, because the purpose of this system is the temporal fit of the biological variations into the rhythmically varying environment. With frequency control (i.e., with an undefined phase relationship to the environmental rhythms), this biological meaning would not be reached. An absent biological rhythmicity, at least, is not worse than a wrongly fitted rhythmicity. The independent proof of phase control, as the mode of zeitgeber action, has some fundamental implications. For instance, it finally allows the ruling out of the possibility of continuous frequency transformation in biological rhythms. This mechanism was discussed to generate, under apparently constant conditions, circadian rhythms with continuously varying periods as an alternative to the self-sustainment of the rhythms under those conditions (Brown, 1972). This mechanism, however, is not compatible with the proven mode of each zeitgeber action (i.e., with phase control). It would presuppose frequency control. The alternative hypothesis for describing free running rhythms, in contrast to self-sustained rhythms running autonomously, therefore, can be rejected by considering zeitgeber actions.

As another example, the proof of the phase control mode of the zeitgeber action allows the discrimination of whether or not

an external periodicity is effective as a zeitgeber. This discrimination may be of interest with regard to the lunar day. It was shown that the periods of rectal temperature rhythms, after separation from activity rhythms by the spontaneous occurrence of internal desynchronization, could not be differentiated significantly from the period of the lunar day [24.88 ± 0.19 hours versus 24.83 hours (cf. 2.3)]. Additional cases of separated rectal temperature rhythms, running autonomously, were found in experiments with forced internal desynchronization (cf. 3.3). Also in these 30 experiments, the periods of the rectal temperature rhythms are close to that of the lunar day (24.78 ± 0.13 hours). A discrimination of whether the coincidence in the periods is only accidental or due to a general synchronization of the separated rectal temperature rhythms to the lunar rhythm, is possible from the consideration of the phase relationships between the two rhythms. If there is a zeitgeber synchronization, this only can act by phase control and, therefore, there must be a preferred phase angle difference between the rectal temperature rhythms and the lunar rhythm.

In the first instance, the phase positions of separated rectal temperature rhythms, relative to the lunar day, are presented for spontaneous and forced internal desynchronization separately (Fig. 101, left and middle). The reason is that there may be differences. In a case of forced internal desynchronization, the starting point of the state of internal desynchronization is predetermined by the experimental conditions. A fixed steady state phase relationship to the lunar day, therefore, would presuppose transients in the periods, in order to reach this fixed phase relationship from the different original phase relationships. These transients necessarily must modify the periods (i.e., they must enlarge the variability of the periods around the mean). There, in fact, are only periods varying very little, with standard deviations even smaller than spontaneous internal desynchronization. This result is an argument against the presence of

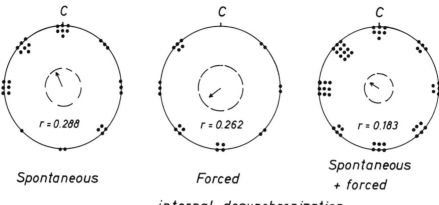

Figure 101. Angular distribution of acrophases of rectal temperature rhythms, as separated during the state of internal desynchronization (grouped within classes of 45°), presented relative to the lunar day. Left: results of experiments performed under constant conditions with spontaneously occurring internal desynchronization. Middle: results of experiments performed under the influence of a strong artificial zeitgeber forcing internal desynchronization. Right: summary of both sets of results, presented in the other diagrams. Each dot represents an acrophase obtained, on the average, from one experiment. C = zeitgeber reference (i.e., culmination of the moon). Inner (dotted) circles: probability references with regard to the mean vector (arrow) with $p = 0.05$. The lengths of the mean vectors are indicated.

transients and, therefore, against a distinct steady state phase relationship to the moon. In a case of spontaneously occurring internal desynchronization, the starting point may be determined by the phase relative to the lunar day and, therefore, a distinct steady state phase relationship could be adjusted without transients. A concentration around a distinct phase relationship to the lunar day, if present at all, must be expected to be stronger with spontaneous than with forced internal desynchronization. If, however, there is a general synchronization of desynchronized rectal temperature rhythms to the lunar day, it must lead to one distinct phase relationship, independent of the reason in the occurrence of internal desynchronization. In a third diagram (Fig. 101, right), therefore, the distributions of phases of the combined separations, spontaneous and forced, are presented. In all cases the phases are grouped into eight classes of 45° each, with the lunar period of 24.83 hours taken for 360°. The effect of grouping on the statistical calculations is considered by introducing a correction factor (Batschelet, 1965).

As can be seen from figure 101, the distribution of phases of desynchronized rectal temperature rhythms, with regard to the lunar day, cannot be differentiated from random distributions. There are no preferred phase positions at any level of significance. Only with spontaneously occurring desynchronization, when considered separately (Fig. 101, left), would a concentration of phases be close to the limit of significance ($0.05 < p < 0.1$). This means that it cannot be excluded with certainty, in cases of spontaneous desynchronization, that the lunar rhythm affects the rectal temperature rhythm, as it can be excluded with forced desynchronization. This difference, indeed, may fit the consideration, given above, concerning the lunar induced occurrence of internal desynchronization. The consideration of the combined modes of internal desynchronization (Fig. 101, right), however, clearly proves that there is no preferred phase relationship between separated rectal temperature rhythms and the lunar day. Considering the mode of zeitgeber action as just deduced, this means that there is no general synchronization of rectal temperature rhythms to the lunar rhythm. This finally means that the coincidence in the periods of separated rectal temperature rhythms and the lunar rhythm is accidental. It is a necessary consequence of this result that the oscillator dominantly controlling the rectal temperature rhythm must be self-sustained. The coincidence in the periods, therefore, does not affect, in any way, the concept deduced from autonomous rhythms, without considering the special values of average periods (i.e., the concept of the separate self-sustainment of all different oscillators involved in the circadian multioscillator system).

The presence of phase control as the mode of zeitgeber action also can be proven, in principle, in experiments of another type, with a single stimuli given during otherwise constant conditions. The reason is that an oscillatory system reacts against a single stimulus, which would exert a zeitgeber effect by phase control when given periodically, with phase shifts where the amount, and partly the direction, depends on the phase of the oscillation which is hit by the stimulus. In other words, the existence of a 'phase response curve' (Aschoff, 1965b; Daan and Pittendrigh, 1976; Pittendrigh, 1960; Pittendrigh and Daan, 1976a) against a distinct stimulus is another manifestation of phase control as the mode of action of the same stimulus, when operating as a zeitgeber. To be precise, the mere existence of a phase response curve is nothing but a consequence of the oscillation becoming excited separately. It is not bound, for instance, to the self-sustainment capacity. Only the special properties of the phase response curve, especially its dependency on the parameters of the rhythm and of the external stimulus, may give complementary information about the details of this separate excitement.

In man, a phase response curve, in its original meaning, has never been measured. Such a measurement would need single stimuli (e.g., of light), given in intervals of at least 10 to 14 days; and at least 12 stimuli, at different phases, have to be used. Such a measurement would require an impracticable duration for an experiment, or an impracticable number of experiments. In a more extended sense, however, phase response curves can be measured in another way, needing shorter spans of time (Aschoff, 1965b). One of these modes is the periodically repeated application of stimuli, but with repetitions being controlled by the rhythm itself. This mode is very similar to the self-control mode as it was applied with different stimuli in human experiments (cf. 2.4). The effect of the self-control mode on autonomous rhythms, therefore, directly proves the existence of a phase response curve in man. Indirectly, but at the same level of validity, this existence already was shown by the proof of phase control as the mode of zeitgeber action in synchronized rhythms.

It has been stated that the consideration of the special course of a phase response curve, beyond its mere existence, gives insight into special properties of the circadian system, which cannot be obtained with synchronized rhythms; therefore, there are many animal studies dealing with phase response curves. If this importance of phase response curves also would be valid in man, there would be a reason to attempt to measure phase response curves in man directly, in spite of the difficulties mentioned. To give some examples for possible implications of phase response curves; the steepness of this curve at a definite phase should indicate the stability of entrainment at this phase (Aschoff, 1965b; Wever, 1964b), or the range of a phase response curve indicates the range of entrainment of the rhythm tested (Pittendrigh, 1974; Pittendrigh and Daan, 1976a; Wever, 1965a). As an example, a range of the response curve covering a full period (type-0 response curve; Winfree, 1970) indicates an unlimited range of entrainment, and hence, a non-self-sustained oscillation or an oscillation the self-sustainment capability of which is completely overridden by the external stimuli so that it behaves like a non self-sustained oscillation. Moreover, the separation of response curves coordinated to specific changes in the external stimulus (e.g., lights-on, or lights off) and to a continuous action of this stimulus may help in the evaluation of what proportions these different aspects of the stimulus contribute to the overall effect of this stimulus (Wever, 1960). These concepts presuppose a constancy of the phase response curve and, above all, its independency of the stimulus applied for its measurement. Such an independency can be guaranteed in linear oscillations (e.g., in non-self-sustained oscillations), but by no means in nonlinear oscillations, which include all self-sustained oscillations (Wever, 1965b, 1972a). In principle, in every self-sustained oscillation, a hypothetical phase response curve temporarily becomes changed by a stimulus which inevitably is necessary in the measurement of the curve. As a consequence, the phase response curve depends strongly on the conditions (e.g., it is

especially different in free running rhythms and in rhythms entrained to a zeitgeber). The same holds true for other response curves (e.g., amplitude response curve; Wever, 1965a). The variability of a response curve of one organism, due to changes in the conditions, may preponderate over the variability among different organisms, or even different species, when measured under equivalent conditions (Wever, 1972a).

As a consequence of the phase control mode of zeitgeber action, not only the external phase relationship between the biological rhythm and zeitgeber changes, with a changing zeitgeber period, but also the internal phase relationship between different biological rhythms within one organism. This was shown with the combined light zeitgeber (Figure 72). The different responsivenesses of different rhythms to a zeitgeber demand different phase response curves. If this is true, these differences also must be recognizable in autonomous rhythms, when run-

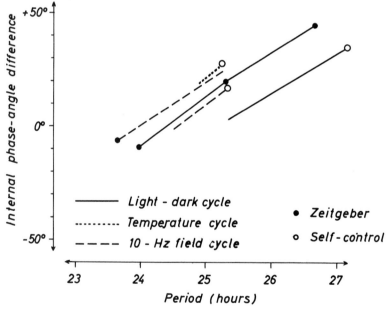

Figure 102. Internal phase angle differences between the rhythms of activity and rectal temperature (i.e., ordinate; increasing angle means increasing phase lead of the rectal temperature rhythm), plotted as a function of the period (i.e., abscissa). Data from experiments with three different external stimuli and, besides free running, two different modes of periodic variations. Average results, originating from one series of experiments, are combined by lines.

ning under self-controlled environmental cycles. This means that changes in the internal phase relationships must occur, not only when the period changes due to a change in the entraining zeitgeber, but also as a consequence of period changes due to self-control (Wever, 1973d). In Figure 102, internal phase relationships between the rhythms of activity and rectal temperature are plotted as functions of the period; they are averaged from five different experimental series where the period was changed either by a zeitgeber or by self-control (i.e., in any case, as a consequence of a periodical change in the controlling environmental conditions). Figure 102 shows that the correlations between internal phase relationship and pe-riod, in all cases, have about equal slopes, close to an advance of the rectal temperature rhythm relative to the activity rhythm of 20° per hour lengthening in period. This similarity in the slopes indicates that each change in the period of a circadian rhythm, which is induced by periodically operating stimuli, affects a change in the internal phase relationship; the amount of which depends only on the amount of the change in period but does not depend on the kind of stimulus operating periodically, or on the mode of application of the external periodicity. In addition, the results included in figure 102 once more independently confirm the fundamental effectiveness of the stimuli applied (e.g., of the artificial electric 10-Hz field).

4
Synthesis

4.1. The One Oscillator Model

In many respects, circadian rhythmicity can be understood as being controlled by only one single oscillator or pacemaker. This is true as long as the different overt rhythms run synchronized internally. The properties of this type of single basic oscillator can be evaluated when the circadian system is operating under conditions experimentally manipulated. In evaluating results of those experiments, it must be differentiated between properties of the overt rhythm, which can be measured, and properties of the hypothetical basic oscillator, or pacemaker, which controls the rhythm. The properties of the overt rhythms, of course, depend on the features of the underlying oscillator, but they also depend on the features of the coupling between the oscillator and the overt rhythm, which also may be affected by the experimental conditions. Finally, the measured variable itself may have features influencing its rhythmicity (e.g., inertia).

The only parameter of an overt rhythm that does not depend on the coupling be-

tween oscillator and overt rhythm is the period of this rhythm which, therefore, must be an equivalent of the oscillator's period. The reason is that the only possible mechanism that could enable a change in period induced by the coupling (i.e., steady frequency transformation) cannot be realized in circadian rhythms as deduced in chapter 3.5. The most reliable information about the basic oscillator, therefore, originates from experiments where period changes are involved. These are experiments, under constant conditions with autonomous rhythms, where the period changes depending on the conditions. These also are experiments under the influence of artificial zeitgebers with varying periods. In general, to evaluate basic properties of the circadian system, experiments are especially suitable when they are performed with subjects isolated from natural time cues. In experiments where the natural day-night cycle is not excluded, many parameters of the overt rhythms, except the period, can be changed experimentally. With all these changes, however, it cannot be decided with certainty whether they are based on changes of the basic oscillator or in the coupling interposed between the oscillator and the overt rhythm.

The most basic features of an oscillator hypothetically underlying circadian rhythmicity are the capacity to run autonomously (i.e., self-sustainment) and the capacity to become synchronized, or entrained, by external periodicities (i.e., separate excitation). Environmental stimuli, which are able to entrain circadian rhythms of man when operating periodically, were shown to have the ability to influence the period of autonomous rhythms when operating continuously (cf. 3.2.4). From this result, it is suggested that parametric excitation is engaged in separate excitation in addition to the common forced (nonparametric) excitation. The assumption of an oscillator, with only these basic features, has consequences that mostly are underestimated. To follow the outline of this book (i.e., to determine basic properties of the circadian system), it is indispensable to deduce the consequences of these features with respect to properties of the measurable overt rhythms.

The most objective way in deriving consequences of oscillator features, with regard to properties of overt rhythms under different conditions, is to develop a mathematical formulation of an oscillation with well defined qualities. Of course, there is an unlimited number of mathematical equations of increasing complexity describing these qualities. It, therefore, is meaningful to apply the specific equation of this variety which is the simplest. The theoretically deduced consequences of these basic features then have to be compared with experimental results. If there are discrepancies, additional basic features must be introduced, and consequences of the extended model then must be compared with experimental results. The features on which the properties of the circadian system are based, therefore, can be evaluated successively by an iterative procedure. In this context, it is evident that only those models which describe not only kinematically the course of the oscillation, but also demonstrate the kinetics of the system,

(i.e., interdependencies in the changes of various oscillation parameters, caused by forces inherent in the system) are useful. Here is not the place to derive the oscillation equation used and to compute solutions of this equation under the different desired conditions. These computations have been presented extensively elsewhere (Wever, 1964a, 1964b, 1965a, 1966b). It is sufficient here to state that the oscillation equation used is based on only some basic features; these being primarily self-sustainment and separate parametric and nonparametric excitations. In the following, some general results of those computations will be compiled.

4.1.1. Autonomous Rhythms

The examination of the oscillation equation, with autonomous rhythms, shows that nearly all measurable parameters of a rhythm mutually depend on each other and, therefore, they depend on the period. Those parameters are, for example, mean value and amplitude and shape of the rhythm. The intra- and interindividual variability of the rhythm, when running under the influence of a distinct "noise," or the duration of transients, after any change in the rhythm, further depend on the period. All these parameters can be measured in human circadian rhythms when running autonomously with a varying period. The measurement of all these parameters and, especially, the interdependencies between these rhythm parameters certainly give more information about the structure of the circadian system than the measure of only the period. Since an electric 10-Hz field was shown to have the capacity to control the period of autonomously running human circadian rhythms regularly, it is referred here to the field experiments (cf. 2.4.5).

Figure 103 presents values of three parameters of rectal temperature rhythms measured separately in experiments including sections with longer and shorter periods (i.e., sections without and with the 10-Hz

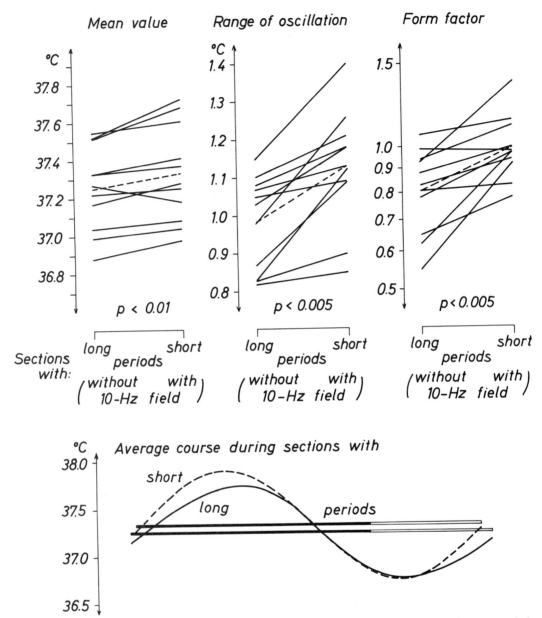

Figure 103. Three parameters of autonomous rectal temperature rhythms depending on period, measured in experiments during which the period was changed regularly by an electric AC field (i.e., 10 Hz square wave, 2.5 V/m; operating continuously in one section). Presented are each the values of the parameters, by lines combining results obtained in the different sections, with long and short periods, of individual experiments. The dotted lines combine the means of the respective sections. Significances are indicated as calculated from the Wilcoxon-test. Left diagram: Mean value (i.e., arithmetic mean of the rectal temperature course). Middle diagram: Range of oscillation (i.e., temperature interval between averaged maximum and minimum values of rectal temperature). Right diagram: Form factor (i.e., ratio between descending and ascending parts of the rectal temperature course during one cycle) presented with a logarithmic scale. In this case, the means (dotted line) are calculated from the logarithms of the individual values. Bottom diagram: Courses of averaged rectal temperature cycles, relative to the activity cycles, presented separately for the sections with long and short periods. After Wever (1971b).

field continuously in operation). The first parameter is the mean value of rectal temperature. It is significantly higher in the sections with short periods than in other sections of the same experiments, but with longer periods. In female subjects, changes in the mean value, due to period changes, may interfere irregularly with changes in the mean value, due to different phases of the menstrual cycle. The only line, in fact, with an aberrant slope originates from a female subject. Consequently, changes in the mean rectal temperature value, due to the transition between the two sections, obtained in experiments with only male subjects, are significant to a higher degree than in those of all subjects, in spite of the decreased number of participants (Wever, 1971b). The second parameter of the rectal temperature rhythm to be considered is the range of oscillation, or the amplitude of this rhythm. In all experiments, without exception, it is larger in the sections with short periods than in other sections. The last parameter change presented in figure 103 is the form factor. This factor describes the shape of the rhythm and is defined by the ratio between the duration of the descending slope and that of the ascending slope within a cycle. This form factor, without exception, is larger in the sections with short periods than in those with long periods. In the two parameters last mentioned, it is not meaningful to consider results for the two sexes separately because neither the amplitude nor the form factor of the rectal temperature rhythm show a dependency on the menstrual cycle in female subjects, as it shows the mean value (Schmidt, 1972). In summary from figure 103, changes of all three parameters, which can be determined independently of each other from the measured course of the rectal temperature rhythm, are correlated negatively to changes in the period to a significant degree. Significances always are calculated from the intraindividual changes of the parameters in order to exclude interindividual variabilities. The lowest diagram of figure 103 shows the average course of the rectal temperature rhythm in the two sec-

tions relative to the activity rhythm. As can be seen from this diagram, the differences are small, but are consistent among the experiments. The interdependencies between all rhythm parameters, which can be determined, are in full agreement, even quantitatively, with postulations derived from the simple mathematical model mentioned (Wever, 1971b). This means all of these interdependencies are nothing more than consequences of the few basic features mentioned.

Figure 104 correspondingly presents changes of three parameters of the activity rhythm, also obtained in the sections with long and short periods. The first parameter is the ratio between activity time and rest time ($\alpha{:}\rho$-ratio). In spite of the generally great interindividual differences of this parameter, it is significantly larger in the sections with short periods than in the other sections. The second parameter of the activity rhythm represents the intraindividual precision of the rhythm. It is determined as the ratio between the value of the period and the standard deviation, which formally is computed from successive onsets and terminations of activity time. The third parameter is given by the ratio between the two standard deviations, when computed separately, for onset and termination of activity, [i.e., "ratio of deviations" ($s_{end}{:}s_{onset}$)]. It is primarily greater than one, indicating a larger variability of activity end than of activity onset. This ratio is significantly greater in the sections with the short periods than in the sections with the long periods. This result means that with a shortening period of the autonomous rhythm, not only the average variability decreases, but also the variability of activity onset decreases more strongly than that of activity termination. It was shown earlier that the interindividual variability of the periods also is correlated positively to the period (Fig. 58, and Table 7). As the consequence, inter- and intraindividual variabilities are correlated positively to each other. In summary, figure 104 shows that changes of all three parameters of the activity rhythm, which can be determined inde-

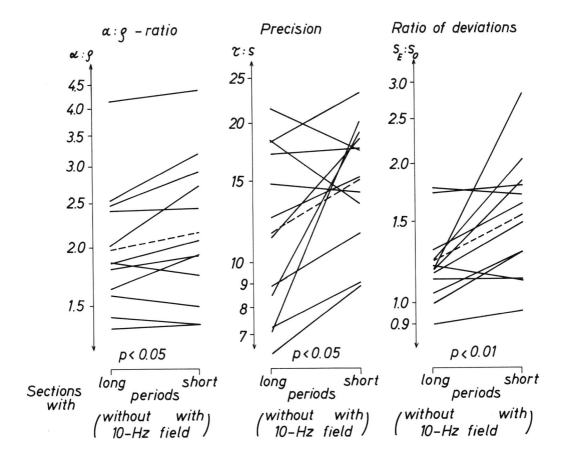

α : ℘ – ratio

Precision

Ratio of deviations

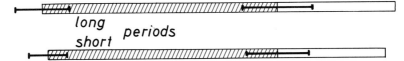

Average activity period during sections with

Figure 104. Three parameters of autonomous activity rhythms depending on period, measured in experiments during which the period was changed regularly by an electric AC field (i.e., 10 Hz square wave, 2.5 V/m; operating continuously in one section). Presented, each in logarithmic scales, are the values of the parameters by lines combining results obtained in the different sections, with long and short periods, of individual experiments. The dotted lines combine the logarithmic means of the respective sections. Significances are indicated as calculated from the Wilcoxon-test. Left diagram: $\alpha{:}\rho$-ratio (i.e., ratio between activity time and rest time). Middle diagram: Precision (i.e., ratio between period and the average of the standard deviations of activity onset and end). Right diagram: Ratio of deviations (i.e., ratio between the standard deviations of activity end and onset). Bottom diagram: Schematic representations of the activity rhythms, as averaged separately from the sections with long and short periods, with activity time (shaded bars) and rest time (white bars). Thick lines: standard deviations of onset and end of activity. All standard deviations are calculated formally and cannot be applied in statistical analyses. After Wever (1971b).

pendently of each other from the measured data, are correlated negatively to changes in the period, to significant degrees, although at lower statistical levels than changes of parameters of rectal temperature rhythms. All interdependencies obtained experimentally again are in agreement with postulations derived from the simple mathematical model (Wever, 1971b).

In the lowest diagram of figure 103, not only average courses of rectal temperature rhythms were presented separately for the sections with long and short periods but, additionally, the phase relationship between the rhythms of rectal temperature and activity can be obtained from this diagram. As can be seen, the maximum of rectal temperature occurs earlier, compared to the activity rhythm, during the sections with the short periods than in the sections with the long periods. The average ($\pm$ standard deviation) is $15° \pm 13°$ (significantly deviating from zero with $p < 0.01$). It can be seen that the minimum of rectal temperature occurs almost simultaneously, compared to the activity rhythm, during both sections. On the average, it is delayed during the sections with short periods, in comparison to the other sections, by $-1.5° \pm 12°$; therefore, not significantly deviating from zero. Because of this inconsistency, considering the different extreme values within a period, the consideration of the computed acrophase may lead to a more reliable estimation. As the result, the acrophases of rectal temperature rhythms occur, during the sections with the short periods, earlier compared to the acrophases of activity rhythms than during the sections with the long periods; on the average, by $7° \pm 9°$ (significantly deviating from zero with $p < 0.05$). This apparent internal phase shift could be interpreted as internal dissociation; however, this deduction would be conclusive only when the shape of the rhythm remains unchanged.

As can be seen in figure 104 (extreme right diagram), the form factor describing the rhythm's shape is different systematically in the two sections with long and short periods. Together with the fact that the α:ρ-

ratio is consistently larger than one (Fig. 104, extreme left diagram), this leads, for pure kinematic reasons, to an apparent phase shift with varying period between the oscillation itself and the rectangular derivative of this oscillation, generated by a threshold (Wever, 1973d). In the model mentioned, the rectal temperature rhythm is represented by the oscillation itself, and the activity rhythm is represented by the rectangular derivative (Wever, 1960) In other words, the model apparently leads to internal phase shifts between two different representations of the same oscillation. The apparent contradiction of this statement is based on the impossibility of stating phase angle differences, in the strict mathematical sense, in oscillations with shapes deviating from the sinusoidal shape. In particular, it is meaningless to compare phase angle differences in oscillations of different shapes. In these oscillations, any statement of phase angles, even if it concerns the maximum value, minimum value, or acrophase, is only meaningful with regard to a special model. Applying the mathematical model which was shown to be successful in many other respects, quantitative estimations, introducing a change in period in an amount as measured experimentally, lead to phase angle differences which coincide with corresponding phase angle differences measured experimentally (Wever, 1973d). Accepting these results, the "true" phase relationship between the rhythms of rectal temperature and activity is the same during the sections with long and short periods; therefore, the phase relationship between the two rhythms is independent of the period. This means that internal phase shifts can be simulated by changes in the shape of the rhythm, even when these two rhythms are assumed to be controlled directly by one single oscillator without an interposed coupling that may vary the phases.

The results presented in figures 103 and 104 demonstrate interdependencies between different parameters of a rhythm. Only for clarity, the values of the different parameters are plotted as functions of the respective section of the experiment. To differentiate between intra- and interindividual interdependencies, the correlation between two parameters should be shown directly. Since the period (Fig. 58) and the range of oscillation of the rectal temperature rhythm (Fig. 103, upper middle diagram) are the parameters most strongly correlated to the experimental conditions (i.e., absence and presence of an artificial electric 10-Hz field), the mutual dependency between these two rhythm parameters is selected as an example. Figure 105 shows that changes in the range of oscillation, without exception, are correlated negatively to changes in the period. The mean regression, computed from the logarithms of the individual regressions, is a $-0.113 \pm 0.054°C$ change in the range per hour change in period. In the statistical analysis, this mean regression deviates from zero with $p < 0.001$ ($t = 6.94$). In contrast to this highly significant intraindividual correlation, the absolute values of the parameters are not correlated mutually interindividually. There is no significant correlation between the individual values of period and range of oscillation; neither during the sections with the long periods (without the field in operation) nor during the sections with the short periods (with the field continuously in operation). The respective coefficients of correlation are r = 0.295, and r = 0.201; both correlations not differing significantly from zero. The same is true with interdependencies between other rhythm parameters. Although there always are significant correlations between intraindividual changes in the different parameters with changing experimental conditions, the individual values of these parameters, measured in one condition, are not correlated mutually (Wever, 1968c). This statement is true only in circadian rhythms of man. In some animal rhythms, there are significant interindividual correlations between period and range of oscillation and other parameters (Aschoff et al., 1971c). A possible solution of this difference between human and animal rhythms may be the fact that the interindividual variations in the different parameters are remarkably small in man but broader in most animals. They, therefore, may undergo random fluctuations in man, but not in animals. With this consideration, it must be expected that there also are significant interindividual correlations between the different rhythm parameters in man when a much larger sample of subjects is considered.

In summary, autonomous circadian rhythms of man, in all respects tested, behave like a simple model oscillation. This is true with different parameters of the rectal temperature rhythm and the activity rhythm, when the rhythms are affected by changes in the experimental conditions. This means that the experimentally discovered properties of the circadian system are nothing but consequences of some basic features (i.e., self-sustainment and separate excitation,

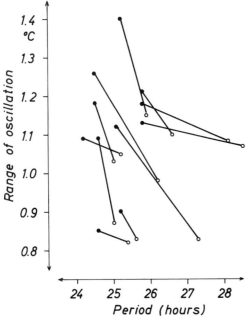

Figure 105. Interdependency between range of oscillation and period in autonomous rectal temperature rhythms, measured in experiments during which the course of the period was changed regularly by an electric AC field (i.e., 10 Hz square wave, 2.5 V/m; operating continuously in one section). ○: parameters in the sections with long periods (i.e., field not in operation). ●: parameters in the sections with short periods (i.e., field in operation). Results from individual experiments are combined by lines.

both parametric and nonparametric). In addition, the results derived from figures 103 and 104 have another aspect. All parameters included in these figures have been calculated independently of each other and of the periods. All these parameters, independently of each other, depend on the experimental conditions. In this special case, the condition was defined by the absence or presence of an artificial electric 10-Hz field. Therefore, there in fact, may be a small possibility that the consistency in the change of one parameter, following a change in the state of this stimulus, is simulated by random fluctuations. The possibility, however, that many parameters, which were calculated independently, may change due to random fluctuations, moving consistently in directions which have been postulated theoretically, is extremely low. Considering the changes of all rhythm parameters collectively, the effect of the artificial electric 10-Hz field on human circadian rhythms (cf. 2.4.5), therefore, is guaranteed at a very high level of significance.

4.1.2. Entrained Rhythms

Human circadian rhythms can be described by simple oscillation laws; not only when running autonomously but also when entrained by a forcing zeitgeber. First, each self-sustained oscillation can be entrained only within limited ranges of entrainment; not only around the natural frequency, but also to a lower extent (i.e., within narrower limits) around multiples and submultiples of the natural frequency. The width of these ranges depends on the ratio of the zeitgeber strength to the oscillatory strength. Outside the ranges of entrainment, relative coordination (v. Holst, 1939a) occurs showing that a zeitgeber effecting the rhythm is present and this zeitgeber is, with its special frequency, too weak to entrain the rhythm. Inside the ranges of entrainment, the phase relationship between the zeitgeber and entrained rhythm depends on the frequency. It changes from one limit to the other by about

180° (Wever, 1964b). All these properties also were found in human circadian rhythms. It was shown in chapter 3.1.1 that human circadian rhythms can be entrained only within limited ranges of entrainment. These ranges are small with weak zeitgebers (cf. 3.2.1) and broad with strong zeitgebers (cf. 3.3.1). Outside the range of entrainment, relative coordination can be demonstrated (Fig. 70) and, inside this range, the phase relationships of all rhythms measured to the zeitgeber vary with the period (Fig. 72). All these experimental results are in agreement with postulations of the simple oscillation model.

When an entraining zeitgeber becomes shifted in phase, the rhythm must follow the shift within several days. The rate of this reentrainment, according to the oscillation model, mainly depends on the ratio of the zeitgeber strength to the oscillatory strength. In the experiments discussed in chapter 3.1.2, the strength of the external zeitgeber can be assumed to be more or less the same in all experiments. Differences in the rate of reentrainment under otherwise similar conditions, therefore, are most probably due to differences in the oscillatory strengths. If this statement is correct, the experimentally discovered positive correlation between the original amplitude of the rhythm and the duration of reentrainment (Fig. 76) means, at the same time, a positive correlation between the original amplitude and the oscillatory strength or the degree of persistence of this rhythm. If this result could be confirmed by further experiments, it would have practical implications. It would enable the determination of the degree of persistence of individual 'internal clocks'; the larger the amplitude of a rhythm, the more persistent, or stronger, is the underlying oscillator or pacemaker.

Beside the oscillatory strength, the autonomous period of a rhythm determines the duration of reentrainment after a phase shift of a definite zeitgeber. In rhythms with autonomous periods being longer than the zeitgeber period, as is generally the case in human circadian rhythms (cf. 2.3), a faster reentrainment after delaying than after advancing shifts could be expected. In the phase shift experiments, however, the direction asymmetry is exactly reversed. Reentrainment consistently is faster after advancing than after delaying phase shifts of the zeitgeber (Figs. 75 and 76). The apparent discrepancy between theoretical expectations and experimental results can be solved by a closer look at the oscillation theory. In its simplest form, this theory only applies to linear oscillations. It needs refinement in cases of self-sustained (nonlinear) oscillations. In particular, the expectation is based on oscillations whose amplitude remains constant during the shift. In self-sustained oscillations, however, the amplitude does not remain constant during the shift, but becomes diminished. This also happens in human circadian rhythms, when they are shifted (Fig. 74). Following the oscillation theory, a temporary diminishing in the amplitude (i.e., a diminishing relative to its steady state value) leads to a temporary acceleration of the oscillation (Wever, 1963a). When applied to reentrainment, this means that advancing shifts, with respect to transients, have preference over delaying shifts when the rhythm's amplitude is diminished during the shift. In general, while the steady state amplitude influences the duration of reentrainment, independent of the direction of the shift (Fig. 76), a deviation of the amplitude from its steady state value during the shift, must be expected to influence the direction asymmetry. In man, also the effect on amplitude is asymmetrical since the amplitude is more reduced in advancing than in delaying phase shifts. This must be expected since, in the 24-hour day, the zeitgeber period does not coincide with the peak of the resonance curve (at about 25 hours). An advance shift leads the period farther from the resonance peak and, therefore, to a smaller amplitude, than a delay shift of the same amount. As the summarizing result of these considerations, the experimental observations concerning reentrainment of human circadian rhythms after phase shifts of the zeitgeber are in full agreement with theoretical postulations. The more the amplitude of an overt rhythm is reduced after a sudden phase shift of the zeitgeber (Fig. 74), the greater the preponderance of the reentrainment rate after an advancing shift over that after a delaying shift (Fig. 75).

A periodic environmental stimulus acts as a zeitgeber only if its periodicity is controlled externally (i.e., independent of the subject). In cases where the environmental conditions are controlled by the subject himself, the resulting environmental periodicity, by definition, does not represent a zeitgeber and, therefore, does not break the autonomy of the oscillation. In this type of a self-control, the oscillation model postulates a period which is longer than it would be under constant conditions of equal average quality. It also postulates a reversal in the dependency of the period on the magnitude of the controlling stimulus (Wever, 1967a). Regarding the behavior under self-controlled conditions, the experimentally observed properties of human circadian rhythms also agree fully with the theoretically derived postulations.

4.1.3. Conclusions

All results discussed clearly show the close coincidence between properties of human circadian rhythms, as measured in isolation experiments of very different modes, and postulations of a simple mathematical oscillation model, derived from the assumption of a single oscillation having the capacity to be self- and separately excited simultaneously. This coincidence primarily concerns the period of the overt rhythms observed, but also the period of the basic oscillator hypothetically underlying the overt rhythm, because the period cannot be changed by the interconnected coupling between the basic oscillator and the overt rhythm. Second, the coincidence discussed also concerns all other measurable parameters of the overt rhythms. These other parameters, in fact, can be changed by the coupling (i.e., the changes of these other parameters do not reflect necessarily only equivalent oscillator changes, but also can be due to changes in the interconnected coupling between the basic oscillator and the overt rhythm). The measured changes of all parameters, nevertheless, agree with the theoretical postulations which ignore any effect of the coupling. The formulated hypothesis, therefore, is the coupling forces between the basic oscillator and the overt rhythms do not affect systematically the possibility of extrapolating measured changes in parameters of overt rhythms to equivalent changes in parameters of the basic oscillator. This hypothesis states that changes in the overt rhythms, depending on environmental stimuli, clearly reflect changes in the basic oscillator, while effects of the interconnected coupling forces on the overt rhythms are negligible (i.e., rather constant and less depending on the environmental conditions).

In summary, the properties of human circadian rhythms can be understood, as long as the rhythms run synchronized internally, on the basis of the assumption that they are controlled by one simple basic oscillator or pacemaker. This is true with respect to properties manifested under the influence of constant environmental conditions with a varying magnitude of the controlling stimuli, and periodically alternating conditions. The basic oscillator must fulfill only the prerequisite that it is self- and separately excited simultaneously, parametric and nonparametric. It would not be useful to extend the features of the basic oscillator to more complicated qualities and to introduce a relevant dependency of the coupling between basic oscillator and overt rhythm on environmental conditions. In both cases, the complication of the hypothesis would not improve the applicability of the hypothesis in any respect nor the agreement between postulations of the hypothesis and experimental results. The statements concluded from the hypothesis, of course, only concern the kinetics of the basic oscillator and not its basic mechanism. The knowledge of the underlying kinetics may help in the search for this basic mechanism, which is still unknown at present.

4.2. The Multioscillator Model

Although human circadian rhythms can be described in many respects with the assumption of one single underlying oscillator, this assumption generally can be shown to be insufficient. All phenomena related to internal desynchronization lead to the conclusion that more than one oscillator or pacemaker must be involved. A multioscillatory system already is suggested by the occurrence of internal dissociation when different overt rhythms adopt different periods temporarily, but it is only by true internal desynchronization that the deduction of a multioscillatory system becomes conclusive.

4.2.1. Internal Dissociation

Internal dissociation first was observed in rhythms changing from the natural synchronized state to the autonomous state where the period consistently is longer than 24 hours (Fig. 17). To the present, the question has not been answered whether this change in internal phase relationship is due to the transition from the synchronized to the autonomous state or the change in period. To give a sufficient answer, three different types of experiments must be compared, considering the occurrence of internal phase shifts. First, experiments where the rhythm passes between the synchronized and the autonomous state, without simultaneously changing the period (Fig. 78). Second, experiments where the period changes during the autonomous state, due to a change in the magnitude of a continuously operating stimulus controlling the rhythm (Fig. 55). Finally, experiments where the period changes during the synchronized state, due to a change in the period of the entraining zeitgeber (Fig. 69). Although all of these experiments already have been discussed separately, in the following summarized results

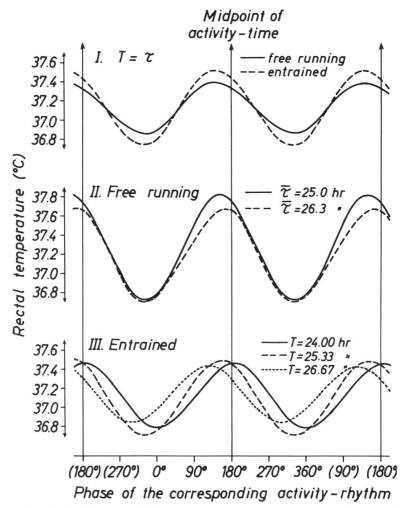

Figure 106. Summary of three types of experiments. Courses of averaged rectal temperature rhythms, relative to the activity rhythms. For clarity, two cycles are plotted successively. *I.* (top diagram). Comparison between rhythms with equal periods, running autonomously and entrained to an artificial zeitgeber (i.e., relative light-dark cycle and regular calling signals) (compare Fig. 78). *II.* (middle diagram). Comparison between autonomous rhythms with different periods, obtained in experiments during which the course of the period was changed regularly by an electric AC field (i.e., 10 Hz square wave, 2.5 V/m; operating continuously in one section) (compare Fig. 55). *III.* (bottom diagram). Comparison between entrained rhythms with different periods, obtained in experiments with an artificial zeitgeber (i.e., relative light-dark cycle and regular calling signals) of a varying period (compare Fig. 69). From Wever (1973d).

of the three types of experiments will be reviewed collectively.

Figure 106 summarizes results of the three experiments mentioned. It presents averaged courses of the rectal temperature rhythms relative to the activity rhythm. The summary of experimental results of the first type (uppermost diagram) shows that the internal phase relationship between the two rhythms is the same when the rhythms are free running and entrained, provided the period is the same under both conditions. Only the range of the rectal temperature rhythm, or its amplitude, is significantly larger in the entrained state than in the autonomous state (Wever, 1973d). The summary of results of experiments of the second type (middle diagram) seems to be less clear. Not only mean value and amplitude, but also the phase of the rectal temperature rhythm relative to the activity rhythm, seem to be different in the two conditions. At least the maximum of rectal temperature occurs significantly earlier in the rhythms with the shorter periods. It, however, was shown earlier (cf. 4.1.1; Fig. 103) that changes in the internal phase relationship, in this special case, are feigned by changes in the shape of the temperature curve; and the "true" internal phase relationship, in this case, is the same in both conditions. In contrast to the two experimental types discussed so far, experiments of the third type (lowermost diagram) clearly show changes in the internal phase relationship between the two rhythms, with a varying zeitgeber period. The amplitude, moreover, may be largest when the zeitgeber period coincides with the autonomous period. In the present experiments, these changes in amplitude, indicating 'resonance', statistically are not significant (Wever, 1973d). As the summarizing result, the comparison of the three types of experiments (Fig. 106) clearly shows that only changes in the period, when induced by an entraining zeitgeber, have the capacity to change the internal phase relationship. In cases of transition between entrained rhythms, with a period of 24.0 hours, and autonomous rhythms, with periods close to 25 hours, not the transition itself, but the change in period due to entrainment to the natural day, is the effective stimulus changing the internal phase relationship.

After knowing the results included in figure 106, the empirically deduced criterion concerning the discrimination between autonomous and synchronized rhythms, based on the internal phase relationship (cf. 2.1.2; Fig. 19), must be discussed once more. The slightly negative, though not significantly deviating from zero, regression between the internal phase relationship and period of autonomously running rhythms now can be understood to be due to changes in the

rhythm's shape, correlated to changes in the rhythm's period. This slight change between the computed acrophases, therefore, does not represent a change of the 'true' phases (Figs. 103; and 106, middle). Figure 19 further includes an apparent contradiction, which must be resolved. The extrapolation of the phase angle differences, between the rhythms of activity and rectal temperature, to an autonomous period of 24 hours, leads to a value greatly deviating from that value belonging to rhythms entrained to 24.0 hours. On the other hand, the transition between autonomous and entrained rhythms without a change in period should not affect the internal phase angle difference (Fig. 106, uppermost diagram). To understand this contradiction, one must remember that entrained rhythms, for which a mean phase angle difference of −42° is given in figure 19, probably would have periods close 25 hours when free running (Fig. 37). Entrainment of these rhythms to 24.0 hours means a considerable change in period and, therefore, considerable changes in the internal phase relationship must be expected. If there would be a subject with a free running period close to 24 hours, entrainment of this subject to 24.0 hours should not result in a change of his internal phase relationship. In this situation, therefore, the temperature cycle should have a leading phase not only during the autonomous run, but also during entrainment. As a consequence, a former statement must be specified. If, under conditions intended to be constant, there is a rhythm with a measured period close to 24 hours, but with a clearly leading phase of the rectal temperature rhythm according to figure 19, it can be stated with certainty that the rhythm has an autonomous period very close to 24 hours. It cannot be stated with certainty, however, the rhythm actually is running autonomously.

Figure 106 primarily shows effects concerning the internal phase relationship between the rhythms of activity and rectal temperature. It secondarily shows effects concerning the amplitude of the rectal temperature rhythm. This amplitude is larger under the influence of an entraining zeitgeber than under constant conditions and is largest when the period of this zeitgeber coincides with the period of the autonomous rhythm. This influence has additional consequences with regard to the internal coupling between different rhythms: the larger the amplitude the stronger is this specific coupling. This means that internal coupling normally is stronger in entrained rhythms than in free running rhythms; or the tendency toward internal desynchronization must be expected to be smaller in entrained than in free running rhythms. This may be the reason why internal desynchronization occurs spontaneously in a considerable part of healthy subjects when living under constant conditions, but very seldom when these subjects are under the influence of an entraining zeitgeber with a period close to 24 hours. It is only under the influence of a very weak zeitgeber, which enlarges the temperature amplitude to only a small amount, that internal desynchronization may occur with an entrained rectal temperature rhythm and a free running activity rhythm (Fig. 81). With an increasing strength of the zeitgeber, not only the entraining action of the external zeitgeber, but also the entraining action of the rectal temperature rhythm on the activity rhythm increases. This statement, of course, only is applicable as long as the rectal temperature rhythm is entrained to the zeitgeber (cf. 3.3.1).

It is the general result of the summary included in figure 106 that internal dissociation occurs exclusively after changes in the period, when induced by an entraining zeitgeber. Neither changes in period of autonomous rhythms, whether spontaneously or as a consequence of changes in the magnitude of a controlling stimulus, nor the transition between entrained and autonomous rhythms, in the steady state, result in internal dissociation. These conclusions can be extended in two directions. First, they are not restricted to the relationship between the rhythms of activity and rectal temperature. Changes in the period of an entraining zeitgeber also induce internal dissociation between all other measurable overt rhythms

(Fig. 72). Second, the result is neither restricted to the stimulus used as the zeitgeber in the experiments underlying figure 106 nor to periodically operating stimuli that act as zeitgebers. It was shown earlier (Fig. 102) that other effective stimuli, when operating periodically, and stimuli operating in a self-control mode also induce internal dissociation for equal amounts per hour change in period.

Internal dissociation does not occur only permanently in the steady state, due to entrainment to different periods, but also temporarily, as a consequence of phase shifts of the zeitgeber. The time necessary to become reentrained to a shifted zeitgeber differs among different overt rhythms (Fig. 75). This means that during reentrainment, the temporal order in the relationship between the various overt rhythms is disturbed and, therefore, internal dissociation is present during reentrainment. After all rhythms have reentrained fully, the original internal phase relationships between the different rhythms usually is reestablished and the temporary internal dissociation is terminated. In summary, internal dissociation, in the meaning commonly used, can occur in two different forms. First, a changed internal phase relationship is maintained, after transients have faded away, in the steady state. This form occurs, for example, after changes in the period of an entraining zeitgeber. Second, a changed internal phase relationship is present only temporarily (i.e., only during transients). This form occurs, for example, after phase shifts of an entraining zeitgeber. To differentiate between these two forms, it is proposed to speak of 'internal phase shift' in the first case and to reserve the term 'internal dissociation' for the second case.

4.2.2. Internal Desynchronization

While internal dissociation, or internal phase shift, does not require necessarily the existence of more than one independent oscillator, internal desynchronization does. Internal dissociation, or internal phase shift, can be described by different coupling forces interconnected between one basic oscillator and the various overt rhythms (i.e., by effects of the "hands of the clock" instead of effects of the "clock itself"). This description, however, cannot be applied to internal desynchronization, except by assuming frequency transformation as a property of the coupling; a theoretical case which already has been ruled out as a possibility in circadian rhythms (cf. 3.5). The difference between internal dissociation and desynchronization also can be expressed in terms of a "phase map", as introduced at the beginning (Fig. 3). During internal dissociation, the phase map is changed, with regard to amplitudes and phases of all rhythms, until the transients have faded. In the final steady state, the same phase map as before the disturbance (e.g., the phase shift of the zeitgeber) is valid. After internal phase shifts, a totally changed phase map is valid in the steady state. For instance, under the influence of a zeitgeber with a varying period, the complete structure of the phase map varies with the period. On the other hand, during the state of internal desynchronization, no stable phase map exists. This is true not only when internal desynchronization occurs spontaneously in autonomously running rhythms (cf. 2.2.1), but also when forced internal desynchronization occurs under the influence of a zeitgeber (cf. 3.3.1).

In the definition used here, internal desynchronization is characterized by different steady state periods of different rhythms, as can be proven only by demonstrating internal phase shifts between these different rhythms by more than 360°. Because of the impossibility of frequency transformation, the different periods of the overt rhythms clearly reflect different periods of the underlying oscillatory system (i.e., they prove the existence of different oscillators underlying the different overt rhythms). The state of internal desynchronization, therefore, shows that the human circadian system cannot be controlled by only one basic oscillator, but by several, This multioscillator hypothesis includes that the different oscillators run primarily synchronously to each other so that they appear outwardly as only one single oscillator, but the system inherently includes the possiblity of separating the different oscillators, either spontaneously or forced by external conditions.

Originally, the multioscillator concept was deduced from the discovery of internal desynchronization between two or more different overt rhythms; for example, between the overt rhythms of activity and rectal temperature. After establishing the regularities of this state, especially by considering the interactions between desynchronized rhythms, this concept was modified. It seems appropriate to speak of internal desynchronization between different oscillators involved in the circadian system instead of desynchronization between different overt rhythms. This follows from the multioscillator model derived earlier. This model is based on the presence of several different oscillators controlling the great variety of overt rhythm in such a manner that each of the oscillators simultaneously controls each of the overt rhythms, or at least many overt rhythms, but for different proportions. Conversely, every overt rhythm of the great variety available, is controlled simultaneously by all existing, or at least several, basic oscillators. As a consequence of this model, the different periods representing the different oscillators, in principle, can be demonstrated in the spectral analyses of every single overt rhythm. The same periods reliably are present in all overt rhythms but, in detail, the dominant of these periods may vary from overt rhythm to overt rhythm. This is true in spontaneously occurring internal desynchronization (e.g., part II of Figs. 25, 27, 28, 30, and 36) and in forced internal desynchronization (e.g., part II of Figs. 81, 86, 87, 91, and 93).

Following the multioscillator hypothesis, it depends on the arbitrary and occasional selection of overt rhythms measured, whether the state of internal desynchronization is indicated by differences in the dominant periods of different overt rhythms or by the presence of different periods within a single overt rhythm. In all examples of internal desynchronization shown so far, this state, in fact, was indicated by different periods of the overt rhythms of activity and rectal temperature. The presence of more than one period in a single overt rhythm has been shown, so far, in only the period analyses. It was never evident in the inspection of the raw data given in the presentations. By applying a dodge, however, the simultaneous presence of two different periods can be seen in the presentation of original data. In the longitudinal presentation, besides a single rhythmicity, only regular fluctuations in the amplitude can be detected, suggesting beat phenomena. Even beat phenomena, however, indicate the presence of a second rhythmicity, at least indirectly, but other causes of regular fluctuations in the amplitude are imaginable. In the vertical presentation, an overt rhythmicity, more or less arbitrarily, always must be selected since the sequence of successive cycles must be presented; and the definition of a cycle depends on the selected period. This normally is the dominant rhythmicity, but the simultaneous presence of a second rhythmicity again cannot be detected. The most promising method of presenting original data, to facilitate the obvious detection of two rhythmicities with different periods being present simultaneously, is the vertical presentation; however, without selecting predetermined periods, but presenting the full time series. This kind of presentation was demonstrated in figure 12/II, with a doubling 24.0-hour scale, and in figure 13/I, with different averaging periods. Because, in this type of presentation, the detectability of a rhythm depends on the deviation of its period from the applied averaging period, the special dodge is to select an averaging period which is the mean to be expected of the two periods.

Figure 107 shows, as a first example, an original computer plot of locomotor activity, presented in the standard manner commonly used in all animal studies where locomotor activity is measured. The plot originates from the experimental results already shown in figure 87. In the second section of this experiment, internal desynchronization was forced by a strong zeitgeber with a period of 28.0 hours. As the results of the period analyses (Fig.87/II), in the activity rhythm two periods are present, with periods of 28.0 and 24.8 hours. For the plot of locomotor activity, an averaging period of 26.5 hours was selected and, for clarity, two cycles of 26.5 hours were plotted successively. As can be seen from figure 107, in the first section of the experiment (i.e., 24.0-hour day; Fig. 87/I), only one rhythmicity was present. As indicated by the flat slope of the activity indications, its period deviated strongly from the averaging period (24.0 hours versus 26.5 hours). In the second section (i.e., 28.0-hour day), two rhythmicities can be recognized, with slopes that are nearly symmetric but less flat than in the first section (24.8 and 28.0 hours, each versus 26.5 hours). The duality of periods is so obvious that guidelines have not been drawn, in order to avoid prejudicing the perception. The two rhythmicities intersect several times, so there can be no doubt that there is a steady state. This is in contrast to apparently similar animal experiment records where 'splitting phenomena' are present (Hoffmann, 1970, 1971; Pittendrigh, 1960, 1967; Pittendrigh and Daan, 1976b). In all these cases, different activity components, in fact, separate from each other, but never by more than about 180°; therefore, they again run synchronously to each other in the steady state. In such cases, internal dissociation evidently is present, but not internal desynchronization.

As another example, figure 108 shows, in a similar manner, the course of rectal temperature obtained in an experiment with constant conditions where internal desynchronization occurred spontaneously. Results of this experiment already were presented in figure 25. Since the period analysis of the rectal temperature rhythm resulted in two relevant periods of 24.8 and 33.5 hours (Fig. 25/II), an averaging period of 29.0 hours has been selected for the presentation of figure 108. Because of the stronger devia-

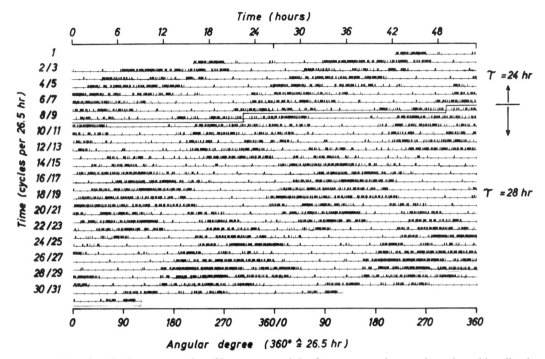

Figure 107.   Standard computer plot of locomotor activity from an experiment where the subject lived under the influence of a strong artificial zeitgeber (i.e., absolute light-dark cycle and regular calling signals) with a period of 24.0 hours, during an initial section, and 28.0 hours, during the main section (Fig. 87). The plotting is based on a repetition period of 26.5 hours, which is about the average of the two periods included in the time series (Fig. 87/II). For clarity, two cycles, of 26.5 hours each, are plotted successively.

tion of the rhythm's periods from the averaging period, five successive cycles, of 29.0 hours each, in addition to the vertical presentation, are drawn longitudinally so each measured point is included in the diagram 5 times. To further facilitate the pursuing of corresponding phases of the rhythm, those sections of the rectal temperature course that are above the mean temperature, as computed from the total experiment (36.85°C), are drawn with solid lines and those sections that are below this mean are drawn with dotted lines. Guidelines within the diagram again have been avoided to avoid prejudicing the perception. To find the slopes belonging to the included periods, arrows are drawn outside the diagram. As seen in figure 108, besides the main period of 24.8 hours, simultaneously a secondary period (33.5 hours) evidently is present. Due to the more complicated course of a continu-

ously recorded variable, the impression of the duality of periods is not as obvious as it is in the activity record (Fig. 107).

The two examples shown (Figs. 107 and 108) should demonstrate that the state of internal desynchronization also can be recognized from the inspection of the course of only one variable. Similar records could be presented from all other 66 experiments where internal desynchronization occurred, either spontaneously or forced by a zeitgeber. Courses of previously presented experiments are shown repeatedly to facilitate understanding. Those presentations reveal the participation of more than one basic oscillator in the control of one only overt rhythm, which was postulated by the multioscillator model proposed. The meaning of the perception gained from those presentations, however, can be understood only after internal desynchronization was studied by analyzing

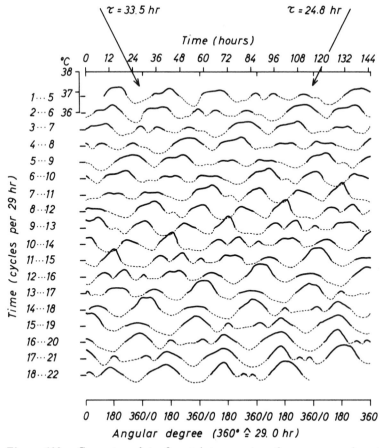

Figure 108. Computer plot of rectal temperature from an experiment where the subject lived under constant conditions (Fig. 25). The plotting is based on a repetition period of 29.0 hours, which is about the average of the two periods included in the time series (Fig. 25/II). The two periods, with respect to their slopes, are indicated by arrows outside the diagram. For clarity, five cycles, of 29.0 hours each, are plotted successively, and the rectal temperature course is given by a solid line, as long as it runs above the experimental mean (i.e., 36.85°C), and by a dotted line, as long as it runs below this mean.

the courses of many different variables comparatively.

4.2.3. Properties of Separated Oscillators

Assuming a multioscillator system, as suggested, two questions arise; are the different oscillators separately self-sustained and are these oscillators separately affected by external stimuli (i.e., separately entrainable by zeitgebers)? As shown earlier, both of these

properties can be ascribed to the basic oscillator.

In autonomously running, internally synchronized rhythms, it must not be presupposed necessarily that the different oscillators involved are separately self-sustained. It also can be assumed that only one of the oscillators is self-sustained and the other oscillators are being driven by the first one. When under constant conditions internal desynchronization occurs spontaneously, the different oscillators continue to run autonomously, but with different speeds. In this case, the running of one oscillator cannot be the direct consequence of the running of another oscillator and, therefore, the different oscillators must run self-sustained separately. It may be argued that the cycle of wakefulness and sleep must not be due necessarily to an underlying self-sustained oscillator, like the overt rhythms of the vegetative variables (e.g., rectal temperature), but may be due to the force of habit (e.g., taking three meals per activity time). In this case, the intervals between the meals may be determined by the capacity of the stomach and the velocity of digestion rather than a superior rhythmicity. Not only the feeding habit, but also other habits, were changed in corresponding experiments without relevant changes in the parameters of the activity-rest cycle. It seems very unlikely that the overt activity rhythm is formed by any learned habits instead of being controlled by an underlying oscillator (cf. 3.3.4). The argument of the habitual origin of the rhythm, which concerns only the activity rhythm but not the rhythms of vegetative variables, nevertheless, cannot be rejected with certainty from results of autonomous rhythms obtained under constant environmental conditions.

Self-sustainment of an oscillator not only can be tested with autonomous rhythms, but also with heteronomous rhythms, which are controlled by external zeitgebers. While non-self-sustained oscillators can be synchronized by external forcing oscillations to anyone frequency, though with largely varying amplitudes, self-sustained oscillators can be entrained only within limited ranges. In internally synchronized circadian rhythms, the limitations of entrainment clearly can be show (Figs. 69 and 70) and, therefore, in these rhythms, self-sustainment is demonstrated independently. This self-sustainment again could concern only one of the oscillators while the other oscillators are driven by the first.

When the rhythms desynchronize internally, being forced by a strong zeitgeber (cf. 3.3), the separated rhythm of rectal temperature free runs in spite of the presence of a zeitgeber (i.e., it is out of its range of entrainment while the separated activity rhythm still is synchronized). This result means that the oscillator dominantly controlling the rectal temperature rhythm has been proven to be self-sustained in heteronomous rhythms, independent of the proof in autonomous rhythms. The limitation of the range of entrainment of the separated activity rhythm was shown only preliminarily with the strong zeitgeber (Fig. 94). In experiments with a weak zeitgeber, however, a free run of the activity rhythm clearly was demonstrated combined with an entrained rectal temperature rhythm (Fig. 81). Since the activity rhythm was shown to be entrainable, even when running desynchronized (s. above), the most likely interpretation of this result is, in this case, the activity rhythm is outside its range of entrainment. This means that self-sustainment also was proven in heteronomous rhythms with regard to the activity rhythm.

With this consideration, separate self-sustainment of the activity rhythm was suggested strongly from the examination of individual experiments under constant conditions as well as under zeitgeber influence. The most relevant evidence for this capacity, however, comes from the summarizing inspection of all experiments performed under constant conditions, with regard to the periods. If the rhythmicity of the alternation between wakefulness and sleep would be due to 'habit', a continuous distribution of periods must be expected, but not the multimodal distribution shown in figure 37 (below). The multimodality, in fact, can be understood only when it is based on the self-sustained origin of the activity rhythm. As will be discussed in detail in the following, the multimodality indirectly reflects the limitations of ranges of entrainment; not only of the primary range with an internal 1:1 synchronization, but also the secondary ranges with a 2:1 and 1:2 synchronization. To understand the deduction from self-sustainment to the multimodality of the period distribution, consideration of the 'strengths' of the different oscillators must be inserted.

It was shown earlier (Fig. 29) that, with the occurrence of internal desynchronization, the periods of the different oscillators change in opposite directions, but for very different amounts. On the average, the change in the period of the overt activity rhythm is about twelve times greater than the change in the period of the rectal temperature rhythm, consistent in the different types of internal desynchronization. According to the definition given by Klotter (1960), the ratio by which the variability of periods differs between two oscillators is a reciproce of the ratio by which the oscillators differ in their degree of persistence. This means that the oscillator controlling dominantly the rectal temperature rhythm (type I oscillator) has a degree of persistence, or an oscillatory strength, which is about 12 times greater than the other oscillator dominantly controlling the activity (type II oscillator; Wever, 1975a). The same 1:12 ratio in the strengths of the different oscillators can be deduced not only from the variabilities connected with the transition between internally synchronized and desynchronized rhythms, but also from the interindividual variabilities. In figure 37 where the measured distributions were given from all overt rectal temperature rhythms (above) and all overt activity rhythms (below), the formally computed normal distributions were indicated by dotted lines. These two normal distributions differ from each other in their parameters, characterizing the interindividual variability, for a factor of 12 (Wever, 1975a).

In figure 109, the two formally computed distributions already discussed are normalized to equal areas. It is the hypothesis, to be discussed, that these two distributions represent the period distributions of all oscillators without mutual interaction. In the real circadian system, however, there is mutual interaction between the two types of oscillators which manifests itself by internal synchronization of free running rhythms. This interaction can be calculated on the basis of the different oscillatory strengths just deduced. It results in mutual entrainment

within only limited ranges of entrainment, because of the self-sustainment of the oscillators. As is common in nonlinear oscillations, entrainment is possible not only to the period of the forcing oscillation (i.e., primary entrainment), but also to multiples and submultiples of this period (i.e., secondary entrainment). The stronger oscillator (type I; rectal temperature) adopts the role of the forcing oscillation and the weaker oscillator (type II; activity) adopts the role of the forced oscillation, because period changes of the stronger oscillator, due to mutual entrainment, are nearly negligible in comparison to those of the weaker oscillator (Fig. 29). Consequently, the arrows in figure 109 indicate the period changes of the activity oscillator which are caused by the mutual interaction with the temperature oscillator. Period changes of the latter oscillator, in this scale, are not recognizable. Since the period distribution of the activity oscillator covers such a wide range including the half and the double period of the mean of the other distribution, these arrows also are arranged symmetrically to half and double the mean rectal temperature period.

As seen in figure 109, the mutual interaction must result primarily in changes of activity periods, in the range between about 20 and 30 hours, to the period of the rectal temperature rhythm, which is always close to 25 hours. Secondarily, activity periods around half and twice this value (i.e., in the ranges between about 10 and 15 hours, and between about 40 and 60 hours respectively) must be changed by the mutual interaction to periods close to 12.5 hours and 50 hours, respectively. There remain other unchanged periods outside the primary and secondary ranges of entrainment. These periods, which are positioned between about 15 and 20 hours and about 30 and 40 hours and, further, if those periods are present, shorter than 10 hours and longer than 60 hours, respectively, must stay with their original periods of the normal distribution. In figure 109, the distribution to be deduced from the normal distribution, after theoretically introducing the mutual interaction, is indicated

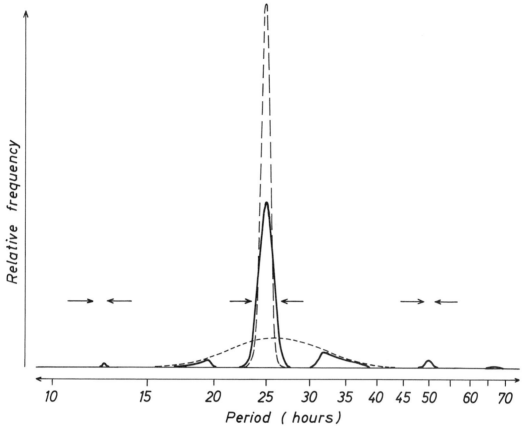

Figure 109. Theoretical synthesis of the multimodal distribution of activity periods in autonomous rhythms, deduced from the hypothetical normal distributions of periods coordinated to the two groups of oscillators (broken lines) taken from figure 37. Arrows: period changes induced by the mutual interaction between the two oscillator groups of different strengths, resulting in mutual entrainment within limited ranges. The solid line gives the resulting distribution of the group of weaker oscillators. From Wever (1975a).

by the solid line. The comparison between this theoretically derived distribution (Fig. 109) and the measured distribution of activity periods (Fig. 37, below) shows a remarkable coincidence. Both distributions equal each other in details [e.g., in the asymmetry of the amounts of the secondary peaks, or in the shapes of the separated peaks, which are partly symmetric (the smaller peaks around 12.5, 25.0 and 50.0 hours) and partly asymmetric (the broader peaks between 15 and 20 hours and between 30 and 40 hours)]. The nice agreement between theoretical and experimental results confirms the validity of the underlying hypothesis. This was based on separate self-sustainment of the two os-

cillators involved, but with different degrees of persistence, and a mutual interaction between the two oscillators. From these basic requirements, the mutual interaction and self-sustainment of the rectal temperature oscillator was proven directly. Only self-sustainment of the other oscillator was, as yet, suggested strongly, but not finally proven. Considering the deduction of figure 109, self-sustainment of the activity oscillator also is shown clearly. It is impossible to deduce the measured multimodal period distribution of this oscillator by the alternative hypothesis, which would state missing self-sustainment of this oscillator and, therefore, unlimited ranges of synchronization.

The next question concerns the capacity of separate excitation of the different oscillators. If internally synchronized rhythms ran entrained to a zeitgeber, it cannot be decided whether or not all involved oscillators are affected separately by the zeitgeber directly, or only one or several oscillators are affected by the zeitgeber directly while other oscillators are synchronized by the first. The observation, with a varying zeitgeber period, that the rectal temperature rhythm changes its external phase relationship to the zeitgeber more than the activity rhythm, coincides with the different sizes of the respective ranges of entrainment, even quantitatively (the ratio in the ranges of entrainment, and likewise in the steepness of the regressions between external phase relationship and zeitgeber period is about the square root of 12; cf. 3.1.1). This result generally fits the hypothesis of two oscillators of different strengths, as deduced above, because the effectiveness of a definite zeitgeber increases with decreasing oscillatory strength of the entrained rhythm. This result however, generally would fit also the assumption that only the activity rhythm is affected directly by the zeitgeber while the rectal temperature rhythm is affected only by the activity rhythm, but not directly by the external zeitgeber. A quantitative analysis of entrainment in internally synchronized rhythms already shows that this assumption is very unlikely. It is a well established fact, within the limits of the range of entrainment, and also in nonself-sustained oscillations where this range is unlimited, that the phase relationship between forced and forcing oscillation varies by about 180° (Wever, 1965a). With the assumption of the external zeitgeber as the forcing oscillation, the measured changes in the external phase relationship result in a range of entrainment of the rectal temperature rhythm of about 4.5 hours, which is in agreement with experimental results (cf. 3.1.1). With the assumption of the activity rhythm as the forcing oscillation, the measured changes in the internal phase relationship would result in a range of entrainment of about 8.5 hours,

which is in sharp contrast to the direct experimental measurements. It only can be argued that the linear extrapolation of the measured phase relationship is a very bad approximation for allowing this conclusion; however, another intricacy arises. Within the measured range of entrainment of the rectal temperature rhythm, the external phase relationship between the activity rhythm and zeitgeber varies by about 90°. If only the activity rhythm entrains the rectal temperature, the internal phase relationship must vary, within the range of entrainment, by 180°. This, however, would mean a variation of the phase relationship between rectal temperature rhythm and zeitgeber by about 270°, which again is in contradiction to the experimental observations.

While in experiments with internally synchronized rhythms, separate response of different oscillators to external zeitgebers only is suggested, it clearly can be shown with internally desynchronized rhythms. In experiments with a strong zeitgeber (cf. 3.3), activity rhythms were entrained to the zeitgeber while rectal temperature rhythms free ran; this means that in these experiments the activity rhythms were excited by the zeitgeber independent of the rectal temperature rhythms. In some experiments with a weak zeitgeber, the rectal temperature rhythms were entrained to the zeitgeber while the activity rhythms free ran (Fig. 81). Here, on the contrary, the rectal temperature rhythms were excited by the zeitgeber, independent of the activity rhythm. In summary, each different oscillator was shown to have the capacity to become entrained by an external zeitgeber, independent of the other oscillators (Wever, 1975e). Finally, this capacity can be demonstrated in group experiments with internally desynchronized rhythms, under constant conditions and zeitgeber influence. When, in a group experiment, internal desynchronization occurs spontaneously, not only the activity rhythms, but also the rectal temperature rhythms of the different subjects stay synchronized to each other (Fig. 67, right). When, under the influence of a strong zeitgeber, internal desynchronization is forced, the activity rhythms of the different subjects are synchronized externally, but independently, the rectal temperature rhythms stay mutually synchronized (Fig. 91). In both cases, even the rectal temperature rhythms must have the capacity to become entrained to those of the other subjects. This, in particular, means that even the rectal temperature rhythm is sensitive to social contacts as zeitgebers when separated from the conscious alternation beween wakefulness and sleep by internal desynchronization.

After the capacity of separated oscillators was established as being entrainable by external zeitgebers, it may be questioned whether or not parametric excitation contributes to the overall excitation, as it does in the control of the internally synchronized system (cf. 4.1). This question cannot be answered sufficiently at the present since only a few pilot experiments have been performed. In these experiments, the activity rhythms were fixed by a strong zeitgeber to periods outside the range of entrainment of the vegetative rhythms. Simultaneously, a continuously operating stimulus is set to influence the free running rectal temperature rhythm, and the magnitude of this stimulus is changed between successive sections of the experiment (Figs. 92 and 93). As the preliminary result of these experiments, the period of the rectal temperature rhythms, in fact, changed with the condition, indicating parametric excitation of these rhythms, even when separated from the activity rhythms by internal desynchronization (Wever, 1976b). This result, if confirmed significantly by further experiments, establishes the fundamental parity of the different oscillators with respect to separate excitation. Not only as long as circadian rhythmicity can be considered sufficiently as being controlled by one oscillator system, but also if a multioscillator system must be assumed, the basic features of each of the different oscillators involved in this system include, beside self-sustainment, parametric and nonparametric modes of separate excitation. These few basic features were shown to be sufficient to consti-

tute a model describing the general properties of circadian rhythms (cf. 4.1).

After fundamentally establishing the parity of the different oscillators involved in the circadian system, with regard to self-sustainment and to separate excitation, the question arises concerning quantitative differences in the parameters of the oscillators. One of these parameters is the oscillatory strength. It already was shown to be different in the different oscillators (i.e., for a factor of about 12 in the 2 main oscillator types). Another parameter is the dependency of the oscillators on external forces. It seems hopeless to evaluate the dependency of desynchronized rhythms on continuously operating stimuli with the other rhythms being fixed by a zeitgeber directly, because of the great number and complexity of experiments necessary for significant results. It seems appropriate to evaluate this dependency indirectly, by determining the dependency of internal phase relationships on changes of period, due to changes in the magnitude of continuously operating external stimuli, in internally synchronized rhythms. The general result of such a consideration, which already was shown in figure 106, is that the internal phase relationship between the rhythms of activity and rectal temperature remains constant when the period changes. This can be shown especially with an artificial electric 10-Hz field as the stimulus. Under the influence of such a field that is continuously in operation, the autonomous period is significantly shorter than without it (Fig. 58). The internal phase relationship between rhythms of activity and rectal temperature, however, is the same in the sections with short and long periods (Fig. 103). The same result was obtained in other experiments. If the period of an autonomously running, internally synchronized rhythm changes, due to the change of any other stimulus operating continuously, the internal phase relationship again remains unchanged (Fig. 64). Since the internal phase relationship was shown in other experiments, with periodically operating stimuli (Fig. 102), to not be a fixed quality, but subject to variations, the constancy in autonomous rhythms proves that in autonomous rhythms the different oscillators are affected by the external stimuli to equal amounts. Generally, the different oscillators involved in the circadian multioscillator system show equal dependencies on external forces.

The statement that different oscillators, when running autonomously, are affected by continuously operating external stimuli for equal amounts, seems to be contradictory to the statement that these different oscillators are affected by periodically operating stimuli for different amounts. This apparent contradiction, however, is nothing more than a consequence of equal dependency of parameters of the different oscillators on external stimuli and different oscillatory strengths. Autonomous rhythms are affected by continuously operating stimuli according to their responsiveness to those stimuli, but independent of their oscillatory strengths. The effectiveness of periodically operating stimuli, especially those of zeitgebers, additionally depends on this strength. In particular, it depends on the ratio between zeitgeber strength and oscillatory strength. The stronger the oscillator, or the more persistent it is, the weaker is the effect of a definite zeitgeber, even when the dependency of the oscillator's parameters on the external stimulus is unchanged.

Oscillatory strength and dependency of the oscillator's parameters on external forces are different features of an oscillator and are independent of each other. In particular, these features depend on very different mechanisms. As an example, if a variety of more or less identical oscillators constitutes a synchronized system, due to mutual coupling forces, this variety outwardly behaves like a single oscillator. The oscillatory strength, or the degree of persistence of this overall oscillator may increase with the number of participating single oscillators, but the dependency of its parameters on external stimuli is independent of this number but equals the dependency of each of the single oscillators.

4.3. Internal Interaction Between Different Rhythms

4.3.1. Oscillatory Interaction

The multioscillator model previously discussed demands a mutual internal coupling between different rhythms. This is obvious especially in autonomously running rhythms where all overt rhythms run synchronously. Since external zeitgebers are absent, synchronization can be only the result of mutual interaction. The possibility of internal desynchronization shows that this mutual synchronization is effective only within limited ranges of periods. The internal coupling between different circadian rhythms, therefore, is comparable to the interaction between an external zeitgeber and a circadian rhythm. The only difference is the directional sense of the interaction, which is bidirectional in a case of the mutual internal coupling but unidirectional in an external zeitgeber effect. This difference, however, is not very great because even the bidirectional internal coupling is not symmetrical with regard in both directions, but shows a considerable directional asymmetry as it recently was derived (cf. 4.2.3). A biological rhythm, therefore, can be conceived, in a more general sense, as an 'internal zeitgeber', in relation to other rhythms, which controls these rhythms in addition to external zeitgebers.

The internal zeitgeber effect can be tested not only under constant conditions, but also with externally synchronized rhythms. For this purpose, one of the overt rhythms must be altered arbitrarily in its course. In this context, the activity rhythm (i.e., the alternation between wakefulness and sleep) generally was considered as determining the phases of other overt rhythms (e.g.: Halberg and Simpson, 1967). The reported exceptional role of the activity rhythm, with regard to control of other rhythms, also was expressed by Webb and Agnew (1974b), "the key behavior schedule was the times for sleeping and waking". The overt activity rhythm occupies a special position in the respect that it is the only overt rhythm which, to the present, was manipulated arbitrarily to evaluate properties of the circadian system. This means that effects of the activity rhythm on other rhythms have been studied, but never direct effects of other rhythms on the activity rhythm. The often repeated statement of the dominant phase setting role of the activity rhythm, therefore, seems to be supported basically by the fact that only this role was studied. Because of the fundamental equivalence of the different oscillators involved in the multioscillator system, however, reversed internal zeitgeber actions also must be expected (i.e., internal actions from the vegetative rhythms to the activity rhythm). It must be the subject of future investigations to look for these interactions. The essential difficulty in the study of internal zeitgeber effects under the remaining influence of external zeitgebers is to differentiate whether an observed effect originates from the internal or external zeitgeber. To elude this difficulty, the internal zeitgeber either must be ceased or changed drastically in one of its parameters.

To analyze the controlling role of the sleep-wake cycle over the other rhythms, a preliminary possibility is given by experiments with sleep deprivation (Halberg et al. 1961). These experiments have been performed frequently, with varying numbers of successive nights without sleep. They all generally agree with the result that the overt rhythms persist, although with partially diminished amplitudes. As an example, figure 110 shows summarized results of a series of experiments with two successive nights of sleep deprivation. The temporal courses of a physiological and a psychological variable are presented, each averaged from 12 subjects. As can be seen in figure 110/I, the diminishing in the amplitude of the rectal temperature rhythm is due to an increase of the minimum values, while the maximum values nearly remain unchanged. Correspondingly, also in the psychomotor performance (i.e., computation speed), the minimum values are higher during the nights without sleep than during those with sleep,

during which the subjects were awakened for the tests. This result, at least for the first day of sleep deprivation, means that the average performance is higher with sleep deprivation than on days with normal sleep. This apparently paradoxical result is due to the especially low performance after awakenings. The subjective scoring of the performance level decreases considerably with the sleep deprivation and, therefore, is in contradiction to the objective measurement (Ringer, 1972).

A closer inspection of the temporal courses of the different rhythms during sleep deprivation shows a clear delay of the phases (Ringer, 1972). Especially, the phases of the minimum values of all rhythms measured are delayed in comparison to the normal days. This result, which coincides with other experimental series with only 1 night (Aschoff et al., 1972), or even 3 successive nights without sleep (Levi, 1966; Fröberg et al., 1972), is more obvious in figure 110/II. It could be argued that this phase delay is a beginning of a free run. This however, can never be confirmed clearly because sleep deprivation cannot be continued for intervals long enough to prove sufficiently the autonomy of a rhythm. It was shown in other experiments that the vegetative rhythms can remain synchronized to normal zeitgebers, independent of the activity rhythm, over a longer period of time (Fig. 81). It, therefore, is more likely that the phase delay during sleep deprivation announces a changed steady state phase position to the zeitgeber. This would mean that the normal phase position of the vegetative rhythms is determined not only by the external zeitgeber, but also the internal 'sleep-wake zeitgeber'. In fact, the phase position which becomes changed by sleep deprivation can be considered as a consequence of the oscillatory properties just derived. The oscillator which dominantly controls the activity rhythm is the weakest and, therefore, is the oscillator most strongly affected by the external zeitgeber. Because the period of the natural zeitgeber always is shorter than the autonomous period of all oscillators, this os-

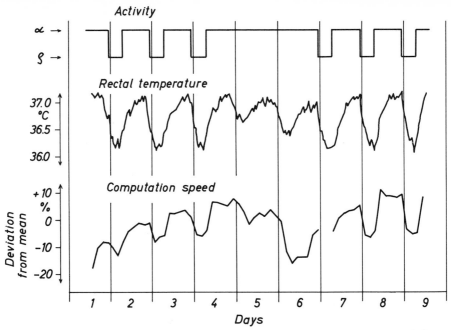

Figure 110. Influence of sleep deprivation on circadian rhythms. Results averaged from twelve subjects, in groups of three, living in standardized conditions under the influence of a strict 24.0-hours routine performed by continuous contacts with an experimenter and, in between, two successive nights without sleep. In the night following the sleep deprivation, the subjects were not awakened for the tests, as was done in the other nights. *I.* Longitudinally presented courses of activity (i.e., alternation between wakefulness α and rest ρ), rectal temperature (measured continuously), and computation speed (i.e., Pauli-test, measured at regular 3.0-hour intervals) averaged from the twelve subjects.

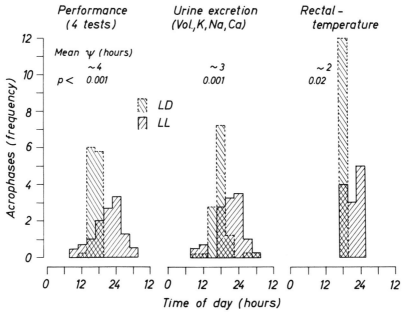

Figure 110/II. Frequency distributions for times of day of mean acrophases, averaged from the rhythms of four different performance tests (left diagram), urine volume and three different urine constituents (middle diagram), and rectal temperature (right diagram) Presented are results from the twelve subjects, averaged from 2 successive days with sleep deprivation and 4 days with sleep (i.e., 2 successive days before and 2 successive days after sleep deprivation). $\Delta\psi$: differences in the temporal positions of the acrophases measured with and without sleep. The statistical significances of the deviations of these differences, from zero, are indicated. Data from Ringer (1972).

cillator necessarily has an earlier phase position relative to the zeitgeber than any other. Because of the mutual coupling between the different oscillators, this early phase position assists in advancing the phase positions of the other oscillators. If the activity oscillator is idle, because of sleep deprivation, this assistance ceases and, therefore, the other oscillators, which are no longer controlled by the activity rhythm as an additional (internal) zeitgeber, necessarily delay their phases with regard to the external zeitgeber.

Another possibile study of effects of internal activity zeitgebers is to search for situations where these zeitgebers conflict with the common external zeitgeber, with respect to the phase. This situation is shift work. Shift workers must shift their activity-rest cycles according to the working schedule, but they remain in social contacts with their unshifted environment. With regard to vegetative rhythms, therefore, the internal sleep-wake zeitgeber does not coincide in its timing with the external social zeitgeber during night shifts as it does during day shifts. Regarding this aspect of conflicting zeitgebers, it must be expected that the phase position of the vegetative rhythms and, therefore, the internal phase relationship between the activity rhythm and the vegetative rhythms, depends on the strength of social contacts. Industrial shift workers, who mostly live with their families and interrupt the shift work during the weekends, have normal contacts which were shown to exert stronger zeitgeber effects than the internal activity zeitgeber. In these shift workers, the phase position of the vegetative rhythms should be determined predominantly by the external social zeitgebers and, therefore, should show normal phase positions nearly being equal in day and night workers, in spite of the reversed living routine in the night workers. Additionally, it must be considered that rectal temperature is higher during activity than rest, reactively (see below). For this reason, unequal amplitudes of rectal temperature, but similar phases (with diminished amplitudes in the night workers) must be expected in day and night workers. In

fact, exactly this situation often was observed (Benedict and Snell, 1902; Benedict, 1904; v.Loon, 1963; Colquhoun et al., 1968, 1969), indicating a predominant zeitgeber effect of the external social contacts, in comparison to the internal zeitgeber action of the shifted activity rhythm. There are some investigations with night nurses, who mostly have limited social contacts with the environment and also continue the night shift during the weekends. In those shift workers, predominance of the internal zeitgeber effect, and, therefore, a reversal of the vegetative rhythms, could be expected rather than in the industrial workers. In night nurses, a nearly complete reversal of the vegetative rhythms, in comparison to their normal phase positions, sometimes were observed (Høyer, 1944; Toulouse et Pieron, 1907). Similar observations were made in mine workers living with strictly limited social contacts in the arctic (Lobban, 1965a). The concept of conflicting interaction between internal and external zeitgebers, therefore, seems to apply to shift work.

A final situation, where this conflict may play a role, is the simulation of transmeridian flights. In experiments with "simulated flights," as discussed earlier (cf. 3.1.2), subjects were not informed about the purpose and schedule of the experiments and they did not perceive the zeitgeber shifts. The circadian system of the subjects, in those experiments, behaved similarly to real flight experiments. It may be argued that, in the real flight experiments, the passengers are very well informed concerning the phase shift of the zeitgeber and, for this reason, simulated and real flights are not comparable regarding the resulting phase shift. Other investigators, therefore, performed simulation experiments where full information was given the subjects concerning the instant and amount of the phase shift (Elliott et al., 1971b, 1972; McCally et al., 1973). These simulation experiments should fit better with the real flight experiments than the other type of simulation experiments; however, there is a handicap with this second type. In the first type, without information, the subjects are convinced they live in temporal coincidence with their environment after as well as before the shift, even when they have no direct contacts to this environment. They, therefore, imagine they are in contact with the environment, although the subjective impression is objectively wrong. In the second type of simulation experiments, with full information, the subjects know that they live, after the shift, temporally in disagreement with their environment, without absolute security that this knowledge is correct. In both types of experiments, the activity rhythms of the subjects adjust immediately to the shifted zeitgeber. In the first type, therefore, there exists a coincidence between the zeitgeber effects of the activity rhythm and the imaged social contacts. In the second type, however, there is no coincidence and, therefore, a conflict between the internal and the imaged external zeitgeber. As a result, the resynchronization must be expected to be faster in the first than in the second type of simulation experiments.

In simulation experiments of the first type, without information, total resynchronization, in fact, was observed in each subject and with each single overt rhythm. The rate of resynchronization (Fig. 75) is similar to that in real flight experiments (Aschoff et al., 1975), indicating the strength of the applied artificial zeitgeber is similar to the strength of the natural zeitgeber. In simulation experiments of the second type, with full information, resynchronization is often irregular and sometimes even incomplete (McCally et al., 1973). On the average of those cases where full resynchronization occurred in the experiments with full information, the rate of resynchronization seems to be smaller than in real flight experiments (Elliott et al., 1972). The agreement in the knowledge concerning the fact of the zeitgeber shift, therefore, seems to be insignificant in comparison to the agreement in the knowledge concerning the temporal coincidence with the environment, even if this coincidence only is based on imagination. It, therefore, must be concluded that the second type of simulation experiments, where the subjects know they

live in temporal disagreement with their environment, simulates shift work rather than a time shift after long distance flights.

4.3.2. Reactive Interactions

From the oscillatory interaction between different rhythms discussed so far, another type of mutual interaction must be discriminated; that being the direct interaction between different variables affecting each other reactively (i.e., 'masking effect'). This reactive interaction essentially is different from the oscillatory interaction, where the controlling oscillators mutually interact. As an example, muscular exercise raises the actual body temperature, independent, or even better being nearly independent, of the phase of the running temperature rhythm (cf. Fig. 30/II). Conversely, an increase in body temperature reactively can force an increase in physical activity, especially in psychomotor performance. A special type of masking effect seems to be the low value in psychomotor performance after awakening from sleep, which again is nearly independent of the phase of the performance rhythm (Rutenfranz et al., 1972; Wever, 1972c). In general some variables interact mutually, additionally to the oscillatory interaction between the respective rhythms, in a manner that changes in one variable affects reactively proportional changes in the other variable, which nearly superimpose additively to the common rhythmic course of this variable.

With sleep deprivation, the phases of all overt rhythms shift generally to later phases, in comparison to the control phase positions during night sleep (Fig. 110). These phase delays were described on the basis of an oscillatory interaction between the rhythms and the activity cycle. At least with regard to some of the rhythms, these phase delays, however, also can be understood as mere consequences of a masking effect. This explanation is based on the fact that, in the 24-hour day, the body temperature rhythm and performance rhythms generally lag behind the activity rhythm (Fig. 17). The masking effect, during the night sleep, must decrease the rectal temperature to a certain amount. Since this additive decrease, on the average, is earlier than the minimum value of rectal temperature, when measured without sleep, it must simulate an advance of the rectal temperature rhythm. The resulting phase of the rectal temperature rhythm, measured with regard to the activity rhythm or local time, therefore, must be earlier with sleep than without sleep, due to only the masking effect. The same consideration is true with regard to the performance rhythms. Performances also were shown to be affected reactively from activity and, especially, from sleep (see above). The phase delay of the performance rhythm during sleep deprivation, therefore, also can be understood merely on the basis of the masking effect.

As the general result, the change in the phase positions of the rhythms of rectal temperature and psychomotor performances, with regard to local time during sleep deprivation in the 24-hour day, can be understood on the basis of direct masking effects and an oscillatory interaction. Since both kinds of mutual interaction between different rhythms must be present, as shown independently in other experiments, both of these types of interaction necessarily participate simultaneously in the internal phase shifts observed during sleep deprivation. The portions where they participate cannot be derived from the presently available results. Because of the practical importance of this problem, the evaluation of the portions mentioned must be subjected to further investigations.

During shift work, the masking effect is of special importance because there exists a constant conflict between the external zeitgeber, which remains unshifted, and the forced activity-rest cycle, which is shifted. This becomes obvious with figure 111 (upper diagram), which presents long term averages of body temperature originating from three subjects, being inexperienced in shift work, working 13 weeks on a night shift with the normal day shift occurring before and after

the night shift. (v. Loon, 1963). At first glance, there is a shift between the two groups of temperature curves. Considering the acrophases of the fundamental periods, the amount of this shift, on the average, is about 5 hours. This may indicate an incomplete adaptation to the sleep time, which is shifted for 8 hours. The amplitudes of the fundamental periods additionally are reduced during night shift, on the average, to only half the value measured during day shift. With a closer inspection of the curves, the difference between the two groups is coordinated strongly to the sleep time, according to the two different schedules. During the sleep of the subjects, body temperature generally is reduced. This is obvious especially during the night shift, where the subjects went to sleep only in the morning, after the body temperature started to increase. The idea of a masking effect of the sleep is suggested here.

In the lower diagram of figure 111, with the same measurements, the hypothetical masking effect was omitted by calculation. For this reason, it is accepted that sleep generally reduces body temperature by about 0.4°C (Fig. 110). Reductions by other amounts (e.g., 0.2 and 0.6°C) essentially do not change the conclusions. Measurements taken during the sleep time, as indicated at the upper border, therefore, are raised arbitrarily for 0.4°C (the day shift values at 7:30, which are taken 0.5 hours after termination of sleep, are raised for 0.2°C). The resulting body temperature curves, purified artificially from the masking by sleep, are presented in the lower diagram of figure 111. The two groups of temperature curves now do not deviate systematically from each other. From the computed fundamental periods, neither the acrophases nor the amplitudes show significant differences. The deviations in the courses of the body temperature rhythms during day and night shift, in this special case, can be stated as merely being simulated by a well-known masking effect.

The result derived from figure 111, of course, can not be generalized to the statement that, with shift work, a true oscillatory

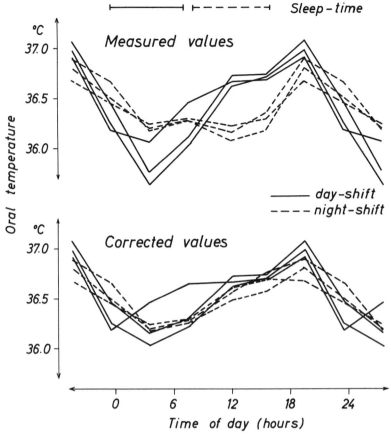

Figure 111. Influence of shift work on body temperature rhythms. Results from three subjects, inexperienced in shift work, working for 13 weeks continuously on a night shift and, before and after, on a day shift. The sleep times, during the respective shifts, are indicated. Presented are courses of body temperature of the three subjects, averaged over many weeks. Upper diagram: Measured values of body temperature. Lower diagram: Values arbitrarily "corrected" by eliminating the hypothetical masking effect of sleep on body temperature. All values taken during sleep time are raised for 0.4 °C. The day shift values at 7:30 which were taken shortly after termination of sleep, are raised for 0.2°C. Measured data from v.Loon (1963).

adaptation of the vegetative rhythms to the shifted work-rest cycle is never possible, but only a simulation of such an adaptation by masking effects. Because a true oscillatory zeitgeber effect of the activity rhythm on other rhythms was shown under other conditions, a more or less complete adaptation thoroughly is possible in shift work. The presentation of the special example at figure 111 should give only a suggestion that masking effects may simulate, in some cases, a

phase shift of vegetative rhythms following a forced phase shift of the activity rhythm. In other words, an observed internal phase shift must not be based necessarily on only a change in the circadian system, but may be based on simulation by a reactive masking effect. This consideration also may be true in cases of time shift experiments, when the resynchronization seems to be incomplete. Especially in experiments where full information is given the subjects (see above), it must be considered carefully to what amount the masking effect simulates the results.

4.3.3. Separation of the Interactions

It is the general result of considerations previously discussed that different rhythms can interact mutually at two different levels, with an oscillatory interaction and a direct, or "masking", interaction. The first type of interaction is effective between controlling oscillators, which influence each other mutually, like an external zeitgeber influences an oscillator. In special cases, there may be an "internal zeitgeber effect" of an overt rhythm on a controlling oscillator. The second type of interaction is effective directly between overt rhythms or variables which influence each other reactively. Not only for practical purposes, but also to understand the properties of the circadian system theoretically, a discrimination between both types of interaction is desirable. For instance, the phase setting role of the activity rhythm on other rhythms, as often stated (see above), indeed, easily can be understood on the basis of a masking effect. It, however, is an interesting question whether or not the activity rhythm also plays a dominant role in the oscillatory interaction, especially after considering it was shown to be controlled by a rather weak oscillator (cf. 4.2.3).

A discrimination between the two types of internal interaction, as discussed, is possible by considering the temporal relations. First, while, with oscillatory interaction, a steady state only can be reached after transients of shorter or longer duration have faded, the steady state is reached immediately with the masking effect. Second, while an effective interaction, with oscillatory interaction, only is possible within a limited range of periods, it is independent of the periods with the masking effect. Finally, a mutual interaction by the masking effect

only can result in parallelity of the rhythm or in equal phases, while any internal phase relationship is possible with the oscillatory interaction. The application of the criteria discussed leads to the result that, in most cases, the masking effect, although present, plays a minor role in comparison with the oscillatory interaction. This becomes clear when the interaction between the rhythms of activity and rectal temperature is considered following a rhythm disarrangement. As can be seen, especially in phase shift experiments (cf. 3.1.2), mutual synchronization between the two rhythms is reached only in the course of several days (i.e., after transients have faded). This can be derived from the differences in the resynchronization rate of the different rhythms (Fig. 75). The possible occurrence of internal desynchronization, either spontaneously (cf. 2.2.1) or forced (cf. 3.3), shows that the two rhythms interact mutually only as long as the periods are close enough together (i.e., only within a limited range of periods). With the transition between synchronized and free running rhythms (Fig. 17) and in experiments with an artificial zeitgeber of varying period (Fig. 72), the internal phase relationship between the two rhythms varies systematically and only results in exact parallelity of the rhythms under exceptional conditions. In summary, all criteria, independent of each other, show that the oscillatory interaction preponderates the reactive interaction, even when the action from the activity rhythm, to the other rhythms, is considered.

A direct separation of the two types of internal interaction between the different rhythms (i.e., oscillatory and reactive) is possible during internal desynchronization of the rhythms. During this state, the oscillatory interaction is ceased because the periods of the different overt rhythms are outside the mutual ranges of entrainment. Only the small remaining interaction, due to relative coordination, can be effective during this state. The reactive interaction, however, is fully present during internal desynchronization because it, by no means, is

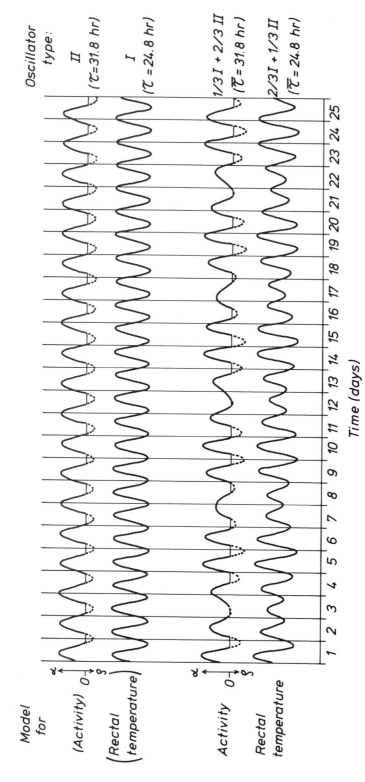

Figure 112. Demonstration of beat phenomena produced by linear superposition of two sine waves (independent of the mechanism of generating the sine waves). *I.* Longitudinal presentation of the two basic sine waves (above) and two different types of mutual linear superposition with different weights (below). The courses of the basic "type II" wave and the representation of the "activity rhythm" is arbitrarily divided by a threshold into "activity" (α; above the threshold) and "rest" (ρ; below the threshold).

Time (hours)

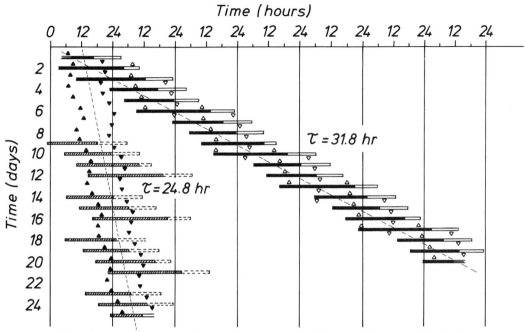

Figure 112/II. Successive presentation of the two superposition models derived in I, in correspondence to the preferred manner of presenting experimental data (cf. Figure 16/I). Bars: representations of the "activity rhythm" (black: sections where the rhythm courses above the threshold; white: sections where the rhythm courses below the threshold); shaded bars: temporally correct redrawings of corresponding full bars. Triangles: representations of the "rectal temperature rhythm", indicating the temporal positions of maximum (▲) and minimum values (▼); empty triangles: temporally correct redrawings of corresponding full triangles. Abscissa: "local time"; ordinate: sequence of successive cycles.

restricted to any relationship of the periods. This means that the reactive interaction cannot be ceased in any way, and the oscillatory interaction can be ceased only when the different rhythms have periods deviating sufficiently from each other. Internal desynchronization, therefore, is the only condition where one of the two types of internal interaction between different rhythms can be measured separately.

Before separating the two types of mutual interaction in internally desynchronized rhythms, it must be considered to what degree the different rhythms interact mutually at all. On the one hand, the scalloping patterns which are obvious in many experiments seem to indicate these interactions; on the other hand, it had been mentioned that beat phenomena, which are independent of any active interaction, contribute to the observed patterns. In order to under-

stand the meaning of beats, it may be helpful to insert a simple theoretical consideration dealing with linear superpositions of sine waves, i.e., excluding any active interaction between the waves. Figure 112/I shows the procedure of superposition. The upper two diagrams should give sine wave representations of the two basic oscillators involved in the system, type I, and type II, with periods corresponding to the averages of many experimental results. The course of the type II oscillator which dominantly represents the "activity-rest cycle," is arbitrarily divided by a threshold into "activity" (α) and "rest" (ρ), according to a "threshold-level model" of activity given earlier (Wever, 1960, 1962). The lower two diagrams should give the results of the superposition procedure; they are simply calculated by adding the two upper sine waves but with differents weights which again are averages of many experimental results. The representation of the "activity-rest rhythm" includes type I with only 50% of the amplitude of type II; its course again is arbitrarily divided by a threshold separating activity (α) and rest (ρ). The representation of the "rectal temperature rhythm" includes, reversely, type II with only half the amplitude of type I; its course demonstrates the regular fluctuations in the amplitude as observed in many human experiments (see Figs. 25/I and 87/I).

Figure 112/II presents the data derived from Figure 112/I in the same manner as experimental data are frequently presented. In the bars, "activity" means sections out of the "activity rhythm" representation of Figure 112/I where this rhythm runs above the threshold, and "rest" means sections below the threshold. The triangles are derived from the "rectal temperature" representation of Figure 112/I as the temporal positions of the extremum values. Figure 112/II demonstrates that, in addition to the amplitude, also the phases of the rhythms undergo regular fluctuations as a consequence of beat phenomena. Both rhythms show clearly scalloping patterns which are similar to many experimentally observed courses of internally desynchronized rhythms (cf. 2.2.1). As it is especially obvious in the redrawings of activity, the mutual phase relationship between the two rhythms seems to indicate mutual interaction; during those cycles where this phase relationship is "normal," an apparent mutual coupling seems to try to hold this phase relationship for some cycles, while the mutual phase relationship changes much faster during cycles where it is "wrong." Of course, in this drawing the mutual relative coordination is only simulated by beat phenomena; by definition, there cannot be any coupling or active mutual interaction between the two rhythms, neither oscillatory nor masking. This formal demonstration of beats should prevent the reader from the general conclusion to mutual interaction in the interpretation of frequently observed phenomena; the scalloping patterns of the rhythms, or the appearance of mutual relative coordination, may be due, also in human circadian rhythms, mainly to

beat phenomena which are independent of any interaction. This demonstration should, however, not deny the presence of mutual interaction; both, oscillatory interaction as well as masking are present in any case of internally desynchronized rhythms, but the contribution of these interactions to the obvious phenomena must not be of great importance.

In considering experiments with internal desynchronization, spontaneously occuring cases will be considered in the first step (cf. 2.2.1). As can be seen in Figures 12/I, 25/I, and especially 30/II, sleep sections can shift over the rectal temperature rhythm more or less continuously, with the result that sleep occurs every day at another phase of the rectal temperature rhythm. In all cases, however, the direct masking influence of sleep on rectal temperature is small compared to the amplitude of circadian rhythmicity in rectal temperature. A more systematic consideration of internal desynchronization is possible in experiments where this state is forced by a strong zeitgeber operating outside the range of entrainment of the physiological rhythms (cf. 3.3). For a closer inspection, see figure 87; in the experiment underlying this figure, the subject, after an initial base line section, lived steadily in an artificial 28-hour day. In this experiment, forced internal desynchronization occurred, which, in this context, must be preferred to internal desynchronization occuring spontaneously under constant conditions, because of the more definite conditions. In the experimental section of this experiment, the alternation between wakefulness and sleep, in fact, followed the artificial zeitgeber though with considerable variations. In all other variables measured, only a small secondary rhythm component was present, showing the zeitgeber period. Only in this small component, 'masking', due to activity, could contribute. The consideration of the internal phase relations, however, shows masking cannot be involved to a relevant amount. Figure 87/III clearly shows the 'morning increase' in rectal temperature is terminated at "lights-on" with this rhythm component when activity is only beginning, and the rectal temperature shows a more or less constant plateau during and after activity onset. The "evening decrease" in rectal temperature again is clearly earlier than the end of activity. Not only a reactive effect of the alternation between wakefulness and sleep on rectal temperature is missed, but also on cortisol excretion. The 28.0-hour component of this rhythm, which, indeed, is not reliable, shows an unusual phase relationship to the activity rhythm, and also to the rectal temperature rhythm. The only recognizable masking effect is the remarkable depression of performance at 'midnight' when the subject always had to be awakened for this measurement. It already was mentioned (cf. 3.3.1) that only this 'midnight value' constitutes a rhythmicity. It now can be concluded that this rhythm component, which, indeed, is reliable, is based on only the masking effect. The same performance data, however, show a rhythmic component with the typical free running period of 24.8 hours, with a larger amplitude and a higher reliability, although this component cannot be masked in any way by the alternation between wakefulness and sleep.

The result of this experiment is confirmed by results of several more experiments of this same type. In no case is the rectal temperature masked by the activity rhythm to a relevant amount. At best, performance is masked partly by sleep. It seems characteristic, however, that in those cases where the dominant component of performance rhythms runs synchronously to the activity rhythm (e.g., 3rd sect, Fig. 86; 3rd sect, Fig. 88; 2nd sect, Fig. 89), the inspection of the averaged course of the performance rhythm contradicts a substantial contribution of a "sleep masking," but also shows rhythmicities that are based on the regular 'day values' (Fig. 86/III). A mutual masking effect, between different vegetative rhythms or physiological and performance rhythms, also cannot be great. The amount of this masking should be independent of the experimental conditions. It, therefore, is not compatible with the masking concept when the performance rhythm, in one experimental condition, runs parallel to rectal temperature but, in another experimental condition, does not during the same experiment (Figs. 86, 88, and 92).

In experiments with forced internal desynchronization discussed so far, in addition to the alternation between wakefulness and sleep, the light-dark cycle was shown to not exert a phase setting effect. In spite of the cooperation of both of these cycles during forced internal desynchronization, they do not have the capacity to entrain other rhythms to a period, for instance, of 28.0 hours. This is true regarding the rectal temperature rhythm, and also to the cortisol rhythm, which was postulated as being controlled especially close to light as an external stimulus and near activity as an internal stimulus. The interaction between the activity rhythm and the other rhythms, which was shown to be effective when the periods are closer together, therefore, is missed in these experiments, even when the influence of the activity rhythm is supported by an external zeitgeber. This gives clear evidence that the interaction mainly is based on an oscillatory effect and not a masking effect, since only the 'internal zeitgeber effect' can be absent outside a limited range of entrainment, as is the effect of external zeitgebers.

Not only in experiments with forced internal desynchronization can a substantial contribution of masking on the mutual interaction between different overt rhythms be excluded, but also when this state occurs spontaneously under constant conditions. It was shown earlier (cf. 2.2.1) that the internal phase relationship between the rhythms of activity and rectal temperature coincide in internally synchronized rhythms and all different rhythm components of internally desynchronized rhythms. This also means that, in the component where the activity is dominant, the rectal temperature rhythm leads the activity rhythm. It can be seen in the averaged courses of the respective rhythm component (Fig. 27/III), that rectal temperature increases before activity onset and decreases before termination of activity. This result again is not compatible with masking, but only with an oscillatory interaction between the different rhythms.

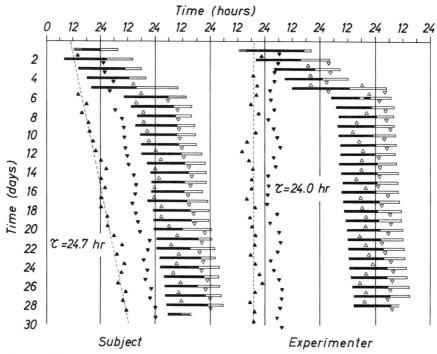

Figure 113.   Autonomous rhythm of a subject (D.M., ♀ 28 y) living under constant conditions without environmental time cues (left diagram) and the rhythm of the experimenter (J.Z., ♂ 29 y) who had to watch during the sleep of the subject, for the complex sleep recording (right diagram). Temporal courses of the rhythms of activity and rectal temperature are presented successively, one period beneath the other. Indications are the same as in figure 27/I.

It is the general result of the experiments discussed in this chapter, that the influence of the activity rhythm on other rhythms is rather weak. This is especially obvious when the "internal activity zeitgeber" conflicts with an external zeitgeber. Such an occasional zeitgeber conflict was observed in an experiment designed for another purpose (Fig. 113). In this experiment, the interaction between the circadian rhythm and the faster rhythm in sleeping behavior with a period of about 90 minutes, should be investigated under constant conditions (Schulz et al., 1975, 1976; Zulley, 1976). This task necessitated the continuous recording of the subject's EEG during sleep time. Because of the complexity of the recording equipment, it necessitated the continuous observation of an experimenter during this time. The experimenter was outside the experimental room and without direct contact with the subject. During the experiment, the subject showed a

normal circadian rhythm, with internal dissociation at the beginning, but with synchronously running rhythms in the steady state with a period of 24.7 hours (Fig. 113, left). In the context to be discussed here, however, the rhythm of the experimenter is of greater interest than that of the subject. Because of the desired task, the experimenter's rest time was restricted to the subject's activity time, when the EEG recording was not running. The experimenter's activity rhythm, therefore, was controlled in its period by that of the subject, in spite of the fact that the experimenter was continuously informed about objective time and deviation of his activity rhythm from the 24-hour day (Fig. 113, right). As a consequence, the other rhythms of the experimenter, which were measured as those of the subject, stood under the conflicting influence of the external (i.e., social) zeitgeber, with a period of 24.0 hours, and of the internal (i.e., activity) zeitgeber, with a period close to 24.7 hours. Figure 113 shows, in the subject, that the rhythm of rectal temperature, and other rhythms measured, ran synchronously to the activity rhythm, but this was not the case for the experimenter. While the rectal temperature rhythm of the subject had a period of 24.7 hours, coinciding with the activity rhythm, the rectal temperature rhythm of the experimenter had a period of 24.0 hours, in spite of his activity rhythm having a period similar to that of the subject (i.e., clearly deviating from 24.0 hours). This means that the rhythms of the subject ran synchronized internally, except for the first several days when they showed internal dissociation. This further means that the rhythms of the experimenter ran desynchronized internally, with an activity rhythm being forced by the subject's rhythm and a rectal temperature rhythm being synchronized to local time. From the two conflicting zeitgebers effecting the vegetative rhythms, the external (i.e., social) predominated the internal zeitgeber (i.e., activity rhythm). As the result, the zeitgeber strength of the activity rhythm on the other rhythms must be concluded to be weak in comparison to the strength of external social zeitgebers.

There are many experiments testing the influence of the activity rhythm on other rhythms, with the activity period fixed experimentally. They all show only a small effect. There are no experiments with fixed rectal temperature rhythms testing the influence of this rhythm on the activity rhythm directly, although the result of those experiments would be of great interest. A much greater effect must be expected, according to the greater strength of the 'rectal temperature oscillator'. The importance of this effect can be deduced only indirectly. A first reference to the 'internal zeitgeber effect' of the rectal temperature rhythm comes from the inspection of the multimodal distribution of autonomous activity periods obtained under constant conditions (Fig. 37). It was shown that the theoretical synthesis of this distribution results in the assumption of a range of entrainment where the activity rhythms are

synchronized to the, more or less, fixed rectal temperature rhythms of not less than ± 4 to 5 hours (Fig. 109). This indicates a remarkable strength of the 'internal zeitgeber' involved. A second reference comes from the inspection of rhythms under the influence of an artificial zeitgeber of a varying period (cf. 3.1.1). From the change in the external phase relationship between the zeitgeber and activity rhythm, a range of entrainment of about 15 hours must be concluded. In the experiments, however, this range is not larger than ± 2 hours (i.e., not exceeding the range of entrainment of the rectal temperature rhythm), except in a few rare cases resulting in forced internal desynchronization (Fig. 71). It is the necessary conclusion that, outside this much smaller range, the 'internal zeitgeber effect' of the rectal temperature rhythm normally predominates the effect of the external zeitgeber. Consequently, these experiments also indicate indirectly a remarkable strength of the "internal rectal temperature zeitgeber."

In summary, different oscillators involved in the human circadian multioscillator system are coupled mutually in a manner that corresponds to the interaction between an external zeitgeber and a circadian oscillator. It, therefore, can be termed a mutual internal zeitgeber effect. Because of the self-sustainment capacity of each single oscillator (cf. 4.2.3), the mutual interaction only is effective within limited ranges of entrainment. Inside these ranges, a steady state in the mutual phase relationship between different oscillators only is reached after transients have faded. Additionally, different overt rhythms interact mutually in a manner corresponding to a direct reaction of a change in one variable to another. This internal masking effect is independent of the periods and superimposes the rhythm nearly additively. Both types of mutual interaction can be understood as mere consequences of simple oscillation laws (Wever, 1964b). As the general result of many different experiments, the oscillatory interaction or the "internal zeitgeber effect" predominates the masking effect in most cases.

5

Conclusions and Speculations

From the results of human isolation experiments discussed in this book, several conclusions can be drawn. These conclusions concern the structure of the human circadian multioscillator system (its "Wirkungsgefüge''; v. Holst, 1939b; Mittelstaedt, 1954; i.e., the cybernetic analysis of this system) and may be helpful in preparing the ground for an analysis of the concrete mechanisms underlying circadian rhythmicity. These conclusions also concern practical implications of the special properties of human circadian rhythms. It was the primary aim of this book to derive basic features of the circadian system. The main emphasis, therefore, was placed on the theoretical aspects. The practical aspects which must be founded on a solid theoretical analysis, however, cannot be ignored and must be touched on in a concluding section. Furthermore, the theoretical and practical considerations are tempting for entering speculations beyond established facts.

Before going into details, it again must be emphasized that all experiments discussed in this book were performed with volunteers. It is evident this selection of subjects limits the validity of generally applicable and quantitative statements derivable from the results of these experiments. Most experiments, therefore, are designed in such a manner that the expected results can be validated qualitatively, and not only quantitatively. As an example, the statement that the human circadian system has the capacity to desynchronize internally is very likely to be generalized, although it is based on experiments with volunteers. Even statements like internal desynchronization occurs more frequently under self-controlled than constant illumination, and more frequently in older than younger subjects can certainly be generalized. Results concerning the fraction of subjects showing internal desynchronization under a certain condition, however, can by no means be generalized. The percentage of these subjects depends on the very special population of subjects (e.g., age distribution) and experimental conditions, which partly cannot be quantified, or even described, in detail (e.g., the special 'atmosphere' of the experiments). The same, of course, is true regarding all other quantitative statements, such as, for instance, the responsiveness to a specified zeitgeber (e.g., as a critical case, the percentage of subjects being synchronized to the natural 24-hour day in spite of the extensive isolation) or the amount of changes in the autonomous period, or other parameters, under the influence of a specified external stimulus.

5.1. Theoretical Aspects

The knowledge gained, with regard to the structure of the human circadian system, is summarized in figure 114. The environment, with equal strengths, affects all different oscillators or pacemakers separately, either by periodically operating stimuli forcing the oscillators as external zeitgebers, or by continuously operating stimuli determining the parameters of autonomously running oscillators. Simultaneously, environmental stimuli directly affect some of the overt rhythms by reactive effects resulting in "masking." The different oscillators, furthermore, affect each other mutually by exerting "internal zeitgeber effects." A small number of oscillators control the multiplicity of overt rhythms in a manner where each of the oscillators controls each of the overt rhythms, or at least many overt rhythms, and each of the overt rhythms is controlled by all oscillators, or at least several oscillators, simultaneously. Only the proportions in the control by the different oscillators vary from variable to variable and with experimental conditions. Finally, some of the overt rhythms mutually interact in a direct manner, exerting "masking effects."

The control of the overt rhythms by several distinct oscillators instead of only one single oscillator, was suggested by that part of the subjects who spontaneously showed internal desynchronization (cf. 2.2.1). The multioscillator hypothesis, however, can be extended to all subjects because it was shown that internal desynchronization can be forced, under appropriate conditions, in every subject tested (cf. 3.3). It is due to the mutual internal zeitgeber action between the different oscillators that, in the majority of

subjects (i.e., in all those with internal synchronization), the separate autonomy of each oscillator cannot be observed; just as the action of external zeitgebers does not allow the observation of autonomy of the total circadian system.

In the scheme of figure 114, the controlling oscillators or pacemakers are only hypothetical because their outputs cannot be observed directly. The consistency in the rhythmic behavior of all different variables, however, compels the assumption that oscillators underlie the overt rhythms. Following this hypothesis, the experimental results discussed in this paper show that the different oscillators have equal properties, except with regard to the oscillatory strength. All properties of the oscillators, as deduced from the different experiments, are consequences of nothing more than the capacity of self-sustainment and of becoming excited separately by driving oscillations, both parametrically and nonparametrically (cf. 4.1; Wever, 1964b, 1965a, 1966b). The oscillators, therefore, obey simple oscillatory laws. These, in the language of mathematics, are characterized by two nonlinearities, the directions of which are determined by stability conditions. Exactly these nonlinearities seem relevant in other fields of living being also [e.g., in homeostasis (Wever, 1963b, 1966b)].

Between the basic oscillators and the overt rhythms, which are observable, coupling forces are interconnected which, on principle, may influence the relation between oscillator and overt rhythms. The only parameter of an overt rhythm, which clearly reflects the corresponding parameter of the underlying oscillator, is the period or frequency. All other parameters (e.g., amplitude or phase) may be affected, more or less, by the coupling forces and, therefore, these parameters can be different in the overt rhythms and the underlying oscillator. All analyses, however, show that systematic changes in the different parameters of overt rhythms, depending on changes in the external conditions, reflect equivalent changes in the corresponding parameters of the under-

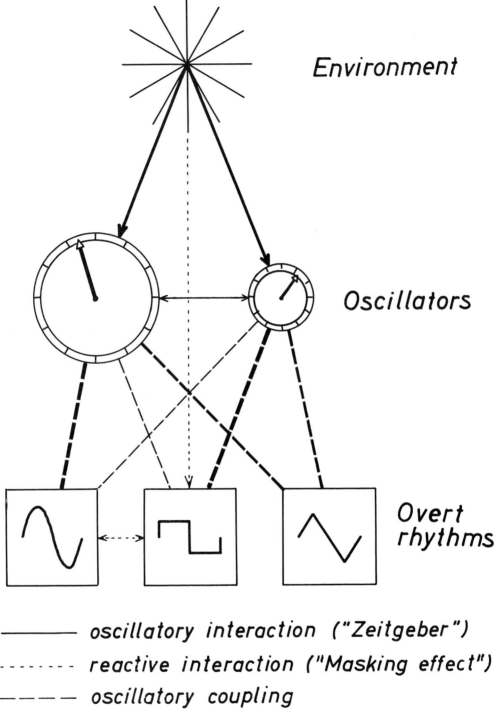

Environment

Oscillators

Overt
rhythms

———————— oscillatory interaction ("Zeitgeber")

- - - - - - - - reactive interaction ("Masking effect")

— — — — oscillatory coupling

Figure 114. Scheme of the interactions between environment, basic oscillators, and overt rhythms. The size of an oscillator represents its degree of persistence or oscillatory strength. The different symbols of the overt rhythms represent their different manifestations. Environmental stimuli operate on all different oscillators with equal strengths; moreover, they operate directly on a part of the overt rhythms. Each of the oscillators controls each of the overt rhythms. The thicknesses of the connection lines represent the strength of the respective coupling force. Between the different oscillators, there are oscillatory interactions, and between a part of the overt rhythms, there are reactive interactions. For clearness, only two different oscillators and three different overt rhythms are presented.

lying oscillators (cf. 4.1). Interdependencies between different rhythm parameters, (including the period), coincide with corresponding interdependencies between parameters of the oscillator. Statements about the coupling forces themselves, indeed, cannot be deduced from experimental analyses. All these analyses, however, show that the coupling forces remain unchanged with varying conditions. Therefore, it, indeed, is impossible to conclude from an observed parameter of an overt rhythm to the corresponding parameter of the basic oscillator, except the period. An observed change in any rhythm parameter, however, reflects a change of an equal amount in the corresponding parameter of the basic oscillator. This is true not only when an overt rhythm is controlled by one single oscillator, but also when controlled simultaneously by several oscillators.

The endogenous oscillators have the capacity to run autonomously. They also have the capacity to become modified by external stimuli. If those stimuli are operating continuously, they determine the parameters of the endogenously generated oscillations. The amount of this exogenous effect on rhythm parameters is the same in the different oscillators (cf. 4.2.3) as indicated in figure 114 by lines of equal gauge. If the external stimuli are operating periodically, they act as zeitgebers (i.e., entrain the oscillator as long as they operate with periods being within the range of entrainment). The relative zeitgeber strength of a distinct periodic stimulus is different in the different oscillators, in spite of the equal effects on the parameters of these oscillators. This difference is due to the different degrees of persistences of the different oscillators. The effectiveness of external stimuli, regarding the oscillators, is not restricted to one mode of the stimulus. There is a variety of stimuli having the capacity to affect the oscillators. Apart from light and temperature, there are subtle ones among the effective overt stimuli, (e.g., weak electric AC fields). The most effective stimuli, specifically in human circadian rhythms, were shown to be of social origin. There, therefore, cannot be a single receptor

of the oscillators sensitive against all these different stimuli. There must be one specific effect which is released by all the different environmental stimuli. In other words, the different external stimuli release an internal stimulus the mode of which is independent of the mode of the releasing condition and affects the circadian oscillator directly. It would be very attractive to assume that this exogenously released stimulus, directly affecting separate excitation, is of the same mode as the endogenous stimulus causing self-sustainment. Perhaps it is not too speculative to observe some support of this assumption in the effectiveness of weak electric AC fields (i.e., external electric stimuli similar to stimuli generated endogenously).

At present, nothing is known about the concrete basis of the oscillatory mechanism. We, however, know that every cell has the capacity to behave like a circadian oscillator. Unicellular organisms were shown to have circadian variations, with regard to metabolism and other variables (e.g., Brinkmann, 1965, 1971; Hastings, 1959; Hastings and Wilson, 1976). Isolated organs and cell cultures obtained from higher organisms, under adequate conditions, have the capacity to continue circadian rhythmicity (Andrews, 1968; Rintoul, 1975; Shiotsuka et al., 1974; Tharp and Folk, 1965). Within the cell, a most plausible hypothesis states membranes are substantial bases of the 'clock mechanism' (Njus et al., 1974, 1976). In a multicellular organism, normally the oscillators of all single cells synchronize mutually with each other. Although, on principle, all cells have virtually equivalent capacities within the network of mutually entraining oscillators, the mechanisms of these interactions prefer certain cells, in a manner that they predominate in the role of pacemakers with regard to other cells. The concept of billions of virtually autonomous oscillators located in the different cells, therefore, does not conflict with the concept of one or several master clocks, driving all cells synchronously. This primary oscillator would consist of a complex of cells functionally coordinated and spatially adjoined. Following this concept, it is reasonable to assume that the oscillatory strength of this primary oscillator is determined by the size of this complex or the number of cells constituting a primary oscillatory center. The different oscillators of the multioscillator system are represented by several of such centers that have different sizes according to the different oscillatory strengths.

The theoretical considerations need supplementation concerning the valuation of the different rhythm parameters. To here, it was determined that the period of an overt rhythm is the most important parameter. This preference was due to the fact that the period is the only parameter of an overt rhythm which clearly reflects the corresponding parameter of the underlying oscillator, without any influence of the coupling between the oscillator and overt rhythm; and also is the parameter that can be determined most precisely and where small changes can be detected most reliably. (Concerning the previous sentence, the second may be based on the first reason.) This preference, for practical reasons, by no means states that the period is the parameter that is controlled by the selective pressure for evolution. It also may be that changes in the period, following changes in the environmental conditions, are side effects which are unavoidable because of the nonlinear characteristics of self-sustained oscillations. Only necessary in the evolutionary sense is the general responsiveness of circadian rhythms to external stimulation; to enable entrainment to the natural alternation between day and night. The capability of external synchronization necessarily need not include any continuous action approach. Such an approach, which indicates parametric excitation, however, may support external synchronization.

From an evolutionary point of view, there would be no use in changing the autonomous period by changing continuously operating external stimuli (e.g., social contacts, electric AC fields, stress) since, under natural conditions, the actual period always is 24.0 hours (i.e., it always is synchronized to the natural day). The external phase relationship of the rhythm to the zeitgeber, which may be a relevant feature under natural conditions, however, is correlated to the autonomous period. Furthermore, parameters like mean value or amplitude, changes of which are correlated to changes of the autonomous period (cf. 4.1.1), also may be of importance under synchronized conditions. It, therefore, may be found that changes of those parameters, due to external stimulation, are the teleonomic goal in the development of mechanisms responding to continuously operating external stimuli. Correlated changes in the autonomous period, with this type of consideration, more or less are artifacts which are unavoidable, due to the nonlinear mechanisms, but which are ineffective totally while the organism is living under natural conditions; therefore, there is no need to eliminate these artifacts.

The amplitude of a rhythm is a parameter that deserves attention. Theoretically, it is the only parameter that clearly is correlated to the variability of a self-sustained oscillation (Wever, 1971b). The period also is correlated to the precision of a rhythm (Fig. 104). In organisms, with a range of autonomous periods being larger than in humans, this correlation, however, is bivalent, i.e., shows highest precision with a medium period and decreasing precision with both a shortening and lengthening period (Aschoff et al., 1971c). Furthermore, the amplitude is the parameter that is pertinent directly to the strength of an oscillator (i.e., the larger the amplitude, the more stable is the oscillator against external perturbations). Finally, the amplitude of a rhythm determines the strength of the coupling to other rhythms (cf. 4.2.1.). The amplitude of a rhythm, therefore, is an indicator for the tendency of the rhythm toward the spontaneous occurrence of internal desynchronization (i.e., the larger the amplitude the smaller this tendency).

From the correlations discussed, that between amplitude and oscillatory strength was tested directly. The duration of reentrainment of a rhythm, after a certain phase shift of a definite entraining zeitgeber, is an indicator of the oscillatory strength (Aschoff et al., 1975; Hoffmann, 1969; Wever, 1966a). This duration was shown to be correlated to the rhythm's amplitude before the shift (Fig. 76). In this case, it is clear that the oscillatory strength is correlated directly to the amplitude, and not indirectly by the correlation between amplitude and period (Fig. 103). After phase shifts in opposite directions, the durations of reentrainment are correlated to the amplitudes with equal regressions. The correlations to the periods, however, must be expected to pass with opposite regressions (Wever, 1966a). The correlation between the tendency toward internal desynchronization and amplitude presently has been confirmed only indirectly. All changes in the experimental conditions, which increase the tendency toward internal desynchronization, also increase the period (cf. 2.4.), and increases in the period always are accompanied by decreases in the amplitude (Fig. 105). The amplitude of a circadian rhythm, therefore, takes a key position in the stability of these rhythms, both inter- and intraindividually, and this stability is greater the larger the amplitude.

If an external stimulus has any effect on the period of autonomously running rhythms, the amount of this effect depends on the initial period. This was shown directly with self-controlled ambient temperature (cf. 2.4.3) and an artificial electric AC-field (cf. 2.4.5) as the stimuli and, indirectly, by the correlation between mean period and interindividual standard deviation, with any stimuli that are effective (cf. 2.4.9). The linear extrapolation of this correlation to periods shorter than those actually observed would lead to effects of these stimuli being opposite to those actually observed. Applying the interdependency between period and amplitude of self-sustained oscillations, as postulated theoretically (Wever, 1964, 1965a, 1966b) and confirmed experimentally in several different respects (see above), the effects of external stimuli also should be correlated in their amounts to the initial amplitude, but unidirectionally within the total range. Depending on its mode, a definite

stimulus should change the amplitude in a direction which is independent of the initial amplitude, but to an amount that is the greater the smaller the amplitude. This means that a definite stimulus always drives an autonomous rhythm into an 'optimum' state, where its amplitude and precision is largest, independent of the initial state of the rhythm. The period of this rhythm then would always be driven to a medium value (i.e., lengthened when it was initially shorter than the optimum state, but shortened when it was initially longer than the optimum state). Another stimulus, operating antagonistically, always would diminish the amplitude and precision, independent of the initial values, and would drive the period away from a medium value.

The hypothesis just derived, which presupposes an 'optimum' state of autonomous rhythms for theoretical reasons, fails to be confirmed directly by human experiments. Following this hypothesis, autonomous rhythms of man always seem to be positioned at the side of the optimum state with the longer periods, but never at the other side. Amplitude and precision, of course, are smaller at both sides of the optimum than at the optimum state. This statement, however, is true only with regard to the rectal temperature rhythms and, therefore, also to all rhythms running synchronized internally. This statement is not true with regard to the activity rhythms when they are separated from the rectal temperature rhythms during internal desynchronization. In some experiments showing this state, the periods of the separated activity rhythms are considerably shorter than those of the rectal temperature rhythms. The spontaneous occurrence of internal desynchronization, with a drastic shortening of the activity period, is released by the same experimental conditions as those with a drastic lengthening. The plausible interpretation of this experimental result must presuppose the 'optimum hypothesis' (cf. 4.2.2). The respective experimental condition or external stimulus affects, in all cases, diminishings in the amplitude and also changes in the period, but in directions that depend on the initial period. When the period is longer than normally (i.e., close to the upper limit of the mutual range of entrainment), it becomes lengthened so it transgresses this limit; and, when the initial period is shorter than normally (i.e., close to the lower limit of the mutual range of entrainment), it becomes shortened so it transgresses the other limit. As the general result of the action of this stimulus, the activity period is out of the range of entrainment of the rectal temperature rhythm and, therefore, internal desynchronization occurs. Since the activity periods, on the average, are longer than the rectal temperature periods (cf. 2.3), crossing of the limit pertinent to longer periods, must be more frequent and, in fact, just this result was obtained (Table 3).

In summary, all considerations generally show that the investigation of human circadian rhythms has a special bearing on the theoretical understanding of circadian rhythmicity. This bearing is based on the evaluation of interdependencies between different parameters of single overt rhythms and of interactions between different overt rhythms when running separately. The last mentioned aspect is of special importance because internal desynchronization (i.e., the state that allows only the study of those interactions), so far, except for a few preliminary findings in animal experiments, is known only from human experiments. Only this state, however, allows the conclusion of the multioscillator system. Although human experiments necessarily are limited in their feasibility, they, therefore, give an insight into the structure of the circadian system which, to the present, cannot be achieved in a similar manner with animal experiments.

5.2. Practical Aspects

5.2.1. Problems of Phase Maps

The practical aspects of circadian investigations, so far, commonly are related to the concept of phase maps, as presented in an example at the beginning of this book (Fig. 3). These phase maps summarize our knowledge of the temporal patterns of organisms. They show the temporal variations of different variables in the course of the day. They include, besides physiological and psychological values which are measurable directly, responsivenesses to drugs and other external stimuli and, therefore, assist in determining optimal dosages in therapy, depending on time of day. A closer inspection of the rules governing human circadian rhythmicity, however, shows that the applicability of phase maps is limited to the special condition where the phase map was measured. It was shown that phase maps, measured by different researchers on different continents using different methods, coincide remarkably (Guenther et al., 1969; Halberg et al., 1969). Most of these measurements were performed with young, healthy subjects. The applicability of phase maps, however, is of special interest when the conditions are 'abnormal' (e.g., when the dosage of a drug to an ill or aged patient must be determined); and such conditions may develop a phase map deviating from 'normal'.

The common phase map is based on a 24-hour scale at the abscissa. It is evident that such a phase map can be valid only with rhythms synchronized to the 24-hour day. As an experimental result, human circadian rhythms can be entrained not only to 24.0 hours, but also to periods slightly deviating from this value. It is meaningful, therefore, to obtain phase maps that are valid, for instance, to a 25-hour or 26-hour day (i.e., phase maps that are based on abscisse with 25-hour or 26-hour scales). As an experimental result, such a phase map differs totally from the common 24-hour phase map (Fig. 72), with regard to phases and amplitudes (Fig. 106). It may be argued that the structure of a phase map, with a base deviating from 24 hours, is without any practical interest since, on this earth, everyone's rhythms are synchronized to the natural 24.0-hour day. The external and internal phase relationships, however, do not depend on the zeitgeber period itself, but on the ratio between zeitgeber period and natural period. When only healthy subjects are considered, the distribution of free running periods is so remarkably small (Fig. 37) that this period can be considered as constant. If, however, the free running period deviates from the normal value (i.e., from a value close to 25 hours) for any reason (e.g., illness), the 24-hour phase map deviates from the normal phase map, in principle, in the same manner as a phase map based on a deviating zeitgeber period, but originating from a subject with a normal free running period.

An evident example of subjects with deviating free running periods, are blind subjects. It was shown that the free running rhythms of the tested blind subjects ran significantly faster than those of sighted subjects (cf. 2.4.1). Consequently, phase maps of the blind subjects correspond to those of sighted subjects when measured in an artificial day distinctly longer than 24 hours, with rectal temperature rhythms significantly earlier, compared to local time, than in sighted subjects (cf. 3.4). Conversely, different phase maps are known from "morning type" and "evening type" subjects. It was shown that the phase position of the rectal temperature rhythm, compared to local time, is about 1 hour earlier in "morning type," than in "evening type" subjects (Blake, 1971; Oestberg, 1976). Consequently, faster free running rhythms in "morning type," than in "evening type" subjects, must be expected. However, a difference in periods of about 0.2 hours must be expected; i.e., a difference which is so small, in relation to the intra- and interindividual differences in period, that it is difficult to be proven significantly. As the general result, even in rhythms synchronized internally and externally, a phase map cannot be considered to be invariable.

Not only among different samples of subjects do different phase maps exist, but a phase map of the same subject also can vary in its structure. This evidently would happen when the subject becomes exposed to days of varying duration (Fig. 72). Moreover, a drastic alteration in the phase map would happen when the subject becomes isolated from natural time cues and, therefore, shows a free running rhythm (Figs. 17 and 18). Both of these changes cannot occur when the subject lives under 'normal' conditions. There, however, may be conditions, even in a healthy subject living in the 24-hour day, which may cause alterations of the phase map. Figure 115 (upper diagram) may give an example. This figure includes rectal temperature recordings of a young and healthy man obtained continuously by use of a small battery operated device. The two temperature curves are each averaged from continuous records of 1 week. One curve was obtained during extreme mountain climbing, in altitudes between 5,000 and 7,000 meters, and the other was obtained several weeks later when the subject was at home pursuing his normal studies (Wever and Zink, 1971). In addition, the average times of activity during both conditions are indicated. For comparison, the lower diagram of figure 115 shows results of an isolation experiment performed 18 months later with the same subject under constant conditions (28 days duration; with remarkably regular, internally synchronized rhythms; with mean period of 25.3 hours). The diagram presents only the longitudinally pooled courses of the rhythms, which can be compared directly with the courses of the upper diagram. As the result, the upper diagram of figure 115 clearly shows a remarkable alteration in the rectal temperature rhythm, with regard to mean value, amplitude, and phase. The latter parameter is altered, not only when related to local time, but also when related to the respective activity time. It is not clear whether this alteration mainly is due to the extremely hard physical exercise, the low ambient temperature, or the low oxygen pressure during the "experimental week." It is clear, however, that the phase map of this subject is changed drastically between the "control" and "experimental" week. In the lower diagram of figure 115, with the abscissa scale in angular degrees instead of

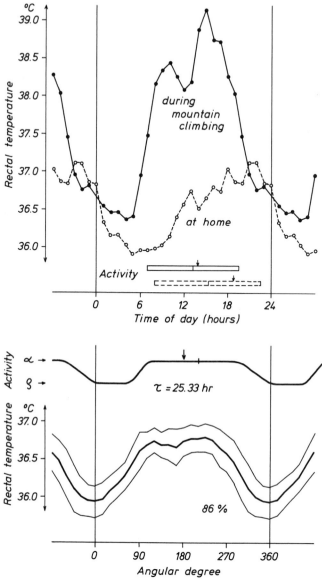

Figure 115. Upper diagram: Rectal temperature rhythm of a subject (U.I., ♂ 23 y), measured continuously in the natural 24-hour day, during extreme mountain climbing in altitudes of 5,000 to 7,000 m (solid line) and at home pursuing normal studies (dotted line). Each curve represents the average of measurements continued for 1 week. Inserted bars: average activity times during the respective sections. Marks within the bars: midpoint of activity time. Arrows at the bars: position of acrophase of the respective rectal temperature rhythm. Lower diagram: Autonomous rhythm of the same subject (25 y) measured during a 4-week experiment under constant conditions without environmental time cues. Presented are the longitudinally pooled courses of the rhythms of activity and rectal temperature, computed with an averaging period of 25.3 hours, derived from a preceding period analysis. Indications are the same as in figure 16/III. Mark at the activity cycle: midpoint of activity time. Arrow at the activity cycle: position of the acrophase of the rectal temperature rhythm. The phase positions within the 360° scale are selected arbitrarily in a manner where the midpoint of activity time coincides with the average of the midpoints of activity time in the upper diagram. Upper diagram from Wever and Zink (1971).

time of day, the phase is normalized in a manner where the activity time coincides with the average of the activity times of the upper diagram. The rectal temperature curve, remarkably enough, is similar in shape to the courses included in the upper diagram, in spite of the very different conditions and the different amplitudes and mean values. This coincidence in shape indicates an individuality of the rectal temperature rhythm which is independent of the conditions (Wever, 1973d). Finally, under constant conditions, the phase of the rectal temperature rhythm is earlier, relative to the activity rhythm, than in the "experimental" week, though the amplitude is smaller than in the "control" week (compare Figs. 78 and 106), and not larger, as it was in the "experimental" week.

As the general result, phase maps of different samples of subjects may be different; and the phase map of one subject may vary in its structure with varying conditions. In all cases, stable phase maps do exist, but they cannot be transferred from one condition to another. A stable phase map can exist, if at all, only as long as the different overt rhythms run synchronized internally. With internally dissociated rhythms, the phase map is temporarily unstable until this state is terminated. For example, after a phase shift of the zeitgeber, no stable phase map exists for several days, and only after terminating reentrainment does the original phase map become valid again. Finally, with internally desynchronized rhythms, a stable phase map does not exist. The internal phase relationships, between the different rhythms, vary from day to day and, therefore, it is impossible to obtain a conclusion from the phase relationships measured in the subject on one day, to the relationships on any other day. Therefore, in a subject showing internal desynchronization, the concept of a phase map is meaningless. It cannot assist, in any way, in determining optimal dosages of drugs in therapy. This statement is valid not only in autonomous rhythms showing spontaneous internal desynchronization under constant conditions, but also

with forced internal desynchronization occurring under the influence of a partially synchronizing zeitgeber. Consequently, if internal desynchronization can occur in the natural 24-hour day, due to partial external synchronization (see below), a stable phase map cannot be expected a priori, even in subjects apparently synchronized to 24.0 hours.

Suggestions of drastic changes in the free running period, connected with the occurrence of forced internal desynchronization, possibly were found in manic-depressives (Atkinson et al., 1975; Pflug, 1976; Pflug et al., 1976). In these cases, the courses of deep body temperature temporarily seemed to follow a rhythm being much faster than the 24-hour rhythm of wakefulness and sleep, although the patients lived under the normal 24-hour routine. The periods or period components of the vegetative rhythms were reported to be much shorter than any ever observed in healthy subjects (i.e., about 22 hours). If this is true, and if drugs must be administered, the instant of maximal and minimal responsivenesses to these drugs must be expected to shift continuously from day to day. The consideration of a phase map, as measured in healthy subjects, therefore, sometimes would lead to serious mistakes, which possibly are more harmful than disregarding any periodic change in the responsiveness. It would be helpful to test this state with healthy subjects. Of course, abnormally short periods cannot be imitated. It, however, is possible, and therefore meaningful, to simulate this state with a transformed time scale. When a healthy subject lives in an artificial 28-hour day, his vegetative rhythms are faster than the overt activity rhythm, for an amount that is similar to the claimed ratio in periods of the manic-depressives living in the 24-hour day. To give an example, the experiment shown in figure 87 again should be referenced. Figure 116 shows the courses of the activity rhythm and the rectal temperature rhythm obtained in the usual manner in this experiment, but with a time base of 28 hours instead of 24 hours. As can be seen during the experimen-

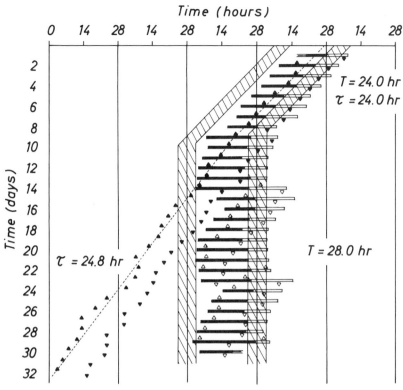

Figure 116.   Rhythm of a subject living without environmental time cues, but under the influence of a strong artificial zeitgeber, with one alteration of the zeitgeber period (same experiment as in figure 87). Temporal courses of the rhythms of activity and rectal temperature are presented successively, one period beneath the other, with a 28-hour time base. Indications are the same as in figure 27/I. Shaded areas: dark time of the zeitgeber.

tal section, the overt activity rhythm is synchronized to the zeitgeber, but with regularly repeated 'sleep disturbances'. The rectal temperature rhythm is not synchronized, but free running, with a period much shorter than the zeitgeber. Of course, the proposed model should only illustrate the possible simulation of pathologic rhythm disorders. The presentation of this model does not depend on whether or not the suggested findings will be confirmed.

In other cases, abnormal phase positions of vegetative rhythms were reported, while the rhythms remained synchronized to the 24-hour day (Menzel, 1962; Papousek, 1975; Richter, 1965). In these cases, it is a reasonable assumption that the natural periods also deviate from their normal values of close to 25 hours. This assumption, in fact, can be

tested only in isolation experiments, but this has never been done. Consequently, in these cases, the actual phase maps must be expected to be shifted for a certain amount, in comparison to the standard phase map. This means that the instants of maximal and minimal responsiveness to any drug are shifted for certain intervals, in comparison to corresponding instants measured in healthy man. It again is unclear whether or not the consideration of a standard phase map would be more helpful than disregarding any circadian variability in responsiveness. The consideration of the individual phase map, of course, would lead to optimal effects, but the measurement of an individual circadian course in the responsiveness to a special drug, even with an ill patient, is a very difficult and time-consuming attempt.

In summary, a phase map is meaningful when applied to a condition that coincides externally and internally with the condition under which the phase map was measured originally. In the natural 24-hour day, this prerequisite usually can be assumed to be fulfilled when healthy subjects are considered to be living in their normal environment. The application of the phase map concept in medicine becomes of special interest, however, in ill or aged patients. In these cases, it cannot be excluded that the phase map is changed or completely does not exist. Alterations in the conditions, corrupting the phase map concept, may consist of changes in the period. The zeitgeber period, aside from very specialized isolation experiments, in fact, is a fixed quantity, but not the natural period of the subjects, which determines the phase map as it does the zeitgeber period. This internal period may be subject to variations as mentioned in the previous examples. Alterations in the conditions, furthermore, may consist of changes in the tendency toward internal desynchronization. It was shown that this tendency depends on various external and internal conditions. Among the internal conditions, old age and an increased tendency toward neuroticism were mentioned (i.e., exactly those conditions, where the application of a phase map may be more important than in young healthy subjects). Finally, alterations in the conditions may be based on changes in the effectiveness of the entraining zeitgeber, either due to changes in the zeitgeber strength or in the oscillatory strength of the entrained rhythm. Especially after knowing the social origin of the primary zeitgeber effect, changes in the responsiveness of a subject to the common 24-hour zeitgeber cannot be excluded, because constancy of the zeitgeber effect would presuppose constancy in the ability and capability to exert social contacts. Nothing is known about the dependency of oscillatory strength on age. Only the independency of free running periods of age was found (Fig. 39). All three modes of alterations in the controlling conditions, which also may occur in combina-

tions, will change the structure of a phase map, as measured under normal conditions, or even repeal its stability.

5.2.2. Problems of rhythm disorders

It was discussed, at the beginning of this book, that circadian rhythmicity is of two-fold importance for biological systems. First, it must guarantee the temporal fit of the biological variables, which always are fluctuating, in the environment, which always undergoes daily periodic variations in all parameters. Second, it must guarantee the temporal order among the various physiological and psychological variables which functionally condition each other. It is evident that the fulfillment of these tasks demands external and internal synchronization. Each disorder of circadian rhythmicity, either due to external or internal desynchronization, disarranges the biological equilibrium and, therefore, must be avoided. After knowing several basic rules governing circadian rhythmicity, it is of practical meaning, therefore, to look for conditions which guarantee the stable synchronization of the intact circadian system.

There are several external conditions raising the tendency toward spontaneously occurring internal desynchronization (e.g., self-control conditions, the absence of stabilizing electromagnetic fields). All these conditions simultaneously have the effect of lengthening the autonomous period (cf. 2.4.9). This normally means that these conditions enlarge the deviation of the free running period from the period of the natural zeitgeber (i.e., from 24.0 hours). Following the 'optimum hypothesis' (cf. 5.1), this would mean that the same stimuli shorten the period in cases where, for any reason, the autonomous period is shorter than 24.0 hours. This reversal in the effect on the period, however, can be correct only with continuously operating stimuli, but not with self-control conditions which, in principle, lengthen the period. Since those considerably short periods, furthermore, seem to appear only in pathologic cases, it must be questioned whether or not the possibility exists that not only the actual period, but also the 'optimum period', is shifted. It further is an unanswered question of practical importance in what direction the tendency toward internal desynchronization is correlated to the period in these pathologic cases. Therefore, the evaluation of regularities of human circadian rhythms, based on healthy subjects, indeed, prepares the ground for applications of these regularities in patients. It, however, must be kept in mind that modifications of these regularities may occur with the transition from healthy to sick subjects.

There are several internal conditions raising the tendency toward internal desynchronization. Among these, especially old age (Fig. 40), and increased scores of neuroticism (Fig. 41) were discussed. These results suggest the assumption that special properties of the subjects, described by these personality data, affect the rhythm. It equally can be assumed, however, that different factors, expressed by these data, commonly affect other properties of the subjects that are controlling directly the tendency toward internal desynchronization. Such a property could be the ability to endure the special experimental condition of isolation studies. It is evident that elder people, or more neurotic subjects, in fact, suffer consciously from these conditions no more than other subjects. It, however, would be reasonable to assume that these subjects, though not consciously, are stressed more by the conditions than other subjects. It was shown earlier (cf. 2.4.7) that psychic burden, or stress, is assumed to affect human circadian rhythms by lengthening the free running period and increasing the tendency toward internal desynchronization. Similar effects were suggested even under zeitgeber influence (Fig. 93).

The question again arises as to in what manner stress would affect a rhythm, the natural period of which, for whatever reason, is shorter than about 24 hours. It was shown, if a rhythm, the period of which is shorter than the average of all autonomous periods, desynchronizes spontaneously, the result always is a drastic shortening of the activity rhythm (Fig. 29). This remains true when the occurrence of internal desynchronization may be due to an increased score of neuroticism (Fig. 28) or old age (Fig. 38). It is the assumption, to be deduced from the multioscillator hypothesis, that the natural period of the activity period, before the spontaneous separation, is considerably shorter than the natural period of the rectal temperature rhythm (i.e., possibly shorter than 24 hours). The state of internal desynchronization would then be released by a further slight shortening of the activity period transgressing the lower limit of the mutual range of entrainment. It would be plausible to assume it is the stress, which increases in these subjects during the progressive course of the isolation experiment, which induces the further shortening of the period. Similar considerations may apply to external conditions raising the tendency toward internal desynchronization. The same stimuli (e.g., absence of definite electromagnetic fields) that tend to release internal desynchronization with lengthened activity periods, release internal desynchronization with shortened activity periods, when the previous period was shorter than the average (Fig. 59). This statement, indeed, is valid to only a limited amount, when the releasing external stimulus is self-control (see above). If internal desynchronization occurs during self-control, a drastic shortening of the activity period is an exception (e.g., it occurs in only 16% of all cases with internal desynchronization under self-controlled illumination, but in 33% of all cases under constant illumination).

It may be argued that the tendency toward internal desynchronization, as discussed so far, is without direct interest. This tendency or changes in this tendency were determined using the unnatural state of constant conditions during complete isolation; and this type of state is never present under natural conditions. The results, however, indirectly reflect tendencies which also may be relevant under zeitgeber conditions. If, under constant conditions, an older subject desynchronizes more easily than a younger subject, or, if under constant conditions, a definite electromagnetic field influences the tendency toward internal desynchronization, it must be expected that similar relationships are true under zeitgeber conditions when partial entrainment, with forced internal desynchronization, can occur.

Not only internal synchronization, but also external synchronization, is necessary to avoid rhythm disorders. The practical importance of this statement is especially based on the observation that, in human circadian rhythms, "social contacts" basically constitute the effective zeitgeber (cf. 3.2.2). Further sophisticated experiments surely are needed to specify the concept of social zeitgebers. A quantification of this effect is handicapped by the great interindividual differences in the subjectively experienced strength of objectively equivalent social signals. In some subjects, the mere knowledge of clock time is a sufficient zeitgeber to entrain their circadian rhythms in an otherwise time free environment. On the other hand, to be in possession of a functioning watch does not lead necessarily to entrainment as long as there remains doubt whether or not the watch is manipulated in any manner. The degree of these doubts cannot be tested. Some subjects seem to be very sensitive to unintentional time cues. In borderline cases, they can be entrained to the 24.0-hour day without identifying the effective zeitgeber (Fig. 21). There are other subjects who are remarkably insensitive to contacts. In some isolation experiments, for example, subjects occasionally, and unintentionally, gained knowledge of the discrepancy between their subjective time and the objective time, accumulated during the experiment. In most of these cases, the courses of their rhythms were not altered, in any way, as a consequence of the contact. It is evident that the motivation of the subjects, or possibly even their knowledge of previous results concerning isolation experiments, influenced the responsiveness to these intended or unintended time cues. Especially in this respect, the limitations of experiments performed with volunteers become obvious.

The result of the basically social nature of effective zeitgebers in man has the consequence, that the possibility as well as the ability to have social contacts become prerequisites for entrainment. These prerequisites always may be fulfilled sufficiently in young and healthy subjects, but perhaps less in old and sick subjects. This means that in these subjects, entrainment to the natural 24-hour day need not be guaranteed under natural conditions. The probability of external desynchronization, therefore, is raised in the same subjects who also have a higher probability for internal desynchronization. In this context, we must refer, once again, to the only known animal experiment that is relevant. Stroebel (1969) produced "psychosomatic" disorder, with impaired performance, in rhesus monkeys by applying "behavioral stress". Part of the animals, during the "stress condition", showed a free running circadian rhythm in brain temperature, under the influence of a persisting 24-hour light-dark cycle, which was effective in entraining the animals before the stress application.

It may be argued that external desynchronization would be detectable obviously and, therefore, actions against this disorder could be taken. This argument, however, concerns only full external desynchronization. It does not concern partial desynchronization because, in this state, the most easily observable rhythms (e.g., activity rhythm) normally are synchronized externally, and only the vegetative rhythms are desynchronized. It was shown earlier, for instance in connection with figure 87, that this state can hardly be detected by measurements covering only a few days, but only by uninterrupted measurements of vegetative variables continued for several weeks. The characteristic of this barely detectable state of partial external desynchronization is its fundamental combination with internal desynchronization (i.e., with another type of rhythm disorder). In summary, even under the influence of a zeitgeber, there is the danger of rhythm disorders, established simultaneously by partial external, and consequently internal, desynchronization. It is evident, in this state, that the biological equilibrium is disarranged in a twofold manner.

To find possible consequences of rhythm disorders, all subjects participating in isolation experiments were tested before and after the experiment. The comparison of results of both of these tests has guaranteed that there are no harmful consequences. This is also true if internal or external desynchronization had occurred, either spontaneously or forced by the conditions. None of the items tested showed a systematic trend during the experiment. This absence of harmful consequences, by all means, is an indispensable precondition in performing isolation experiments. There seems to be only one report suggesting harmful disturbances after a long term cave experiment, with the investigator himself as the subject (Siffre, 1975). The result, however, only means that the organism of a healthy young subject normally has the capacity to cope with short term rhythm disorders; short in comparison to lifespan. This result does not state the same results are expected, in any way, with long term rhythm disorders in an old or sick subject whose organism is debilitated. Harmful consequences, therefore, cannot be excluded in these subjects, on the basis of the experimental results available.

Experiments with long term rhythm disorders were performed with flies that were exposed to different kinds of rhythm disorders during their total lifespan. As the result, the lifespan was drastically reduced in comparison to undisturbed controls (Aschoff et al., 1971a; Pittendrigh and Minis, 1972; Wever, 1968d, 1975d). These results, of course, cannot be applied directly to man. It, however, must be taken in account that, also in man, long lasting disorders of circadian rhythms, especially when occurring with a previously sick subject, may leave permanent complaints. If this is true, and if similar effects as those in flies are suspected, the special danger of a chain reaction is present. Rhythm disorders lead to faster aging. Old age, however, leads to an increased tendency toward rhythm disorders (Wever, 1975d).

In contrast to permanent complaints, transitory alterations in the behavior of human subjects, following short term rhythm disorders, can be detected well enough (e.g., in psychomotor performance). It was deduced that rhythms in performance, and even average levels of performance, can be determined only in zeitgeber experiments where test data are available at regular intervals (i.e., even during rest time of the subjects without a "night-gap" in data). The same is true with respect to rhythms in subjective self-rating scores. To separate alterations in the performance level, induced by rhythm disorders, from regular temporal trends and random fluctuations, the consideration of well defined rhythm disorders or regularly recurring disorders is preferred. These conditions are realized during internal desynchronization, when forced by a strong zeitgeber. In these experiments, sections with internally synchronized and desynchronized rhythms can alternate at the desire of the experimenter; and, further, during sections with internal desynchronization, days showing "right" internal phase relationships regularly alternate with days showing "wrong" internal phase relationships.

Following this concept, we again will consider the course of the experiment which was shown in figures 87 and 116. In the presentation of figure 117, the courses of the variables are condensed and smoothed, by moving averages, to a degree where circadian rhythmicity disappears; so, only the course of the mean value, or of the average level, is left (solid lines). The courses of the amplitude of each variable additionally are presented (dotted lines). For reference, the standardized internal phase relationship between the two oscillators involved in this system (i.e., in section A with equal periods of 24.0 hours; in section B with periods of 24.8 and 28.0 hours; compare figure 87/II) is presented (upper border). Those instants where both oscillators just run counterphased are indicated. As a preliminary re-

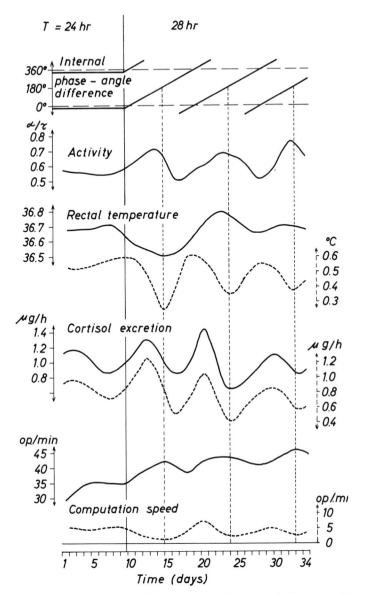

Figure 117. Rhythm of a subject living without environmental time cues but under the influence of a strong artificial zeitgeber with one alteration of the zeitgeber period (same experiment as in figure 87). Presented longitudinally are the compressed courses, smoothed by moving averages (solid lines), and the amplitudes of the fundamental periods (dotted lines) of the four rhythms shown in figure 87, in comparison to the internal phase angle difference between the two oscillators involved (top border). The dotted vertical lines indicate those instances when the two oscillators exactly ran counterphased.

sult, the amplitudes of all rhythms regularly fluctuate with the internal phase relationship, showing sharply marked minimum values when the oscillators run counterphased. This observation confirms a conclusion drawn earlier (Fig. 26), regarding rectal tem-

perature rhythm, and extends it to other rhythms. It obviously suggests the assumption of beat phenomena between the two oscillations (Fig. 112). In the context to be discussed here, the mean values are of greater interest than the amplitudes. The

250 Conclusions and Speculations

mean value of rectal temperature seems to fluctuate randomly, without recognizable correlation to the internal phase relationship. The mean value of cortisol excretion oscillates strictly parallel to the amplitude. This coincidence is due to the fact that the minimum excretion always is very small and only the amounts of maximum excretion are free to change. The most interesting mean value of the psychomotor performance (i.e., computation speed) primarily shows a drastic 'learning increase', apparently lasting during the total experiment. A closer inspection shows that this trend levels off toward the end of the first section (24-hour day) but reappears during the second section (28-hour day). Moreover, the mean performance level seems to fluctuate regularly; with maximum values, during the second section, when the two oscillators run counterphased. The course of the mean performance level, therefore, oscillates opposite to the amplitude of the same variable.

At first glance, the results derived from figure 117, regarding the performance level, seem to be paradoxical. If the circadian system has any biological relevance, one could expect that optimum conditions demand mutual synchronization of all oscillators involved and, in particular, coinciding phases when they control equal variables. In this experiment, however, the psychomotor performance of the subject is objectively higher when the oscillators run internally desynchronized and, in particular, is highest at those instants when the oscillators run counterphased. Although confirmed by performance data of other comparable experiments, this result could be simulated by a temporal trend. Experiments with other sequences of the different sections, therefore, were performed.

Figure 118 shows results from an experiment with three different sections in an arrangement where internal synchronization is not present at the beginning, but during the middle section. The results originate from the experiment the course of which was shown in figure 88. The general result equals that of the other example in figure 117. The

amplitudes of all overt rhythms again accept minimum values when the oscillators involved in this system run counterphased; and the mean value of rectal temperature again fluctuates independent of the internal phase relationship. The courses of all mean values and amplitudes pass more smoothly during the middle section, with internally synchronized rhythms, than during the other sections, with internally desynchronized rhythms. The mean performance level again shows the "learning increase", which seems to be completed during the 24-hour section, but shows a secondary increase during the last section, beginning 1 full month after the beginning of the experiment. The performance level again fluctuates regularly during sections with internal desynchronization, with maximum values when the oscillators run counterphased. As the experiment underlying figure 117, the experiment shown in figure 118 is, in its temporal course, not a unique case, but one of several experiments with equivalent results.

In a third example, shown in figure 119, the temporal sequence of the different sections again is altered. The course of this experiment was shown in figure 89. In figure 118, the circadian system was desynchronized internally during the first and third section, but synchronized internally during the second (i.e., middle) section. In figure 119, the circadian system, conversely, is synchronized internally during the first and third section but desynchronized internally during the second (i.e., middle) section. The result, however, is basically the same as in the other examples. The increase in the performance level, except for the first section of each experiment, is steeper when internal desynchronization takes place than when the circadian system runs synchronized internally. The temporal course of the performance level also shows maximum values when, during the state of internal desynchronization, the oscillators run counterphased.

Finally, in the diagrams of figures 117 to 119, the mean courses of the activity level are included, indicating the duration of the

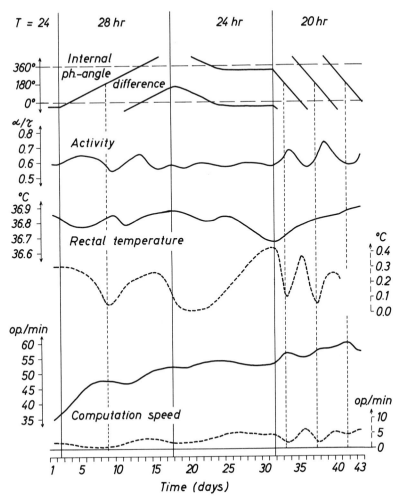

Figure 118.   Rhythm of a subject living without environmental time cues but under the influence of a strong artificial zeitgeber with two alterations of the zeitgeber period (same experiment as in figure 88). Presented longitudinally are the compressed courses, smoothed by moving averages (solid lines), and the amplitudes of the fundamental periods (dotted lines) of the three rhythms presented in figure 88, in comparison to the internal phase angle difference between the two oscillators involved (top border). The dotted vertical lines indicate those instances when the two oscillators exactly ran counterphased.

activity time per period or, conversely, the amount of sleep per period. The first consistent result is the activity level is rather constant during the sections with internally synchronized rhythms but oscillates, correlated to the internal phase relationship, during the sections with internally desynchronized rhythms. Second, the activity level, on the average, is higher during the sections with internal desynchronization, indicating a smaller need for sleep than in those sections where the rhythms run internally synchro-

nized (the fraction of 'night time', compared to the full period, is the same in all sections). Third, during the sections showing internal desynchronization (i.e., with oscillating activity level), this level decreases at instants when the oscillators run counterphased if the zeitgeber period is longer than 24 hours, or the period of the overt activity rhythm is longer than the free running overt rectal temperature rhythm; and it increases at the instants when the oscillators run counterphased if the zeitgeber period is shorter than

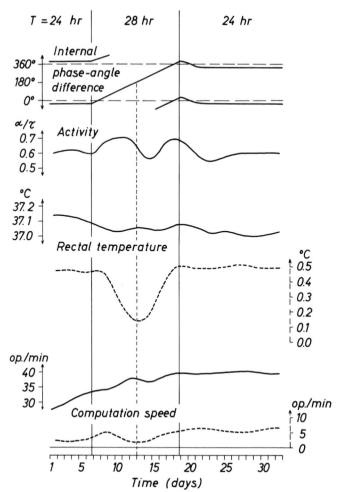

Figure 119.   Rhythm of a subject living without environmental time cues but under the influence of a strong artificial zeitgeber with two alterations of the zeitgeber period (same experiment as in figure 89). Presented longitudinally are the compressed courses, smoothed by moving averages (solid lines), and the amplitudes of the fundamental periods (dotted lines) of the three rhythms presented in figure 89, in comparison to the internal phase angle difference between the two oscillators involved (top border). The dotted vertical line indicates those instances when the two oscillators exactly ran counterphased.

24 hours. It follows, from this result, that the apparently paradoxical course of the performance level cannot be due to a sleep deficit of a changing amount. During the sections where the circadian system is desynchronized internally, the average sleep fraction, on the contrary, is smaller than in the other sections, but the average performance level is higher or the increase in performance is steeper, than in the other sections. The alterations in the activity and performance levels are correlated with opposite signs in sections with zeitgeber periods being longer and shorter than 24 hours. Compare, for example, the first and third section in figure 118.

The results, shown in figures 117 to 119, do not agree with the expectation that internal desynchronization should cause deleterious effects. The findings concerning the objectively measured psychomotor performance, however, are supported by an analysis of subjective statements of the subjects, as recorded on standardized self-rating questionnaires (Goertzen, 1976). With each test session, the subjects scored themselves regarding six items at continuous scales. The questionnaires were removed after each test, so successive scorings largely were independent of each other. Figure 120 shows, as an example, results originating from the experiment where the temporal course was shown in Fig. 88. The objective performance measured in this experiment was shown in figure 118. The subjective scores of four different items are presented separately for the three sections of this experiment. The scores are pooled longitudinally with the respective zeitgeber period as the averaging period. The presentation of only this averaging period does not mean that the subjective scores always oscillated synchronously to the zeitgeber. Partially clear free running components of the subjective scorings are included (Goertzen, 1976). For comparison, figure 120 includes the activity courses during the three sections, with the same type of presentation. The last column of the diagrams includes results pooled from all sections, but separated with respect to the internal phase relationship between the rhythms of activity and rectal temperature. Cycles with a "right" phase relationship (i.e., with the temperature maximum during activity time) are separated from those cycles where the internal phase relationship is "wrong" (i.e., where the temperature maximum fell into sleep time).

Figure 120 preliminarily demonstrates the "oscillatory" behavior of the activity rhythm. Its phase position, relative to the zeitgeber, is earlier the longer the period. The item "contentment" ("Zufriedenheit"), which mainly represents the well-being of the subject, also shows a clear circadian course, and the phase position of this rhythm changes according to oscillation laws. The regular variations in the phase of this rhythm, however, are larger than those of the activity rhythm (i.e., not only the external phase relationship of this rhythm to the zeitgeber varies, depending on period, but also the internal phase relationship to the activity rhythm). This indicates that the rhythm of well-being does not reflect only

reactively the state of activity. The average scores additionally are indicated in figure 120. As can be seen, the well-being is scored higher during the first and third sections, where the rhythms ran desynchronized internally, than during the middle section, where they ran synchronized internally. The well-being further is scored higher during those days when the two oscillators involved ran counterphased (right diagram, dotted line) than on days when they ran with equal phases (solid line). Similar results were obtained with regard to the items "power of concentration" ("Konzentrationsfähigkeit") and "need for mental activity" ("Bedürfnis nach geistiger Aktivität"), which may be understood as subjective correlates to the objectively measured psychomotor performance (Fig. 118). Finally, "fatigue" ("Müdigkeit") takes a circadian course, being reversed in comparison to those of the other items. It always is lowest around noon, and on the average, lowest during the third section, where internal desynchronization is marked most strongly (Fig. 118). With the two other items tested, the subject always scored such extreme values (e.g., "nervousness" always extremely low) that obvious variations could not be detected (i.e., there were neither relevant circadian variations nor differences between the different sections). The scores of the different items, therefore, continue to be in agreement with each other. They generally indicate that the subject is subjectively in a better state when the circadian system is in internal disorder than in its "normal" order. This apparently paradoxical result confirms the result derived from objective performance measurements, which also indicate a better state of the subject when the circadian system is in internal disorder than when in the right order.

The result obtained from the self-rating scales, as presented in figure 120, by no means is unique. It, rather, is confirmed by results of many comparable experiments with several different sequences of the different sections. In summary, in most, but not all, subjects, the objectively measured

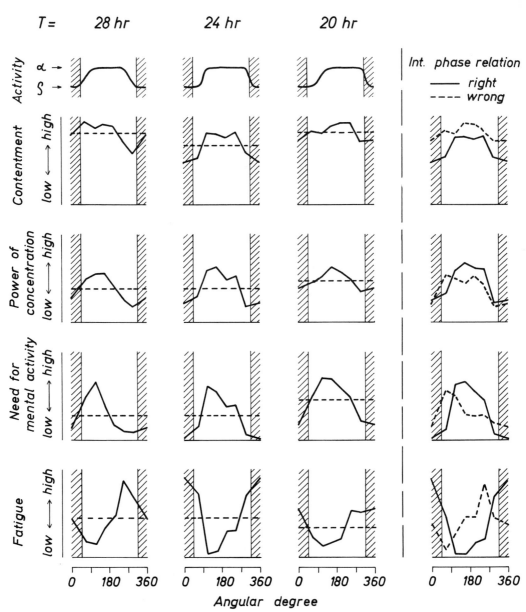

Figure 120. Longitudinally pooled courses of the rhythms of activity and of four subjectively scored items, taken from continuous self-rating scales, scored seven times per period, obtained in the same experiment as in figures 88 and 118. The average cycles are computed separately for the three different sections of the experiment, with each of the different zeitgeber periods as the averaging period (columns 1 to 3). The average scores, during the different sections, are indicated by dotted lines. In the fourth column, longitudinally pooled courses of the four items are presented, separately with respect to opposite internal phase angle differences between the two oscillators involved. Solid lines (i.e., "right internal phase relationship"): average of those cycles where the rectal temperature maximum fell into activity time. Dotted lines (i.e., "wrong internal phase relationships"): average of those cycles where the rectal temperature maximum fell into rest time of the subject. All pooling computations are based on the zeitgeber period as the averaging period. Data from Goertzen (1976).

performance and the subjectively scored well-being are better when the circadian system is desynchronized internally than when synchronized internally. This statement remains true not only regarding averages of different sections, lasting 1 to 2 weeks, but also regarding instantaneous internal phase relationships, when varying within several days. It is worth noting that the differences in the condition did not become conscious to the subjects. No subject could determine whether or not he was in better or worse shape during certain sections. This unawareness which is discrepant from the results of the scorings, may be due to habituation.

It is evident that the experimentally obtained positive effects of internal desynchronization is in strict opposition to the commonly accepted and reasonable assumption that rhythm disorders should have deleterious effects on an organism. This discrepancy between expectation and result, may be solved by considering the fact that the apparently paradoxical results were obtained with young, healthy subjects living for short term experiments (i.e., short in comparison to life span) in a very special environment. It need not be a discrepancy that a definite irritation, which deleteriously affects the organism in the long run, operates as a stimulating agent, when effective only for short term intervals, to a subject whose organism is otherwise intact. Especially during isolation experiments, where the environment of the subjects is rather poor in stimuli, additional stimuli, originating from disorders of the circadian system, may be advantageous to the organism. It is well known that a deprivation of stimuli can be as stressing as an inundation of stimuli.

Following this suggestion, it is evident that the result discussed, though significant, is even less transferable from the experimental condition to the normal condition than other results, and may be less transferable from subjects volunteering in isolation experiments to other people. This unexpected result, therefore, cannot affect the general

meaning that disorders of the circadian system must be avoided. It clearly does show rhythm disorders must not be harmful in any case. It even may be possible that this result will constitute, in the future, a stimulation therapy in special cases. At present, the results discussed justify the conduct of experiments where the state of internal desynchronization is provoked experimentally.

These conclusions and speculations show that the investigation of human circadian rhythms is not only of theoretical interest, but also of increasing practical importance. With regard to the theoretical conclusions drawn, human experiments cannot be replaced, to relevant amounts, by animal experiments, but they can even less with regard to practical consequences. This is due to the fact that besides physiological variables, psychological variables and performances especially are involved, to considerable amounts, in the temporal structure of human beings. This is due also to the fact that the multioscillatory structure of the circadian system especially motivates relevant practical applications. This multioscillatory structure, however, has been proven exclusively, to the present, in human circadian rhythms.

In summary, regarding theoretical and practical conclusions, investigations of human circadian rhythms are of growing interest in the general exploration of the circadian system. In spite of the special expenditures of human experiments, and the great limitations in the practicability of these experiments, circadian experiments with humans are indispensable, in many respects, and are not replaceable by experiments with animals. It was the aim of this book to state some basic features of the human circadian system. It is evident, in trying to give answers to basic questions, that many additional, but even more relevant, questions are challenged. The exploration of the human circadian system, therefore, will gain increasing priority in the future. In formulating relevant problems, this book may be helpful.

6
References

Adey, W. R., Bawin, S. M.: Brain interactions with weak electric and magnetic fields. Neurosci. Res. Progr. Bull. *15/1* (1977).

Andrews, R. V.: Temporal secretory response of cultured hamster adrenals. Comp. Biochem. Physiol. *26*, 179–193, 479–488 (1968).

Apfelbaum, M., Nillus, P.: Evolution de la conductance physiologique chez les femmes vivant à 11°C pendant quinze jours. Rev. Fr. Etud. Clin. Biol. *12*, 80–85 (1967).

Apfelbaum, M., Reinberg, A., Nillus, P., Halberg, F.: Rythmes circadiens de l'alternance veille-sommeil pendant l'isolement souterrain de sept jeunes femmes. Presse Méd. *77*, 879–882 (1969).

Appel, W.: Uber die Tagesschwankung der Eosinophilen. Z. Gesamte Exp. Med. *104*, 15–21 (1938).

Appel, W., Hansen, K. J.: Lichteinwirkung, Tagesrhythmik der eosinophilen Leukozythen und Hypophysennebennierenrindensystem. Dtsch. Arch. klin. Med. *199*, 530–537 (1952).

Aschoff, J.: Der Tagesgang der Körpertemperatur beim Menschen. Klin. Wochenschr. *33*, 545–551 (1955).

Aschoff, J.: Gesetzmässigkeiten der biologischen Tagesperiodik. Dtsch. Med. Wochenschr. *88*, 1930–1937 (1963a).

Aschoff, J.: Comparative Physiology: Diurnal Rhythms. Annu. Rev. Physiol. *25*, 581–600 (1963b).

Aschoff, J.: Circadian rhythms in man. Science *148*, 1427–1432 (1965a).

Aschoff, J.: Response curves in circadian periodicity. In: Circadian Clocks. Aschoff J. (ed.) Amsterdam: North-Holland Publ. Comp. 1965b, pp. 95–111.

Aschoff, J.: Physiologie biologischer Rhythmen. Ärztliche Praxis *18*, 1569, 1593–1597 (1966).

Aschoff, J.: Human circadian rhythms in activity, body temperature and other function. Life Sci. Space Res. *5*, 159–173 (1967a).

Aschoff, J.: Adaptive cycles: Their significance for defining environmental hazards. Int. J. Biometeor. *11*, 255–278 (1967b).

Aschoff, J.: Circadiane Periodik als Grundlage des Schlaf-Wach-Rhythmus. In: Ermüdung, Schlaf und Traum. Baust, W. (ed.) Stuttgart: Wiss. Verlagsges. 1970, pp. 59–98.

Aschoff, J.: Eigenschaften der menschlichen Tagesperiodik. In: Aktuelle Probleme der Arbeitsumwelt, Rutenfranz, J. (ed.) Stuttgart: A. W. Gentner Verlag 1971.

Aschoff, J.: Das circadiane System. Grundlagen der Tagesperiodik und ihrer Bedeutung für angewandte Physiologie und Klinik. Verh. Dtsch. Ges. Inn. Med. *79*, 19–31 (1973).

Aschoff, J., Wever, R.: Spontanperiodik des

Menschen bei Ausschluss aller Zeitgeber. Naturwissenschaften *49*, 337–342 (1962a).

Aschoff, J., Wever, R.: Biologische Rhythmen und Regelung. Bad Oeynhausener Gespräche *5*, 1–15 (1962b).

Aschoff, J., Wever, R.: Über Phasenbeziehungen zwischen biologischer Tagesperiodik und Zeitgeberperiodik. Z. Vergl. Physiol. *46*, 115–128 (1962c).

Aschoff, J., Wever, R.: Resynchronisation der Tagesperiodik von Vögeln nach Phasensprung des Zeitgebers. Z. Vergl. Physiol. *46*, 321–335 (1963).

Aschoff, J., Wever, R.: Circadian period and phase-angle difference in chaffinches (Fringilla coelebs L.). Comp. Biochem. Physiol. *18*, 397–404 (1966).

Aschoff, J., Klotter, K., Wever, R.: Circadian vocabulary. In: Circadian Clocks. Aschoff J. (ed.) Amsterdam: North-Holland Publ. Comp. 1965, pp. 10–19.

Aschoff, J., Gerecke, U., Wever, R.: Phasenbeziehungen zwischen den circadianen Perioden der Aktivität und der Kerntemperatur beim Menschen. Pflügers Arch. *295*, 173–183 (1967a).

Aschoff, J., Gerecke, U., Wever, R.: Desynchronization of human circadian rhythms. Jap. J. Physiol. *17*, 450–457 (1967b).

Aschoff, J., v. Saint Paul, U., Wever, R.: Circadiane Periodik von Finkenvögeln unter dem Einfluss eines selbstgewählten Licht-Dunkel-Wechsels. Z. Vergl. Physiol. *58*, 304–321 (1968).

Aschoff, J., Poeppel, E., Wever, R.: Circadiane Periodik des Menschen unter dem Einfluss von Licht-Dunkel-Wechseln unterschiedlicher Periode. Pflügers Arch. *306*, 58–70 (1969).

Aschoff, J., v. Saint Paul, U., Wever, R.: Die Lebensdauer von Fliegen unter dem Einfluss von Zeit-Verschiebungen. Naturwissenschaften *58*, 574 (1971a).

Aschoff, J., Fatranska, M., Giedke, H., Doerr, P., Stamm, D., Wisser, H.: Human circadian rhythms in continuous darkness: entrainment by social cues. Science *171*, 213–215 (1971b).

Aschoff, J., Gerecke, U., Kureck, A., Pohl, H., Rieger, P., v. Saint Paul, U., Wever, R.: Interdependent parameters of circadian activity rhythms in birds and man. In: Biochronometry. Menaker M. (ed.) Washington D.C.: Nat. Acad. Sciences 1971c, pp. 3–27.

Aschoff, J., Giedke, H., Poeppel, E., Wever, R.: The influence of sleep-interruption and of sleep-deprivation on circadian rhythms in human performance. In: Aspects of Human Efficiency. Colquhoun, W. P. (ed.) London: The English Univ. Press Lim. 1972, pp. 135–149

Aschoff, J., Fatranska, M., Gerecke, U., Giedke, H.: Twenty-four-hour rhythms of rectal temperature in humans: effects of sleep-interruptions and of test-sessions. Pflügers Arch. *346*, 215–222 (1974a).

Aschoff, J., Ceresa, F., Halberg, F. (eds.): Chronobiological aspects of endocrinology. Symposia Medica Hoechst 9. Stuttgart-New York: F. K. Schattauer-Verlag, 1974b.

Aschoff, J., Hoffmann, K., Pohl, H., Wever, R.: Re-entrainment of circadian rhythms after phase-shifts of the zeitgeber. Chronobiologia *2*, 23–78 (1975).

Atkinson, M., Kripke, D. F., Wolf, S. R.: Autorhythmometry in manic-depressives. Chronobiologia *2*, 325–335 (1975).

Autenrieth, J. H.: Handbuch der empirischen menschlichen Physiologie. Tübingen 1801/02.

Baade, W.: Experimentelle und kritische Beiträge zur Frage nach den sekundären Wirkungen des Unterrichtes insbesondere auf die Empfänglichkeit des Schülers. Paedagog. Monogr. Bd. III, Leipzig 1907.

Batschelet, E.: Statistical Methods for the Analysis of Problems in Animal Orientation and Certain Biological Rhythms. Washington D.C.: Am. Inst. Biol. Sciences, 1965.

Benedict, F. G.: Studies in body temperature. I. Influence of the inversion of the daily routine; the temperature of night-workers. Am. J. Physiol. *11*, 145–150 (1904).

Benedict, F. G., Snell, J. F.: Körpertemperatur-Schwankungen mit besonderer Rücksicht auf den Einfluss, welchen die Umkehrung der täglichen Lebensgewohnheiten beim Menschen ausübt. Pflügers Arch. *90*, 33–72 (1902).

Bjerner, B., Swensson, A.: Schichtarbeit und Rhythmus. Acta Med. Scand. [Suppl.] *278*, 102–107 (1953).

Blake, M. J. F.: Temperament and Time of day. In: Biological Rhythms and Human Performance. Colquhoun W. P. (ed.) London-New York: Acad. Press, 1971, pp. 109–148.

Bodenheimer, S., Winter, J. S. D., Faiman, C.: Diurnal rhythms of serumgonadotropins, testosterone, estriadol and cortisol in blind men. J. Clin Endocrinol. Metab. *37*, 472 (1973).

Brengelmann, J. C., Brengelmann, L.: Deutsche Validierung von Fragebogen der Extraversion, neurotischen Tendenz und Rigidität. Z. Exp. Angew. Psychol. 7, 291–331 (1960).

Brinkmann, K.: Temperatureinfluss auf die circadiane Rhythmic von *Euglena gracilis* bei Mixotrophie and Autotrophie. Planta Med. 70, 344–389 (1965).

Brinkmann, K.: Metabolic control of temperature compensation in the circadian rhythm of *Euglena gracilis*. In: Biochronometry. Menaker, M. (ed.) Washington D.C.: Nat. Acad Sciences 1971, pp. 567–593.

Brown, F. A. Jr.: The 'clock' timing biological rhythms. Am. Sci. 60, 756–766 (1972).

Browne, R. C.: The day and night performance rhythm in industry. 5th Conf. Soc. Biol. Rhythm, Stockholm 1955, pp. 61–64 Aco-Print, Stockholm 1961.

Chouvet, G., Mouret, J., Coindet, J., Siffre, M., Jouvet, M.: Periodicité bicircadienne du cycle veille-sommeil dans des conditions hors du temps. Etude polygraphique. Electroencephalogr. Clin. Neurophysiol. 37, 367–380 (1974).

Clegg, B. R., Schaefer, K. E.: Measurement of periodicity and phase shift of physiological functions in isolation experiments by cross-correlation techniques using synthesized periodicities. Aerosp. Med. 37, 271 (1966).

Colin, J., Timbal, J., Boutelier, C., Houdas, Y., Siffre, M.: Rhythm of the rectal temperature during a 6-month free-running experiment. J. Appl. Physiol. 25, 170–176 (1968).

Colquhoun, W. P. (ed.): Biological Rhythms and Performance. London-New York: Academic Press 1971.

Colquhoun, W. P. (ed.): Aspects of Human Efficiency. London: The English Univ. Press Lim. 1972.

Colquhoun, W. P., Blake, M. J. F., Edwards, R. S.: Experimental studies of shift-work. I. A comparison of 'rotating' and 'stabilized' 4-hour shift systems. Ergonomics 11, 437–453 (1968). II. Stabilized 8-hour shift systems. Ergonomics 11, 527–546 (1968). III. Stabilized 12-hour shift systems. Ergonomics 12, 865–882 (1969).

Conroy, R. T. W. L., Mills, J. N.: Human Circadian Rhythms. London: Churchill, J. & A. 1970.

Curtis, G. C., Fogel, M. L.: Circadian periodicity of plasma cortisol levels: effect of random living schedule in man. Space Life Sci. 3, 125–134 (1971).

Daan, S., Pittendrigh, C. S.: A functional analysis of circadian pacemakers in nocturnal rodents. II. The variability of phase response curves. J, comp. Physiol. 106, 253–266 (1976).

D'Allesandro, B.: Circadian rhythms of cortisol secretion in elderly and blind subjects. Br. Med. J. 2, 274 (1974).

Doerrscheidt, G. J., Beck, L.: Advanced method for evaluating characteristic parameters (τ, α, ρ) of circadian rhythms. J. Math. Biology 2, 107–121 (1975).

Elliott, A. L., Mills, J. N., Waterhouse, J. M.: A man with too long a day. J. Physiol. (Lond.) 212, 30–31 P (1971a).

Elliott, A. L., Mills, J. N., Minors, D. S., Waterhouse, J. M.: Effects of simulated time zone shifts upon plasma corticosteriod rhythms. J. Physiol (Lond) 217, 50–51 P (1971b).

Elliott, A. L., Mills, J. N., Minors, D. S., Waterhouse, J. M.: The effect of real and simulated time zone shifts upon the circadian rhythms of body temperature, plasma 11-hydroxycorticosteroids, and renal excretion in human subjects. J. Physiol. (Lond) 221, 227–257 (1972).

Engelmann, W.: Lithium slows down the Kalanchoe clock. Z. Naturforschg. 27b, 477 (1972).

Engelmann, W.: A slowing down of circadian rhythms by Lithium ions. Z. Naturforschg. 28c, 733–736 (1973).

Enright, J. T.: The search for rhythmicity in biological time-series. J. Theor. Biol. 8, 426–468 (1965).

Fahrenberg, J.: Ein item-analysierter Fragebogen funktionell körperlicher Beschwerden (VELA). Diagnostica 11, 141–153 (1965).

Ferin, M., Halberg, F., Richart, R. M., Vande-Wiele, R. L.: Biorhythms and Human Reproduction. New York—London—Sidney—Toronto: J. Wiley & Sons 1974.

Findley, J. D., Migler, B. M., Brady, J. V.: A long-term study of human performance in a continuously programmed experimental environment. Techn. Report (Univ. of Maryland, Dep. of Psychol.) 1963.

Fraisse, P., Siffre, M., Oberon, G., Zuili, N.: Le rythme veille-sommeil et l'estimation du temps. In: Cycles Biologiques et Psychiatrie. Ajuriaguerra, J. de (ed.) Paris: Masson & Cie. 1968, pp. 257–265.

Fröberg, J., Karlsson, C. C., Levi, L., Lidberg, L.: Circadian variations in performance, psychological ratings, catecholamine excretion, and diuresis during prolonged sleep deprivation. Int. J. Psychobiol. *2*, 23–36 (1972); and In: Aspects of Human Efficiency. Colquhoun, W. P. (ed.) London: The English Univ. Press Lim. 1972, pp. 247–253.

Gauquelin, F.: Terrestrial modulations of the daily cycle of birth. J. Interdiscipl. Cycle Res. *2*, 211–217 (1971).

Gerritzen, F.: Influence of light on human circadian rhythms. Aerosp. Med. *37*, 66–70 (1966).

Ghata, J., Halberg, F., Reinberg, A., Siffre, M.: Rythmes circadiens désynchronisés du cycle social (17-hydroxycorticosteroides, température rectale, veille-sommeil) chez deux sujets adultes sains. Ann. Endocrinol. (Paris) *30*, 245–260 (1969).

Giedke, H., Fatranska, M., Doerr, P., Hansert, E., Stamm, D., Wisser, H.: Tagesperiodik der Rectaltemperatur sowie der Ausscheidung von Elektrolyten, Katecholaminmetaboliten und 17-Hydroxycorticosteroiden mit dem Harn beim Menschen mit und ohne Lichtzeitgeber. Int. Arch. Arbeitsmed. *32*, 43–66 (1974).

Gierse, A.: Quaemiam sit ratio caloris organici. Dissertation Halle 1842.

Goertzen, C.: Synchronisation und Desynchronisation verschiedener psychophysiologischer Variablen. Ber. 30. Kongr. Dtsch. Ges. Psychol., pp. 387–388 (1976).

Guenther, R., Knapp, E., Halberg, F.: Referenznormen der Rhythmometrie; circadiane Acrophasen von 20 Körperfunktionen. Z. Angew. Bäder- Klimaheilk. *16*, 123–153 (1969).

Gwinner, E.: Entrainment of a circadian rhythm in birds by species-specific song cycles. Experientia *22*, 765 (1966).

Halberg, F.: Physiologic 24-hour periodicity: general and procedural considerations with reference to the adrenal cycle. Z. Vitamin- Hormon- Fermentforsch. *10*, 225–296 (1965).

Halberg, F.: Chronobiology. Annu. Rev. Physiol. *31*, 675–725 (1969).

Halberg, F., Reinberg, A.: Rythmes circadiens et rythmes de basses fréquences en physiologie humaine. J. Physiol. (Paris) *59*, 117–200 (1967).

Halberg, F., Simpson, H.: Circadian acrophases of human 17-hydroxycorticosteroids excretion referred to midsleep rather than midnight. Hum. Biol. *39*, 405–413 (1967).

Halberg, F., Frank, G., Harner, R., Matheys, J., Aaker, H., Gravem, H., Melby, J.: The adrenal cycle in men on different schedules of motor and mental activity. Experientia *17*, 282 (1961).

Halberg, F., Siffre, M., Engeli, M., Hillmann, D., Reinberg, A.: Etude en librecours des rythmes circadiens du pouls, de l'alternance veille-sommeil et de l'estimation du temps pendant les deux mois de séjour souterrain d'un homme adulte jeune. C. R. Acad. Sci. (Paris) *260*, 1259–1262 (1965).

Halberg, F., Reinhardt, J., Bartter, F. C., Delea, C., Gordon, R., Reinberg, A., Ghata, J., Halhuber, M., Hofmann, H., Günther, R., Knapp, E., Pena, J. C., Garcia Sainz, M.: Agreement in endpoints from circadian rhythmometry on healthy human beings living on different continents. Experientia *25*, 107–112 (1969).

Harth, W.: VLF-Atmospherics—Ihre Messung und ihre Interpretation. Z. Geophysik *38*, 815–849 (1972).

Harth, W.: Atmospherics oder Sferics—Die elektromagnetische Impulsstrahlung atmosphärischen Ursprungs. Inn. Med. *2*, 82–88 (1975).

Hartman, E.: The Biology of Dreaming. Springfield Ill.: Charles C. Thomas, 1967.

Hastings, J. W.: Unicellular clocks. Annu. Rev. Microbiol. *13*, 297–312 (1959).

Hastings, J. W., Wilson, T.: Bioluminescence and chemiluminescence. Photochem. Photobiol. *23*, 461–473 (1976).

Hildebrandt, G.: Die Bedeutung der Umweltreize für den Tagesrhythmus des Menschen. Z. Angew. Bäder- Klimaheilk. *13*, 626–644 (1966).

Hildebrandt, G. (ed.): Biologische Rhythmen und Arbeit. Wien—New York: Springer-Verlag 1976.

Hildebrandt, G., Lowes, E. M.: Tagesrhythmische Schwankungen der vegetativen Lichtreaktion beim Menschen. J. Interdiscipl. Cycle Res. *3*, 289–301 (1972).

Hildebrandt, G., Engel, P., Voigt, E.-D.: Rhythmologische Probleme der Raumfahrt. Bundesminst. Wiss. Forsch., Forschungsber. W 68-30: 285–303 (1968).

Hoffmann, K.: Zum Einfluss der Zeitgeberstärke auf die Phasenlage der synchronisierten circadianen Periodik. Z. vergl. Physiol. *62*, 93–110 (1969).

Hoffmann. K.: Circadiane Periodik bei Tupajas (Tupaia glis) in konstanten Bedingungen. Zool. Anz. Suppl. *33*, 171–177 (1970).

Hoffmann, K.: Splitting of the circadian rhythm as a function of light intensity. In: Biochronometry. Menaker, M. (ed.) Washington D.C.: Nat. Acad. Sciences 1971, pp. 134–146.

Holleck, M.: Zur Frage der Persistenz der 24-Stunden-Rhythmik in den Wasser- und Elektrolytausscheidungen des Menschen bei Zeitgeberausschluss. Dissertation Marburg 1972.

Hollwich, F., Dieckhues, B.: Circadian rhythms in blind. J. Interdiscipl. Cycle Res. *2*, 291–302 (1971).

Holst, E. v.: Die relative Koordination als Phänomen und als Methode zentralnervöser Funktionsanalyse. Ergeb. Physiol. *42*, 228–306 (1939a).

Holst, E. v.: Die Funktionsstruktur des rhythmisch tätigen Fischrückenmarks. Pfluegers Arch. *241*, 569–611 (1939b).

Høyer, K.: Physiological variations in the iron content of human blood serum. II. Further studies of the intra diem variations. Acta Med. Scand. *119*, 562–576 (1944).

Jouvet, M.: Phylogénèse et ontogénèse du sommeil paradoxal: son organisation ultradienne. In: Cycles Biologiques et Psychiatrie. Ajuriaguerra, J. de (ed.) Paris: Masson & Cie. 1968, pp. 185–203.

Jouvet, M., Mouret, J., Chouvet, G., Siffre, M.: Towards a 48-hour Day: Experimental Bicircadian Rhythm in Man. Neurosciences Res. Progr., 3rd Intensive Study Progr. Schmitt, F. O. (ed.) Cambridge: MIT Press 1974, pp. 491–497.

Juergensen, T.: Die Körperwärme des gesunden Menschen. Leipzig 1873.

Kendall, K. G.: Contribution to the Study of Oscillatory Time-Series. London: Cambridge Univ. Press 1946.

Kess, E.: Aktivitätszeit, Zeitschätzung, subjektive Vigilanz und akustische Reaktionszeit bei frei laufender Circadianrhythmik unter Zeitgeberausschluss. Dissertation, Marburg 1972.

Klein, K. E.: East-west and west to east desynchronization. In: Aerospace Med. Ass. Scientific Meeting, Paneel: The desynchronosis syndrome. Las Vegas, Nevada, U.S.A. May 1973.

Klein, K. E., Wegmann, H.-M.: The resynchronization of human circadian rhythms after transmeridian flights as a result of flight direction and mode of acitivity. In: Chronobiology. Scheving, L. E., Halberg, F., Pauly, J. E. (eds.) Tokyo: Igaku Shoin Ltd., 1974, pp. 564–570.

Klein, K. E., Wegmann, H.-M., Hunt, B. I.: Desynchronization of body temperature and performance circadian rhythms as a result of outgoing and homegoing transmeridian flight. Aerosp Med. *43*, 119–132 (1972).

Klotter, K.: General properties of oscillating systems. Cold Spring Harbor Symp. Quant. Biol. *25*, 185–187 (1960).

König. H.: Atmospherics geringster Frequenzen. Z. Angew. Physik *11*, 264–274 (1959).

Kriebel, J.: Die Phasenbeziehungen zwischen den circadianen Periodizitäten von Aktivität, Körpertemperatur und Nebennierenhormonen beim Menschen bei Isolation und bei Synchronisation. Pfluegers Arch. *319*, R 123 (1970).

Kriebel, J.: Circadiane Periodik der Nebennierenmark- und Nebennierenrindenhormone beim Menschen mit und ohne Zeitgeber. Dissertation, München 1971.

Krieger, D. T.: Biorhythms in central nervous system disease (primarily those of pituitary-adrenal hormones). In: Biorhythms and Human Reproduction. Ferin, M., Halberg, F., Richart, R. M., VandeWiele, R. L. (eds.) New York—London—Sidney—Toronto: Wiley & Sons 1974, pp. 621–649.

Krieger, D. T., Krieger, H. P.: Circadian variation of the plasma 17-hydroxycorticosteroids in central nervous system disease. J. Clin. Endocrinol. Metab. *26*, 929–940 (1966).

Krieger, D. T., Glick, S.: Absent sleep peaks of growth hormone release in blind subjects: Correlation with sleep EEG stages. J. Clin. Endocrinol. Metabol. *33*, 847–850 (1971).

Krieger, D. T., Rizzo, F.: Circadian periodicity of plasma 11-hydroxycorticosteroid levels in subjects with partial and absent light perception. Neuroendocrinology *8*, 165–179 (1971).

Krieger, D. T., Kreuzer, J., Rizzo, F. A.: Constant light: effects on circadian pattern and phase reversal of steroid and electrolyte levels in man. J. Clin. Endocrinol. Metab. *29*, 1634–1638 (1969).

Krieger, D. T., Allen, W., Rizzo, F., Krieger, H. P.: Characterization of the normal temporal pattern of plasma corticosteroid levels. J. Clin. Endocrinol. Metab. *32*, 266–284 (1971).

Lamprecht, G., Weber, F.: Eine neue Methode zur Bestimmung von Periodenlängen rhythmisch ablaufender physiologischer Prozesse. Pfluegers Arch. *315*, 262–272 (1970).

Levi, L.: Physical and mental stress reactions during experimental conditions simulating combat. Försvarsmedicin *2*, 1–7 (1966).

Lewis, P. R., Lobban, M. C.: Dissociation of diurnal rhythms in human subjects living in abnormal time routines. Q. J. Exp. Physiol. *42*, 371–386 (1957).

Lobban, M. C.: Dissociation in human rhythmic functions. In: Circadian Clocks. Aschoff, J. (ed.) Amsterdam: North Holland Publ. Comp. 1965a, pp. 219–227.

Lobban, M. C.: Time, light and diurnal rhythms. In: The Physiology of Human Survival. Edholm, O. G., Bacharach, A. L., (eds.) London: Acad. Press Inc. 1965b, pp. 351–386.

Lobban, M. C., Tredre, B.: Renal diurnal rhythms in blind subjects. J. Physiol. (Lond.) *170,* 29 P (1964).

Lobban, M. C., Tredre, B. E.: Perception of light and the maintenance of human renal diurnal rhythms. J. Physiol. (Lond.) *189*, 32–33 P (1967).

Lohmann. M.: Phase-dependent changes of circadian frequency after light steps. Nature (Lond.) *213*, 196–197 (1967).

Loon, J. H. van: Diurnal body temperature curves in shift workers. Ergonomics *6*, 267–273 (1963).

Lucas, R.: Untersuchungen über den Nachtschlaf des Menschen bei circadian freilaufendem Schlaf-Wachzyklus. Dissertation Marburg 1973.

Lund, R.: Circadiane Periode physiologischer und psychologischer Variablen bei 7 blinden Vpn mit und ohne Zeitgeber. Dissertation München 1974a.

Lund, R.: Personality factors and desynchronization of circadian rhythms. Psychosom. Med. *36*, 224–228 (1974b).

McCally, M., Wegmann, H.-M., Lund, R., Howard, J.: Effects of simulated time zone shifts on human circadian rhythms. Proc. XXIst Int. Congr. Aviation Space Med., Munich: 260–263 (1973).

McClintock, M. K.: Menstrual synchrony and suppression. Nature (Lond.) *229*, 244–245 (1971).

Meddis, R.: Human circadian rhythms and the 48-hour day. Nature (Lond.) *218*, 964–965 (1968).

Menzel, W.: Menschliche Tag-Nacht-Rhythmik und Schichtarbeit. Basel—Stuttgart: B. Schwabe & Co. 1962.

Migéon, C. J., Tyler, F. H., Mahoney, J. P., Florentin, A. A., Castle, H., Bliss, E. L., Sammels, L. T.: The diurnal variation of plasma levels and urinary excretion of 17-hydroxycorticosteroids in normal subjects, nightworkers and blind subjects. J. Clin. Endocrinol. Metabol. *16*, 622–633 (1956).

Mills, J. N.: Diurnal rhythms during three months underground. J. Physiol. (Lond.) *171*, 12 P (1964a).

Mills, J. N.: Circadian rhythms during and after three months in solitude underground. J. Physiol. (Lond) *174*, 217–231 (1964b).

Mills, J. N.: Human circadian rhythms. Physiol. Rev. (Wash.) *46*, 128–171 (1966).

Mills, J. N.: Sleeping habit during four months in solitude. J. Physiol. (Lond) *189*, 30–31 P (1967a).

Mills, J. N.: Keeping in step—away from it all. New Scientist *9*, 350–351 (1967b).

Mills, J. N.: Air travel and circadian rhythms. J. R. Coll. Phycus Lond. *7*, 122–131 (1973).

Mills, J. N., Minors, D. S., Waterhouse, J. M.: Periods of different components of human circadian rhythms in free-running experiments. Int. J. Chronobiol. *1*, 344 (1973).

Mills, J. N., Minors, D. S., Waterhouse, J. M.: The circadian rhythms of human subjects without timepieces or indication of the alternation of day and night. J. Physiol. (Lond.) *240*, 567–594 (1974).

Mills, J. N., Minors, D. S., Waterhouse, J. M.: Urinary and temperature rhythms on days of abnormal length. J. Physiol. (Lond) *257*, 54–55 P (1976).

Mittelstaedt, H.: Regelung in der Biologie. Regelungstechnik *2*, 177–181 (1954).

Moore-Ede, M. C.: Circadian rhythms of drug effectiveness and toxicity. Clin. Pharmacol. Ther. *14*, 925–935 (1973).

Moore-Ede, M. C., Schmelzer, W. S., Kass, D. A., Herd, J. A.: Internal organization of the circadian timing system in multicellular animals. Fed Proc. *35*, 2333–2338 (1976).

Nillus, P.: Etude de quelques conséquences biophysiologiques de l'isolement souterrain de sept jeunes femmes bien portantes. Dissertation, Paris 1967.

Njus, D., Sulzman, F. M., Hastings, J. W.: Membrane model for the circadian clock. Nature (Lond.) *248*, 116–120 (1974).

Njus, D., Gooch, Van D., Mergenhagen, D., Sulzman, F., Hastings, J. W.: Membranes and molecules in circadian systems. Fed Proc. *35*, 2353–2357 (1976).

Oestberg, O.: Zur Typologie der circadianen Phasenlage: Ansätze zu einer praktischen Chronohygiene. In: Biologische Rhythmen und Arbeit. Hildebrandt, G. (ed.) Wien—New York: Springer-Verlag 1976, pp. 117–137.

Orth, D. N., Island, D. P.: Light synchronization of the circadian rhythm in plasma cortisol (17-OHCS) concentration in man. J. Clin. Endocrinol. Metabol. *29*, 479–486 (1969).

Orth, D. N., Island, D. P., Liddle, G. W.: Experimental alteration of the circadian rhythm in plasma cortisol (17-OHCS) concentration in man. J. Clin. Endocrinol. Metabol. *27*, 549–555 (1967).

Papousek, M.: Chronobiologische Aspekte der Zyklothymie. Fortschr. Neurol. Psychiatr. *53*, 381–440 (1975).

Pflug, B.: Methodische Probleme der klinischen Rhythmusforschung bei Depressiven. Arzneim. forsch. *26*, 1065–1068 (1976).

Pflug, B., Erikson, R., Johnsson, A.: Depression and daily temperature, a long-term study. Acta Psychiatr. Scand. *54*, 254–266 (1976).

Pittendrigh, C. S.: Circadian rhythms and the circadian organization of living systems. Cold Spring Harbor Symp. Quant. Biol. *25*, 159–184 (1960).

Pittendrigh, C. S.: Circadian rhythms, space research and manned space flight. Life Sci. Space Res. *5*, 122–134 (1967).

Pittendrigh, C. S.: Circadian oscillations in cells and the circadian organization of multicellular systems. In: The Neurosciences: Third study progr., Schmitt, F. O., Worden, F. G. (eds.). Cambridge, Mass.: MIT Press 1974, pp. 437–458.

Pittendrigh, C. S., Daan, S.: Circadian oscillations in rodents: a systematic increase of their frequency with age. Science *186*, 548–550 (1974).

Pittendrigh, C. S., Daan, S.: A functional analysis of circadian pacemakers in nocturnal rodents. IV. Entrainment: Pacemaker as clock. J. comp. Physiol. *106*, 291–331 (1976a).

Pittendrigh, C. S., Daan, S.: A functional analysis of circadian pacemakers in nocturnal rodents. V. Pacemaker structure: A clock for all seasons. J. comp. Physiol. *106*, 333–355 (1976b).

Pittendrigh, C. S., Minis, D. H.: Circadian systems: longevity as a function of circadian resonance in Drosophila melanogaster. Proc. Natl. Acad. Sci. U.S.A. *69*, 1537–1539 (1972).

Poeppel, E.: Desynchronisation circadianer Rhythmen innerhalb einer isolierten Gruppe. Pfluegers Arch. *299*, 364–370 (1968).

Prout, W.: Observations on the quantity of carbonic acid gas emitted from lungs during respiration, at different times and during different circumstances. Thomsons Ann. Phil. *2*, 328 (1813).

Radnot, M., Wallner, E., Hönig, M.: Die Wirkung des Lichtes und des Hydergins auf die eosinophilen Leukozyten des Blutes. Wien. Klin. Wochenschr. *72*, 101–105 (1960).

Reil, C.: Über die Ausdünstung und die Wärmeentwicklung zur Tages- und Nachtzeit. Wäge- und Thermometerversuche. Dtsch. Arch. Physiol. *7*, 359 (1822).

Reinberg, A.: Hours of changing responsiveness in relation to allergy and the circadian adrenal cycle. In: Circadian Clocks. Aschoff J. (ed.) Amsterdam: North-Holland Publ. Comp. 1965, pp. 214–218.

Reinberg, A.: The hours of changing responsiveness or susceptibility. Perspect. Biol. Med. *11*, 111–128 (1967).

Reinberg, A.: Chronopharmacology in man. In: Chronobiological Aspects of Endocrinology. Aschoff, J., Ceresa, F., Halberg, F. (eds.) Symp. Med. Hoechst *9*, 305–337. Stuttgart–New York: Schattauer-Verlag (1974).

Reinberg, A.: Advances in human chronopharmacology. Chronobiologia *3*, 151–166 (1976).

Reinberg, A., Halberg, F.: Circadian chronopharmacology. Annu. Rev. Pharmacol. *11*, 455–492 (1971).

Reinberg, A., Halberg, F., Ghata, J., Siffre, M.: Spectre thermique (rhythme de la température rectale) d'une femme adulte avant, pendant et après son isolement souterain de trois mois. C. R. Acad. Sci. (Paris) *262*, 782–785 (1966).

Reinberg, A., Zagula-Mally, Z. W., Ghata, J., Halberg, F.: Circadian rhythms in duration of salicylate excretion referred to phase of excretory rhythms and routine. Proc. Soc. Exp. Biol. Med. *124*, 826–832 (1967).

Remler, O.: Untersuchungen an Blinden über die 24-Std-Rhythmik. Klin. Monatsbl. Augenheilkd. *113*, 116–140 (1948).

Richter, C. P.: Biological Clocks in Medicine and Psychiatry. Springfield Ill: Thomas Ch. C. Publ. 1965.

Ringer, C.: Circadiane Periodik psychologischer und physiologischer Parameter bei Schlafentzug, Dissertation, München 1972.

Rintoul, D.: Enzyme oscillations in cultured rat liver cells. Physiol. and Biochem. Aspects of Circadian Rhythms. 59th Ann. meet. Fed. Amer. Soc. Exp. Biol. 1975.

Rohles, F. H. Jr., Osbaldiston, G.: Social entrainment of biorhythms in rhesus monkey. In:

Circadian Rhythms in Nonhuman Primates. Rohles, F. H. (ed.) Bibl. Primatol. *9*, 39–51. Basel-New York: S. Karger 1969.

Rutenfranz, J.: Arbeitsphysiologische Aspekte der Nacht- und Schichtarbeit. Arbeitsmed. Sozialmed. Arbeitshyg. *2*, 17–23 (1967).

Rutenfranz. J., Hellbruegge, T.: Über Tagesschwankungen der Rechengeschwindigkeit bei 11-jährigen Kindern. Z. Kinderheilkd. *80*, 65–82 (1957).

Rutenfranz, J., Aschoff, J., Mann, H.: The effects of a cumulative sleep deficit, duration of preceding sleep period and body temperature on multiple choice reaction time. In: Aspects of Human Efficiency. Colquhoun W. P. (ed.) London: The English Univ. Press Lim. 1972, pp. 217–229.

Schaefer, K. E., Clegg, B. R., Carey, C. R., Dougherty, J. H., Weybrew, B. B.: Effects of isolation in a constant environment on periodicity of physiological functions and performance levels. Aerosp. Med. *38*, 1002–1018 (1967).

Scheving, L. E., Halberg, F., Pauly, J. E. (eds.): Chronobiology. Tokyo: Igaku Shoin Ltd. 1974.

Schmidt, T. H.: Thermoregulatorische Grössen in Abhängigkeit von Tageszeit und Menstrualzyklus. Dissertation, München 1972.

Schulz, H., Dirlich, G., Zulley, J.: Phase shift in the REM sleep rhythm. Pfluegers Arch. *358*, 203–212 (1975).

Schulz, H., Dirlich, G., Zulley, J.: Untersuchungen zur Stabilität ultradianer Rhythmen beim Menschen. Arzneim. forsch. *26*, 1055–1058 (1976).

Schumann, W. O.: Über die strahlungslosen Eigenschwingungen einer leitenden Kugel, die von einer Luftschicht und einer Ionosphärenhülle umgeben ist. Z. Naturforsch. [A] *7*, 149–154 (1954).

Schuster, A.: On the investigation of hidden periodicities with application to a supposed 26-day period of meteorological phenomena. Terrest. Magnetism *3*, 13–41 (1898).

Sharp, G. W. G.: The effect of light on diurnal leucocyte variations. J. Endocrinol. *21*, 213–218 (1960a).

Sharp, G. W. G.: The effect of light on the morning increase in urine flow. J. Endocrinol. *21*, 219–223 (1960b).

Shiotsuka, R., Jovonovich, J., Jovonovich, J. A.: In vitro data on drug sensitivity: circadian and ultradian corticosteron rhythms in adrenal organ cultures. In: Chronobiological Aspects of Endocrinology. Aschoff, J., Ceresa, F., Halberg, F., (eds.) Symp. Med. Hoechst *9*: 255–267. Stuttgart-New York: Schattauer-Verlag 1974.

Sieber, W.: Synchronisierte und autonome circadiane Periodik physiologischer Funktionen bei Blinden unter besonderer Berücksichtigung des freien Urin-Cortisols. Dissertation, München 1976.

Siffre, M.: Hors du Temps. Tuillard, Paris 1963.

Siffre, M.: Expériences Hors du Temps. Fayard, Paris 1972.

Siffre, M.: Six months alone in a cave. Nat. Geographics *147*, 426–435 (1975).

Siffre, M., Reinberg, A., Halberg, F., Ghata, J., Perdriel, G., Slind, R.: L'isolement souterain prolongé. Etude de deux sujet adultes sains avant, pendant et après cet isolement. Presse Méd. *74*, 915–919 (1966).

Simpson, H. W., Lobban, M. C.: Effect of a 21-hour day on the human circadian excretory rhythms of 17-hydroxycorticosteroids and electrolytes. Aerosp. Med. *38*, 1205–1213 (1967).

Simpson, H. W., Lobban, M. C., Halberg, F.: Arctic chronobiology. Urinary near-24-hour rhythms in subjects living on a 21-hour routine in the arctic. Arctic anthropology *7*, 144–164 (1970).

Stroebel, C. F.: Biologic rhythms correlates of disturbed behavior in the Rhesus monkey. In: Circadian Rhythms in Nonhuman Primates. Rohles, F. H. (ed.) Bibl. Primatol. *9*: 91–105. Basel-New York: S. Karger 1969.

Szafarczyk, A., Nouguier-Soule, J., Assenmacher, I.: Diurnal locomotor and plasma corticosterone rhythms in rats living on photoperiodically lengthened days, Int. J. Chronobiology *2*, 373–382 (1974).

Takebe, K., Setaishi, C., Hirami, H., Yamamoto, M., Horiuchi, Y.: Effects of a bacterial pyrogen on the pituitary-adrenal axis at various times in the 24 hours. J. Clin. Endocrinol. Metabol. *26*, 437–442 (1966).

Tharp, G. D., Folk, G. E. Jr.: Rhythmic changes in rate of the mammalian heart and heart cells during prolonged isolation. Comp. Biochem. Physiol. *14*, 255–273 (1965).

Toulouse, E., Pieron, H.: Le mechanisme de l'inversion chez l'homme du rythme nychthéméral de la température. J. Physiol. Pathol. Gén. *9*, 425–440 (1907).

Webb, W. B., Agnew, H. W. Jr.: Sleep and

waking in a time-free environment. Aerosp. Med. *45*, 617–622 (1974a).

Webb, W. B., Agnew, H. W. Jr.: Regularity in the control of the free-running sleep-wakefulness rhythm. Aerosp Med. *45*, 701–704 (1974b).

Webb, W. B., Agnew, H. W. Jr.: Sleep efficiency for sleep-wake cycles of varied length. Psychophysiology *12*, 637–641 (1975).

Weitzman, E. D.: Temporal patterns of neuro-endocrine secretion in man: relationship to the 24-hour sleep-waking cycle. In: Chronobiological Aspects of Endocrinology. Aschoff, J., Ceresa, F., Halberg, F. (eds.) Symp. Med. Hoechst *9*: 169–184. Stuttgart: Schattauer-Verlag 1974.

Wever, R.: Possibilities of phase-control, demonstrated by an electronic model. Cold Spring Harbor Symp. Quant. Biol. *25*, 197–201 (1960).

Wever, R.: Zum Mechanismus der biologischen 24-Stunden-Periodik. Kybernetik *1*, 139–154 (1962).

Wever, R.: Zum Mechanismus der biologischen 24-Stunden-Periodik. II. Mitteilung. Der Einfluss des Gleichwertes auf die Eigenschaften selbsterregter Schwingungen. Kybernetik *1*: 213–231 (1963a).

Wever, R.: Zum Problem der Regelung in der Biologie. Pfluegers Arch. *278*, 89–90 (1963b).

Wever, R.: Ein mathematisches Modell für biologische Schwingungen. Z. Tierpsychol. *21*, 359–372 (1964a).

Wever, R.: Zum Mechanismus der biologischen 24-Stunden-Periodik. III. Mitteilung. Anwendung der Modell-Gleichung. Kybernetik *2*, 127–144 (1964b).

Wever, R.: A mathematical model for circadian rhythms. In: Circadian Clocks. Aschoff, J. (ed.) Amsterdam: North-Holland Publ. Comp. 1965a, pp. 47–63.

Wever, R.: Einzel-Organismen und Populationen im circadianen Experiment. Z. Vergl. Physiol. *51*, 1–24 (1965b).

Wever, R.: The duration of re-entrainment of circadian rhythms after phase shifts of the zeitgeber. A theoretical investigation. J. Theor. Biol. *13*, 187–201 (1966a).

Wever, R.: Ein mathematisches Modell für die circadiane Periodik. Z. Angew. Math. Mech. *46*, T 148–157 (1966b).

Wever, R.: Gesetzmässigkeiten circadianer Aktivitäts-Rhythmen bei Tier und Mensch. In: La Distribution Temporelle des Activités Ani-

males et Humaines. Médioni, J. (ed.) Paris: Masson & Cie. 1967a, pp. 3–17.

Wever, R.: Zum Einfluss der Dämmerung auf die circadiane Periodik. Z. Vergl. Physiol. *55*, 255–277 (1967b).

Wever, R.: Über die Beeinflussung der circadianen Periodik des Menschen durch schwache elektromagnetische Felder. Z. Vergl. Physiol. *56*, 111–128 (1967c).

Wever, R.: Einfluss schwacher elektro-magnetischer Felder auf die circadiane Periodik des Menschen. Naturwissenschaften *55*, 29–32 (1968a).

Wever, R.: Mathematical models of circadian rhythms and their applicability to men. In: Cycles Biologiques et Psychiatrie. Ajuriaguerra, J. de, (ed.) Paris: Masson & Cie. 1968b, pp. 61–72.

Wever, R.: Gesetzmässigkeiten der circadianen Periodik des Menschen, geprüft an der Wirkung eines schwachen elektrischen Wechselfeldes. Pfluegers Arch. *302*, 97–112 (1968c).

Wever, R.: Das Problem des Alterns unter den Bedingungen des Weltraumfluges. Bundesminst. Wiss. Forsch., Forschungsber. W 68-30, 328–331 (1968d).

Wever, R.: Autonome circadiane Periodik des Menschen unter dem Einfluss verschiedener Beleuchtungs-Bedingungen. Pfluegers Arch. *306*, 71–91 (1969a).

Wever, R.: Untersuchungen zur circadianen Periodik des Menschen mit besonderer Berücksichtigung des Einflusses schwacher elektrischer Wechselfelder. Bundesminst. Wiss. Forsch., Forschungsber. W 69-31, 1969b.

Wever, R.: The effects of electric fields on circadian rhythms in men. Life Sci. Space Res. *8*, 177–187 (1970a).

Wever, R.: Die gegenseitige Kopplung zwischen den circadianen Periodizitäten verschiedener vegetativer Funktionen beim Menschen. Pfluegers Arch. *319*, R 122 (1970b).

Wever, R.: Zur Zeitgeber-Stärke eines Licht-Dunkel-Wechsels für die circadiane Periodik des Menschen. Pfluegers Arch. *321*, 133–142 (1970c).

Wever, R.: Circadian rhythms of some psychological functions under different conditions. AGARD Conf. Proc. *74*, 1/1–1/8 (1970d).

Wever, R.: Die circadiane Periodik des Menschen als Indikator für die biologische Wirkung elektromagnetischer Felder. Z. Physik. Med. *2*, 439–471 (1971a).

Wever, R.: Influence of electric fields on some

parameters of circadian rhythms in man. In: Biochronometry. Menaker, M. (ed.) Washington D.C.: Nat. Acad. Scienc. 1971b, pp. 117–132.

Wever, R.: Virtual synchronization towards the limits of the range of entrainment. J. Theor. Biol. *36*, 119–132 (1972a).

Wever, R.: Mutual relations between different physiological functions in circadian rhythms in man. J. Interdiscipl. Cycle Res. *3*, 253–265 (1972b).

Wever, R.: Circadian Rhythms in human performance. In: Proc. NATO-Symp. on Drugs, Sleep, and Performance. pp. 11/1–11/12 (1972c).

Wever, R.: Hat der Mensch nur eine "innere Uhr"? Umschau in Wissensch. Technik *73*, 551–558 (1973a).

Wever, R.: Human circadian rhythms under the influence of weak electric fields and the different aspects of these studies. Int. J. Biometeorol. *17*, 227–232 (1973b).

Wever, R.: Die biologische Tagesperiodik und ihre Besonderheiten beim Menschen. Ber. Physik.-Med. Ges. Würzburg *81*, 13–30 (1973c).

Wever, R.: Internal phase-angle differences in human circadian rhythms: causes for changes and problems of determinations. Int. J. Chronobiol. *1*, 371–390 (1973d).

Wever, R.: Der Einfluss des Lichtes auf die circadiane Periodik des Menschen. I. Einfluss auf die autonome Periodik. Z. Physik. Med. *3*, 121–134 (1973e).

Wever, R.: Different aspects of the studies of human circadian rhythms under the influence of weak electric fields. In: Chronobiology. Scheving, L. E., Halberg, F., Pauly, J. E. (eds.) Tokyo: Igaku Shoin Ltd. 1974a, pp. 694–699.

Wever, R.: The influence of self-controlled changes in ambient temperature on autonomous circadian rhythms in man. Pfluegers Arch. *352*, 257–266 (1974b).

Wever, R.: Der Einfluss des Lichtes auf die circadiane Periodik des Menschen. II. Zeitgeber-Einfluss. Z. Physik. Med. *3*, 137–150 (1974c).

Wever, R.: ELF-effects on human circadian rhythms. In: ELF and VLF Electromagnetic Field Effects. Persinger, M.A. (ed.) New York-London: Plenum Press 1974d, pp. 101–144.

Wever, R.: Influence of light on human circadian rhythms. Nordic Council Arct. Med. Res. Rep. *10*, 33–47 (1974e).

Wever, R.: The circadian multi-oscillator system of man. Int. J. Chronobiol. *3*, 19–55 (1975a).

Wever, R.: Autonomous circadian rhythms in man: singly versus collectively isolated subjects. Naturwissenschaften *62*, 443–444 (1975b).

Wever, R.: The direction asymmetry in the duration of resynchronization of human circadian rhythms after phase shifts of the Zeitgeber. Pfluegers Arch. *359*, R 143 (1975c).

Wever, R.: Die Bedeutung der circadianen Periodik für den alternden Menschen. Verh. Dtsch. Ges. Pathol. *59*, 160–180 (1975d).

Wever, R.: Quantitative studies of the interaction between different circadian oscillators within the human multi-oscillator system. Chronobiologia *2*, Suppl. 1, 77 (1975e).

Wever, R.: Probleme der circadianen Periodik und ihrer Störungen. Arzneim. forsch. *26*, 1050–1054 (1976a).

Wever, R.: Effects of weak 10 Hz fields on separated vegetative rhythms involved in the human circadian multi-oscillator system. Arch. Met. Geoph. Biokl. Ser.B, *24*, 123–124 (1976b).

Wever, R., Zink, R. A.: Fortlaufende Registrierung der Rectaltemperatur des Menschen unter extremen Bedingungen. Pfluegers Arch. *327*, 186–190 (1971).

Whittaker, E., Robinson, G.: The Calculus of Observations. London: Blackie & Son 1924.

Wigand, R.: Der Tod des Menschen an inneren Krankheiten in seiner Beziehung zu den Tages- und Jahreszeiten. Dtsch. Med. Wochenschr. *1934*, 1709–1711 (1934).

Winfree, A. T.: Integrated view of resetting a circadian clock. J. Theoret. Biol. *28*, 327–374 (1970).

Winget, C. M.: Circadian rhythms in human subjects. Chronobiologia *2*, Suppl. *1*, 78 (1975).

Wisser, H., Doerr, P., Stamm, D., Fatranska, M., Giedke, H., Wever, R.: Tagesperiodik der Aussecheidung von Electrolyten, Katecholaminmetaboliten und 17-Hydroxycorticosteroiden im Harn. Klin. Wochenschr. *51*, 242–246 (1973).

Wurtman, R. J.: The effect of light on the human body. Sci. Am. *233/1*, 69–77 (1975).

Zulley, J.: Schlaf und Temperatur unter freilaufenden Bedingungen. Ber. 30. Kongr. Dtsch. Ges. Psychol., pp. 398–399 (1976).

Glossary*

Acrophase. Phase angle of the maximum in a sinusoidal oscillation; **acrophase of a rhythm.** acrophase of the corresponding fundamental period.

Amplitude. Difference between maximum value and mean value, or between minimum value and mean value, in a sinusoidal oscillation; **amplitude of a rhythm.** amplitude of the corresponding fundamental period.

Desynchronization. Steady state in which different rhythms run with different periods.

—External. Steady state in which a biological rhythm runs with another period than an external zeitgeber.

—Internal. Steady state in which different biological rhythms within one organism, or different components of the same biological rhythm run with different periods.

Dissociation, internal. State in which different biological rhythms within one organism, or different components of the same biologi-

cal rhythm temporarily change their mutual phase relationship.

Entrainment. Steady state in which a self-sustained (i.e., endogenously generated) rhythm runs synchronously to another rhythm (i.e., zeitgeber), with an equal period and a temporally constant phase relationship.

Extremum value. Highest or lowest value of a rhythmic valiable within one period.

Frequency. Reciprocal of period.

Fundamental period. Sinusoidal oscillation which best fits a rhythm, computed as the first harmonic by a harmonic analysis, or a least square fit.

Maximum. Phase angle of the maximum value.

Maximum value. Highest value of a rhythmic variable within one period.

Mean value. Arithmetic mean of all instantaneous, equidistantly ranged values of a rhythmic variable within one period, or within several full periods.

*This glossary follows, when possible, the terminology recommended by Aschoff et al., 1965; and Wever, 1969b.

Minimum. Phase angle of the minimum value.

Minimum value. Lowest value of a rhythmic variable within one period.

Oscillator. Mechanism generating a rhythm, characterized by a feed-back system guaranteeing the self-sustainment capacity.

Period. Time after which a definite phase of an oscillation reoccurs; **period of a rhythm.** Average time after which an arbitrarily defined state (e.g., maximum value) reoccurs, defined only by using a sufficient number of cycles.

—Autonomous. Period of an autonomously running rhythm.

—Free running. Period of a free running rhythm.

—Fundamental. See **Fundamental period.**

—Natural. Hypothetical period of an entrained rhythm which would be adopted after removal of the zeitgeber.

Phase. Instantaneous state of an oscillation within a period, represented by the value of the variable and all its time derivatives. In a looser sense, used for phase angle.

Phase angle. Value of the abscissa (i.e., time scale) corresponding to a point of the curve (i.e., phase), given either in angular degrees, or in units of time, if the length of the period is stated.

Phase angle difference. Difference between two corresponding phase angles in different oscillations.

—External. Phase angle difference between a biological rhythm and a zeitgeber.

—Internal. Phase angle difference between different biological rhythms within one organism.

Phase relationship. Phase angle difference between different rhythms.

—External. Phase relationship between a biological rhythm and a zeitgeber.

—Internal. Phase relationship between different biological rhythms within one organism.

Range of entrainment. Range of periods, or frequencies, within which a self-sustained oscillation can be entrained by a zeitgeber.

Range of oscillation. Difference between maximum and minimum value of a rhythmic variable within one period. In a sinusoidal oscillation, it is twice the amplitude.

Reentrainment. Transient state of an endogenously generated rhythm after a phase shift of the entraining zeitgeber, lasting until a temporally constant phase relationship to the zeitgeber again is reached.

Resynchronization. Transient state of a rhythm after a phase shift of a synchronizing rhythm, lasting until a temporally constant phase relationship between the two rhythms again is reached.

Rhythm. Oscillation superimposed by random noise, and of a shape which normally deviates from the sinusoidal one.

—Autonomous. Rhythm running self-sustained without being forced by any external periodicity.

—Circadian. Endogenously generated biological rhythm with a period of about (lat.: circa) 1 day (lat.: dies), either freerunning or entrained to a zeitgeber.

—Entrained. Endogenously generated rhythm running entrained to a zeitgeber.

—Free running. Rhythm running autonomously, either under constant conditions or under the influence of an external periodicity which can be shown to not exert a zeitgeber effect.

—Heteronomous. Rhythm running forced by an external periodicity.

—Synchronized. Rhythm running synchronously to another rhythm.

Self-sustainment. Capacity of an oscillation to obtain the periodic input of energy, which is necessary for maintaining, from a constant source of energy.

Separate excitation. Periodic external influencing of a rhythm, with the result the rhythm becomes synchronized.

Steady state. State of a rhythm during which all parameters undergo only random fluctuations (i.e., show neither temporal trends nor any other systematic changes in the long run).

Synchronization. Steady state in which two, or more, rhythms run with an equal period and a temporally constant phase relationship.

—External. Steady state in which a biological rhythm runs synchronously (i.e., en-

trained) to a zeitgeber (i.e., with an equal period and a temporally constant external phase relationship).

—Internal. Steady state in which different biological rhythms within one organism run synchronously (i.e., with an equal period and a temporally constant internal phase relationship).

Transient. Temporally limited state of a rhythm during which parameters undergo systematic changes, normally between two steady states.

Zeitgeber. External, and, also, in a looser sense, internal, periodicity with the capacity to entrain an endogenously generated biological rhythm.

Author Index

*Numbers in italic refer to pages in which complete references are listed.

Subject Index